ELEVENTH EDITION

WEST'S RESPIRATORY PHYSIOLOGY

THE ESSENTIALS

John B. West, MD, PhD, DSc

Professor of Medicine and Physiology
School of Medicine
University of California, San Diego
La Jolla, California

Andrew M. Luks, MD

Professor of Medicine
School of Medicine
University of Washington
Seattle, Washington

. Wolters Kluwer

Philadelphia · Baltimore · New York · London
Buenos Aires · Hong Kong · Sydney · Tokyo

Not authorised for sale in United States, Canada, Australia, New Zealand, Puerto Rico, and U.S. Virgin Islands.

Acquisitions Editor: Crystal Taylor
Development Editor: Andrea Vosburgh
Editorial Coordinator: LaPorscha Rodgers
Manufacturing Coordinator: Margie Orzech
Marketing Manager: Phyllis Hitner
Design Coordinator: Stephen Druding
Production Services: SPi Global

Eleventh Edition

Cataloging-in-Publication Data available on request from the Publisher
ISBN: 978-1-9751-3918-6

This work is provided "as is," and the publisher disclaims any and all warranties, express or implied, including any warranties as to accuracy, comprehensiveness, or currency of the content of this work.

This work is no substitute for individual patient assessment based upon healthcare professionals' examination of each patient and consideration of, among other things, age, weight, sex, current or prior medical conditions, medication history, laboratory data and other factors unique to the patient. The publisher does not provide medical advice or guidance and this work is merely a reference tool. Healthcare professionals, and not the publisher, are solely responsible for the use of this work including all medical judgments and for any resulting diagnosis and treatments.

Given continuous, rapid advances in medical science and health information, independent professional verification of medical diagnoses, indications, appropriate pharmaceutical selections and dosages, and treatment options should be made and healthcare professionals should consult a variety of sources. When prescribing medication, healthcare professionals are advised to consult the product information sheet (the manufacturer's package insert) accompanying each drug to verify, among other things, conditions of use, warnings and side effects and identify any changes in dosage schedule or contraindications, particularly if the medication to be administered is new, infrequently used or has a narrow therapeutic range. To the maximum extent permitted under applicable law, no responsibility is assumed by the publisher for any injury and/or damage to persons or property, as a matter of products liability, negligence law or otherwise, or from any reference to or use by any person of this work.

shop.lww.com

To P.H.W.—John B. West

To P.A.K., R.W.G., and E.R.S.—Andrew M. Luks

————————————

PREFACE

This book was first published over 40 years ago and has served several generations of students. It has been translated into 15 languages. This new 11th edition incorporates a number of changes. First, there are many more multiple choice questions, all written to better test reasoning rather than factual recall. An extensive appendix provides detailed answers to the questions. Learning objectives have been added to every chapter and a number of topics in the text have been expanded to improve the meaning. The fourteen 50-minute YouTube lectures closely based on the material in the book have been retained, and these have proved to be popular with students. The URL is http://meded.ucsd.edu/ifp/jwest/resp_phys/index.html.

In spite of these new features, the objectives of the book have not changed. First, the book is intended as an introductory text for medical students and allied health students. As such, it will normally be used in conjunction with a course of lectures, as is the case at UCSD. Indeed, the first edition was written because I believed that there was no appropriate textbook at that time to accompany the first-year physiology course.

Second, the book is written as a review for residents and fellows in such areas as pulmonary medicine, critical care, anesthesiology, and internal medicine, particularly to help them prepare for licensing and other examinations. Here, the requirements are somewhat different. The reader is familiar with the general area but needs to have his or her memory jogged on various points, and the many didactic diagrams are particularly important.

It might be useful to add a word or two about how the book meshes with the lectures to the first-year medical students at UCSD. We are limited to about twelve 50-minute lectures on respiratory physiology supplemented by two laboratory demonstrations, three small discussion groups, and a review session with the whole class present. The lectures follow the individual chapters of the book closely, with most chapters corresponding to a single lecture. The exceptions are that Chapter 5 has two lectures (one on normal gas exchange, hypoventilation, and shunt; another on the difficult topic of ventilation-perfusion relationships), Chapter 6 has two lectures (one on blood-gas transport and another on acid-base balance), and Chapter 7 has two lectures (on statics and dynamics). There is no lecture on Chapter 10, "Tests of Pulmonary Function," because this is not part of the core course. It is included partly for interest and partly because of its importance to people who work in pulmonary function laboratories.

The present edition has been updated in many areas including blood-tissue gas exchange, mechanics, control of ventilation, and the respiratory system under stress. In addition to the answers to the multiple choice questions, Appendix B contains discussions of the answers to the questions associated with the end-of-chapter clinical vignettes. There are several animations expanding sections of the text, and these are indicated by the symbol . Great efforts have been made to keep the book lean in spite of enormous temptations to fatten it. Occasionally, medical students wonder if the book is too superficial. Not so. If pulmonary and critical care fellows beginning their training in intensive care units fully understood all of the material on gas exchange and mechanics, the world would be a better place.

Many students and teachers have written to query statements in the book or to make suggestions for improvements. We respond personally to every point that is raised and very much appreciate the input.

John B. West
jwest@health.ucsd.edu
Andrew M. Luks
aluks@uw.edu

ANIMATIONS

CONTENTS

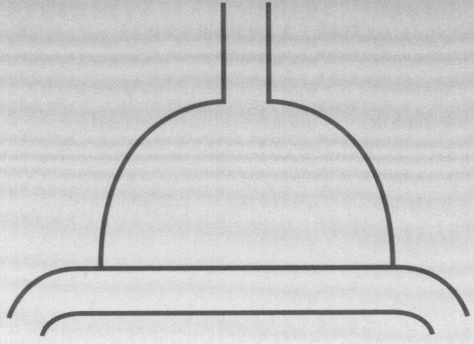

Structure and Function

1

How the Architecture of the Lung Subserves Its Function

- **Blood-Gas Interface**
- **Airways and Airflow**
- **Blood Vessels and Flow**
- **Stability of Alveoli**
- **Removal of Inhaled Particles**
- **Removal of Material from the Blood**

This first chapter of the book provides a short review of the relationships between structure and function in the lung. First, we look at the blood-gas interface, where the exchange of the respiratory gases occurs. Next we look at how oxygen is brought to the interface through the airways and then how the blood removes the oxygen from the lung. Finally, several challenges the lung must overcome are briefly addressed: how alveoli maintain their stability, how the lung is kept clean in a polluted environment, and how the capillaries filters material from the blood. At the end of this chapter, the reader should be able to:

- Describe the functional implications of the thin blood-gas interface
- Outline changes in airway structure and function as one moves from the trachea to the alveolar spaces
- Describe the effect of the branching airway pattern on the cross-sectional area for airflow
- Explain the differences in function between the pulmonary circulation and bronchial circulation
- Describe the functional roles of cilia and surfactant in the healthy lung

1

The lung is for gas exchange. Its primary function is to allow oxygen to move from the air into the venous blood and carbon dioxide to move out. The lung does other jobs too. It metabolizes some compounds, filters unwanted materials from the circulation, and acts as a reservoir for blood. But its cardinal function is to exchange gas, and we shall therefore begin at the blood-gas interface where the gas exchange occurs.

BLOOD-GAS INTERFACE

Oxygen and carbon dioxide move between air and blood by simple diffusion, that is, from an area of high to low partial pressure,* much as water flows downhill. Fick's law of diffusion states that the amount of gas that moves across a sheet of tissue is proportional to the area of the sheet but inversely proportional to its thickness. The blood-gas barrier is exceedingly thin (**Figure 1.1**) and has an area of between 50 and 100 m². It is therefore well suited to its function of gas exchange.

How is it possible to obtain such a prodigious surface area for diffusion inside the limited thoracic cavity? This is done by wrapping the small blood vessels (capillaries) around an enormous number of small air sacs called *alveoli* (**Figure 1.2**). There are about 500 million alveoli in the human lung, each about 1/3 mm in diameter. If they were spheres,† their total surface area would be 85 m² but their volume only 4 liters. By contrast, a single sphere of this volume would have an internal surface area of only 1/100 m². Thus, the lung generates this large diffusion area by being divided into a myriad of units.

Gas is brought to one side of the blood-gas interface by *airways*, and blood is brought to the other side by *blood vessels*.

AIRWAYS AND AIRFLOW

The airways consist of a series of branching tubes, which become narrower, shorter, and more numerous as they penetrate deeper into the lung (**Figure 1.3**).

---

* The partial pressure of a gas is found by multiplying its concentration by the total pressure. For example, dry air has 20.93% O_2. Its partial pressure (P_{O_2}) at sea level (barometric pressure 760 mm Hg) is $20.93/100 \times 760 = 159$ mm Hg. When air is inhaled into the upper airways, it is warmed and moistened, and the water vapor pressure is then 47 mm Hg, so that the total dry gas pressure is only $760 - 47 = 713$ mm Hg. The P_{O_2} of inspired air is therefore $20.93/100 \times 713 = 149$ mm Hg. A liquid exposed to a gas until equilibration takes place has the same partial pressure as the gas. For a more complete description of the gas laws, see Appendix A.

† The alveoli are not spherical but polyhedral. Nor is the whole of their surface available for diffusion (see Figure 1.1). These numbers are therefore only approximate.

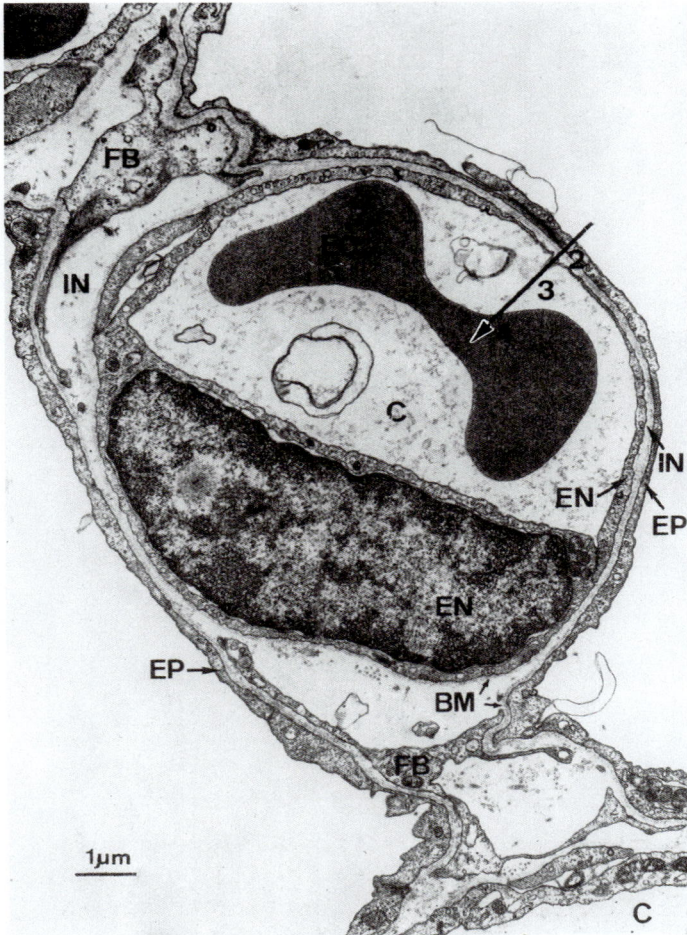

Figure 1.1. Electron micrograph showing a pulmonary capillary (C) in the alveolar wall. Note the extremely thin blood-gas barrier of about 0.3 μm in some places. The *large arrow* indicates the diffusion path from alveolar gas to the interior of the erythrocyte (EC) and includes the layer of surfactant (not shown in the preparation), alveolar epithelium (EP), interstitium (IN), capillary endothelium (EN), and plasma. Parts of structural cells called fibroblasts (FB), basement membrane (BM), and a nucleus of an endothelial cell are also seen. (Reprinted from Weibel ER. Morphometric estimation of pulmonary diffusion capacity: I. Model and method. *Respir Physiol*. 1970;11(1):54-75.Copyright © 1970 Elsevier. With permission.)

The *trachea* divides into right and left main bronchi, which in turn divide into lobar and then segmental bronchi. This process continues down to the *terminal bronchioles*, which are the smallest airways without alveoli. All of these bronchi make up the *conducting airways*. Their function is to lead inspired air to the gas-exchanging regions of the lung (**Figure 1.4**). The larger proximal airways are lined by a ciliated columnar epithelium and

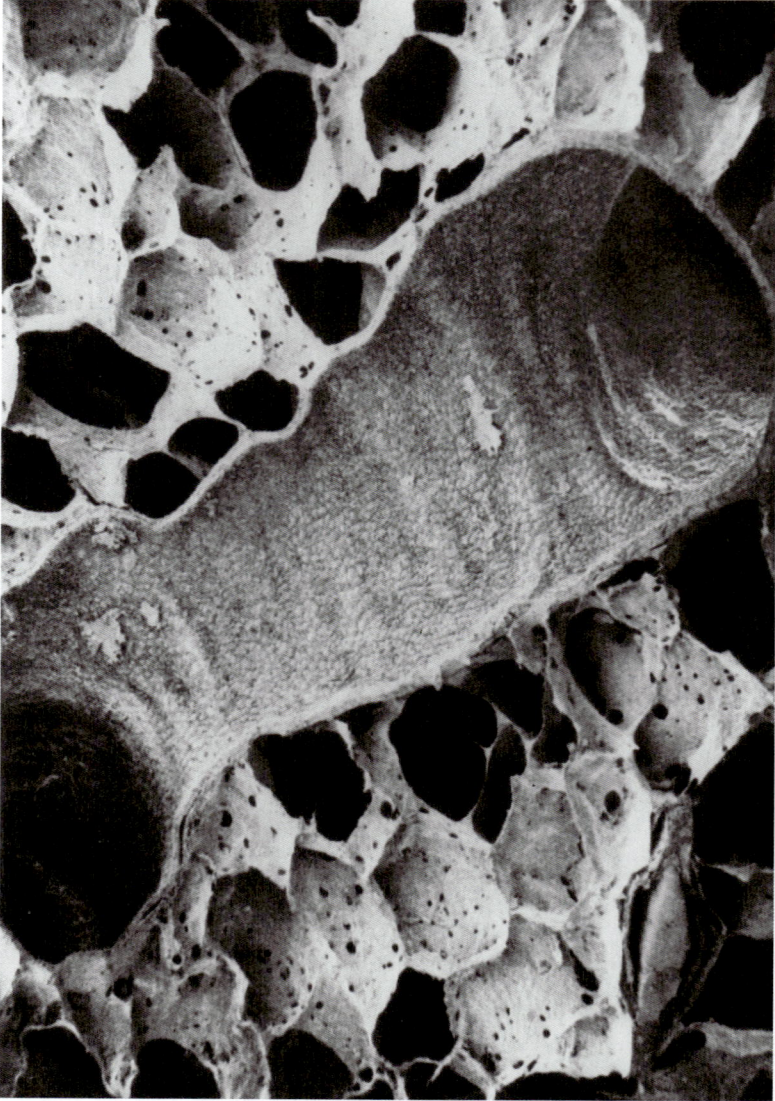

Figure 1.2. Section of lung showing many alveoli and a small bronchiole. The pulmonary capillaries run in the walls of the alveoli (Figure 1.1). The holes in the alveolar walls are the pores of Kohn. (Scanning electron micrograph by Nowell JA, Tyler WS.)

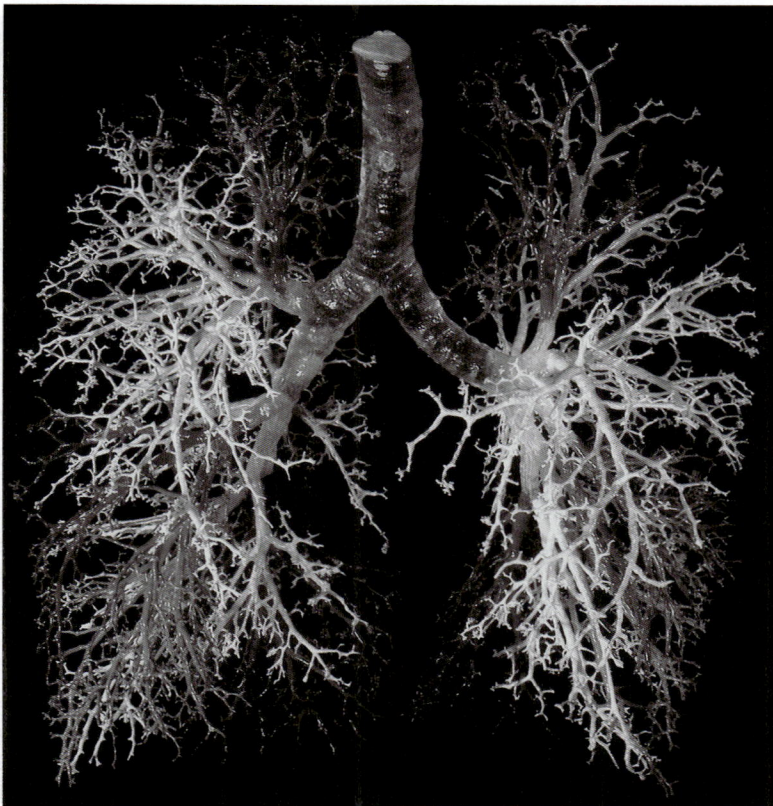

Figure 1.3. Cast of the airways of a human lung. The alveoli have been pruned away, allowing the conducting airways from the trachea to the terminal bronchioles to be seen.

have a lot of cartilage in their walls. As the airways progress distally, the proportion of cartilage decreases and smooth muscle increases such that the very small distal airways are composed mostly of smooth muscle. Because the conducting airways contain no alveoli and therefore take no part in gas exchange, they constitute the *anatomic dead space*, where the term "dead space" refers to areas of lung that receive ventilation but no blood flow. Its volume is about 150 ml.

The terminal bronchioles divide into *respiratory bronchioles*, which have occasional alveoli budding from their walls. Finally, we come to the *alveolar ducts*, which are completely lined with alveoli. This alveolated region of the lung where the gas exchange occurs is known as the *respiratory zone*. The portion of lung distal to a terminal bronchiole forms an anatomical unit called the *acinus*. The distance from the terminal bronchiole to the most distal alveolus is only a few millimeters, but the respiratory zone makes up most of the lung, its volume being about 2.5 to 3 liters during rest.

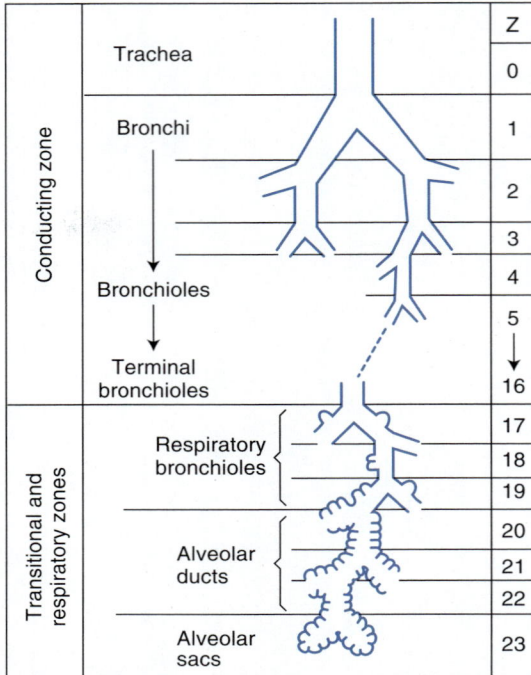

Figure 1.4. Idealization of the human airways according to Weibel. Note that the first 16 generations (Z) make up the conducting airways, and the last 7 make up the respiratory zone (or the transitional and respiratory zones). (Modified from Weibel ER. *The Pathway for Oxygen*. Cambridge, UK: Harvard University Press; 1984:275.)

During inspiration, the volume of the thoracic cavity increases and air is drawn into the lung. The increase in volume is brought about partly by contraction of the diaphragm, which causes it to descend, and partly by the action of the intercostal muscles, which raise the ribs, thus increasing the cross-sectional area of the thorax. Inspired air flows down to about the terminal bronchioles by bulk flow, like water through a hose. Beyond that point, the combined cross-sectional area of the airways is so enormous because of the large number of branches (**Figure 1.5**) that the forward velocity of the gas becomes small. Diffusion of gas within the airways then takes over as the dominant mechanism of ventilation in the respiratory zone. The rate of diffusion of gas molecules within the airways is so rapid and the distances to be covered so short that differences in concentration within the acinus are virtually abolished within a second. However, because the velocity of gas falls rapidly in the region of the terminal bronchioles, inhaled dust frequently settles out there.

The lung is elastic and returns passively to its preinspiratory volume during resting breathing. It is remarkably easy to distend. A normal breath of about 500 ml, for example, requires a distending pressure of less than 3 cm

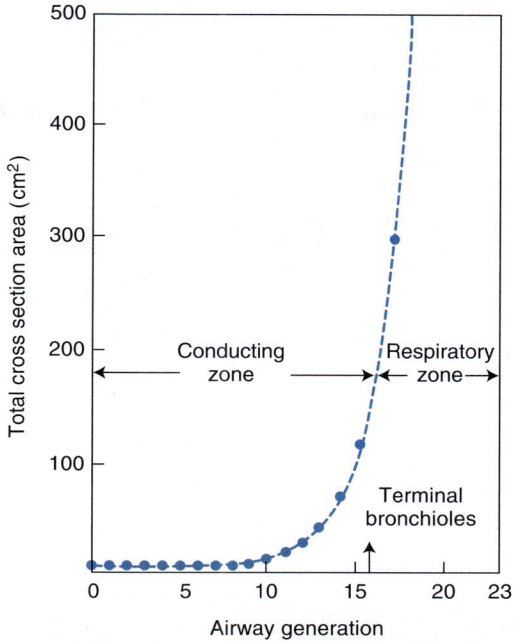

Figure 1.5. Diagram to show the extremely rapid increase in total cross-sectional area of the airways in the respiratory zone (compare Figure 1.4). As a result, the forward velocity of the gas during inspiration becomes very small in the region of the respiratory bronchioles, and gaseous diffusion becomes the chief mode of ventilation.

water. By contrast, a child's balloon may need a pressure of 30 cm water for the same change in volume.

The pressure required to move gas through the airways is also very small. During normal inspiration, an air flow rate of 1 liter·s^{-1} requires a pressure drop along the airways of less than 2 cm water. This can be compared to drinking through a soda straw, which may need a pressure of about 500 cm water for the same flow rate.

Airways

- Divided into a conducting zone and a respiratory zone.
- Volume of the anatomic dead space is about 150 ml.
- Volume of the alveolar region is about 2.5 to 3.0 liters.
- Gas moves by bulk flow down a pressure gradient in the conducting zone.
- Gas movement in the alveolar region is chiefly by diffusion.

BLOOD VESSELS AND FLOW

The pulmonary blood vessels also form a series of branching tubes from the *pulmonary artery* to the *capillaries* and back to the *pulmonary veins*. Initially, the arteries, veins, and bronchi run close together, but toward the periphery of the lung, the veins move away to pass between the lobules, whereas the arteries and bronchi travel together down the centers of the lobules in what is often referred to as the bronchovascular bundle. The capillaries form a dense network in the walls of the alveoli (**Figure 1.6**). The diameter of a capillary segment is about 7 to 10 μm, just large enough for a red blood cell. The lengths of the segments are so short that the dense network forms an almost continuous sheet of blood in the alveolar wall, a very efficient arrangement for gas exchange. Alveolar walls are not often seen face on, as in Figure 1.6. The usual, thin microscopic cross section (**Figure 1.7**) shows the red blood cells in the capillaries and emphasizes the enormous exposure of blood to alveolar gas, with only the thin blood-gas barrier intervening (compare Figure 1.1).

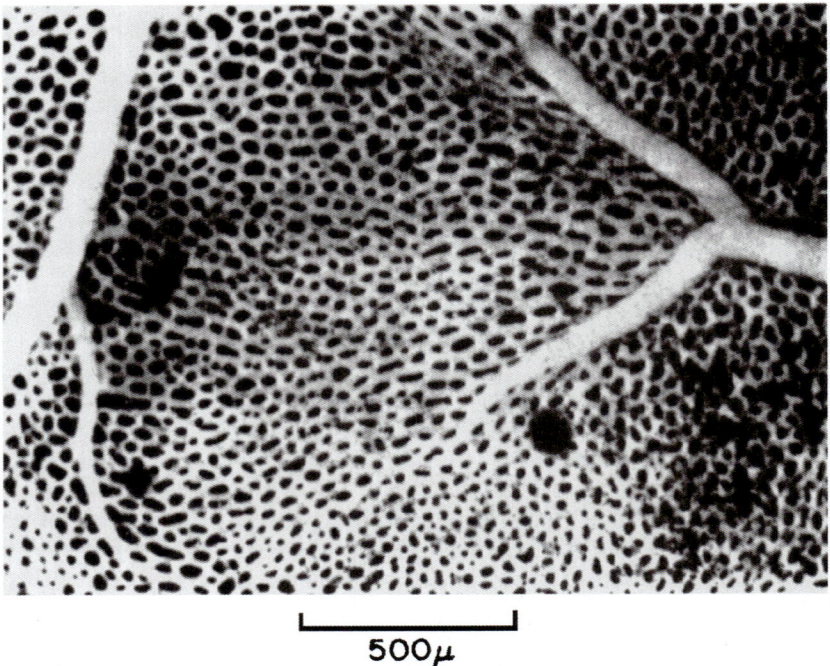

500μ

Figure 1.6. View of an alveolar wall (in the frog) showing the dense network of capillaries. A small artery (*left*) and vein (*right*) can also be seen. The individual capillary segments are so short that the blood forms an almost continuous sheet. (Reprinted from Maloney JE, Castle BL. Pressure-diameter relations of capillaries and small blood vessels in frog lung. *Respir Physiol*. 1969;7(2):150-162. Copyright © 1969 Elsevier. With permission.)

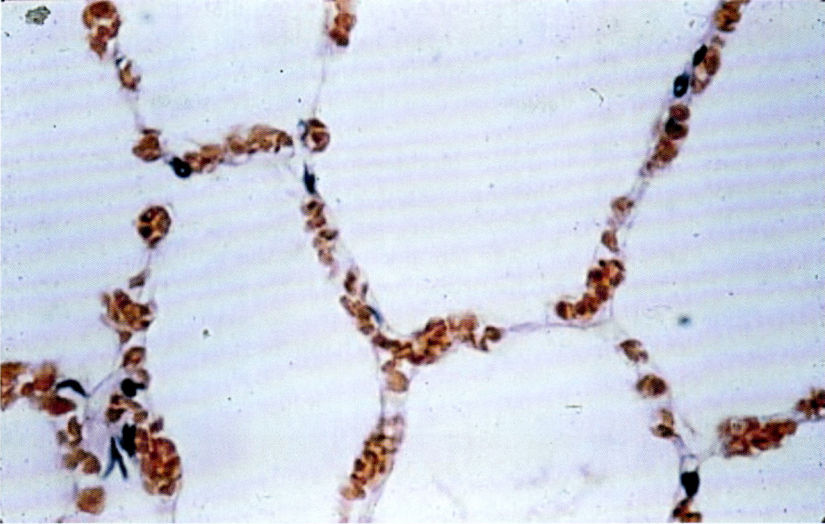

Figure 1.7. Microscopic section of dog lung showing capillaries in the alveolar walls. The blood-gas barrier is so thin that it cannot be identified here (compare Figure 1.1). This section was prepared from lung that was rapidly frozen while being perfused. (Reproduced with permission from Glazier JB, Hughes JM, Maloney JE, et al. Measurements of capillary dimensions and blood volume in rapidly frozen lungs. *J Appl Physiol*. 1969;26(1):65-76. Copyright © 1969 the American Physiological Society. All rights reserved.)

Because the blood-gas barrier is extremely thin, the capillaries are easily damaged. Increasing the pressure in the capillaries to high levels or inflating the lung to high volumes, for example, can raise the wall stresses of the capillaries to a point at which ultrastructural changes can occur. The capillaries then leak plasma and even red blood cells into the alveolar spaces.

The pulmonary artery receives the whole output of the right heart, but the resistance of the pulmonary circuit is astonishingly small. A mean pulmonary arterial pressure of only about 20 cm water (about 15 mm Hg) is required for a flow of 6 liter·min^{-1} (the same flow through a soda straw needs 120 cm water). The mechanisms by which the lung maintains low pressures in the pulmonary circulation and protects the delicate capillaries is discussed further in Chapter 4.

Blood-Gas Interface

- Extremely thin (0.2 to 0.3 μm) over much of its area
- Enormous surface area of 50 to 100 m²
- Large area obtained by having about 500 million alveoli
- So thin that large increases in capillary pressure can damage the barrier

Each red blood cell spends about 0.75 s in the capillary network and during this time probably traverses two or three alveoli. So efficient is the anatomy for gas exchange that this brief time is sufficient for virtually complete equilibration of oxygen and carbon dioxide between alveolar gas and capillary blood.

The lung has an additional blood supply, the bronchial circulation, which provides blood to the conducting airways down to about the terminal bronchioles. Most of this blood is carried away from the lung via the pulmonary veins, while a small amount reaches the left side of the heart and enters the systemic circulation. The flow through the bronchial circulation is a mere fraction of that through the pulmonary circulation, and the lung can function fairly well without it, as happens, for example, following lung transplantation.

Blood Vessels

- The whole of the output of the right heart goes to the lung.
- The diameter of the capillaries is about 7 to 10 μm.
- The thickness of much of the capillary walls is less than 0.3 μm.
- Blood spends about 0.75 s in the capillaries.

To conclude this brief account of the functional anatomy of the lung, let us glance at three problems that the lung has overcome.

STABILITY OF ALVEOLI

The lung can be regarded as a collection of 500 million bubbles, each 0.3 mm in diameter. Such a structure is inherently unstable. Because of the surface tension of the liquid lining the alveoli, relatively large forces develop that tend to collapse alveoli. Fortunately, some of the cells lining the alveoli secrete a material called *surfactant* that dramatically lowers the surface tension of the alveolar lining layer and markedly increases the stability of the alveoli (see Chapter 7). Collapse of small airspaces is always a potential problem, however, and frequently occurs in disease.

REMOVAL OF INHALED PARTICLES

With its surface area of 50 to 100 m^2, the lung presents the largest surface of the body to an increasingly hostile environment. Various mechanisms for dealing with inhaled particles have been developed (see Chapter 9). Large particles are filtered out in the nose, while smaller particles that deposit in the conducting airways are removed by a moving staircase of mucus that continually sweeps debris up to the epiglottis, where it is swallowed or expectorated. The mucus, secreted by mucous glands and also by goblet cells in the bronchial walls, is propelled by millions of tiny cilia, which move rhythmically under normal conditions but are paralyzed by some inhaled toxins.

The alveoli have no cilia, and particles that deposit there are engulfed by large wandering cells called macrophages. The foreign material is then removed from the lung via the lymphatics or the blood flow. Other immune cells, such as neutrophils, participate in the defense against foreign material.

REMOVAL OF MATERIAL FROM THE BLOOD

Just as the lungs eliminate foreign material from the airways and airspaces, the branching network of very small blood vessels traps small pieces of infected material or blood clots that form in or enter the venous circulation. This prevents such material from getting to the left, or systemic, side of the circulation where they could then travel to various organs and cause problems such as stroke, myocardial infarction, or infected fluid collections known as abscesses.

KEY CONCEPTS

1. The blood-gas barrier is extremely thin with a very large area, making it ideal for gas exchange by passive diffusion.

2. The conducting airways extend to the terminal bronchioles, with a total volume of about 150 ml. All the gas exchange occurs in the respiratory zone, which has a volume of about 2.5 to 3 liters.

3. Convective flow takes inspired gas to about the terminal bronchioles; beyond this, gas movement is increasingly by diffusion in the alveolar region.

4. The pulmonary capillaries occupy a huge area of the alveolar wall, and a red cell spends about 0.75 s in them.

5. Surfactant maintains the stability of alveoli, while cilia are important for eliminating foreign material from the airways, and the smallest pulmonary blood vessels trap foreign material in the blood.

CLINICAL VIGNETTE

A 50-year-old man, who has smoked two packs of cigarettes per day since the age of 18, was well until a year ago when he developed hemoptysis (coughing up blood). At bronchoscopy during which a lighted tube with a camera on the end was passed down into his airways, a mass lesion was seen in the left main bronchus, the main airway supplying the left lung. When this was biopsied, it was shown to be malignant. A computed tomography (CT) scan revealed that the cancer had not spread. He was treated by left pneumonectomy in which the entire left lung was removed.

When he was assessed 6 months later, the volume of his lung was found to be reduced by one-third of the preoperative value. The ability of his lung to transfer gases across the blood-gas barrier was reduced by 30% compared with the preoperative value. (This test is known as the diffusing capacity for carbon monoxide and is discussed in Chapter 3.) The pulmonary artery pressure was normal at rest but increased more during exercise than preoperatively. His exercise capacity was reduced by 20%.

- Why was lung volume reduced by only one-third when one of his two lungs was removed?
- How can the 30% reduction in the ability of the blood-gas barrier to transfer gases be explained?
- Why did the pulmonary artery pressure increase more on exercise than preoperatively?
- Why was the exercise capacity reduced?

QUESTIONS

For each question, choose the one best answer.

1. Two healthy women (Subjects A and B) ascend to a mountain hut at 4,559 m in elevation as part of a research project on acute altitude illness. Twelve hours following arrival at the hut, catheters are inserted in each of their pulmonary arteries and used to estimate the pressure in their pulmonary capillaries. Subject A has a pulmonary capillary pressure of 18 mm Hg compared to only 10 mm Hg in Subject B. For which of the following problems is Subject A at greater risk than Subject B?
   A. Decreased alveolar surface tension
   B. Decreased bronchial circulation blood flow
   C. Increased volume of the anatomic dead space
   D. Leakage of plasma and red blood cells into the alveolar space
   E. Delayed airway closure on exhalation

2. A newborn infant is hospitalized for tachypnea and hypoxemia for several days following birth and is subsequently determined to have a genetic defect affecting the primary structural elements of the cilia. For which of the following problems is this newborn infant at risk as a result of this genetic defect?
   A. Decreased airway mucous clearance
   B. Decreased pulmonary blood flow
   C. Decreased surfactant production
   D. Increased diffusion distance across the blood-gas interface
   E. Thickening of the alveolar basement membrane

3. A 30-year-old woman presents to the emergency department in premature labor and gives birth to a baby boy at only 28 weeks of gestation, when surfactant production remains very low. Which of the following would you expect to occur in the lungs of this newborn infant as a result of the premature delivery?
   A. Decreased ciliary function
   B. Increased cross-sectional area for pulmonary blood flow
   C. Increased red blood cell transit time in the pulmonary capillaries
   D. Increased surface tension of the alveolar lining layer
   E. Thickening of the alveolar-capillary barrier

4. Which of the following changes in airway structure and function is seen as air flow transitions from the respiratory bronchioles to the terminal bronchioles on exhalation?
   A. Decreased cross-sectional area for airflow
   B. Decreased proportion of cartilage in the airway walls
   C. Decreased velocity of expired gas
   D. Increased movement of gas by diffusion
   E. Increased number of alveolar ducts

5. A 28-year-old woman with cystic fibrosis is admitted to the hospital with massive hemoptysis (expectoration of blood). As part of her treatment, the interventional radiologist inserts a catheter into two bronchial arteries that provide blood to the right upper lobe and injects a material that stops blood flow through these vessels (referred to as "embolization"). Which of the following changes in pulmonary function would you expect as a result of this intervention?
   A. Decreased blood flow to right upper lobe segmental bronchi
   B. Decreased cross-sectional area for blood flow in the pulmonary circulation
   C. Decreased surfactant production by type II alveolar epithelial cells
   D. Increased blood flow through the pulmonary artery
   E. Slower diffusion of gas from the alveoli to pulmonary capillaries

6. A 65-year-old man complained of worsening dyspnea on exertion over a 6-month period. A lung biopsy was done because of changes seen on chest imaging. The pathology report states that the thin side of the blood-gas barrier is greater than 0.8 μm in thickness in most of the alveoli. Which of the following would you expect?

A. Decreased alveolar surfactant concentrations
B. Decreased rate of diffusion of oxygen into the pulmonary capillaries
C. Increased risk of rupture of the blood-gas barrier
D. Increased volume of individual red cells
E. Slower diffusion of gas from the distal airways to the alveoli

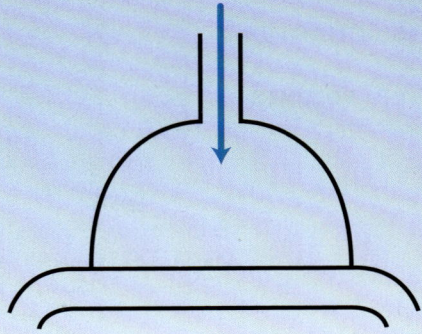

Ventilation

How Gas Gets to the Alveoli

2

- **Lung Volumes**
- **Ventilation**
- **Anatomic Dead Space**
- **Physiologic Dead Space**
- **Regional Differences in Ventilation**

In this chapter, we look in more detail at how oxygen is brought to the blood-gas barrier by the process of ventilation. After briefly reviewing lung volumes, we then discuss total ventilation, with an emphasis on two important concepts, alveolar ventilation, which is the amount of fresh gas getting to the alveoli, and dead space ventilation, the portion of the ventilation that does not participate in gas exchange. Finally, we discuss the distribution of ventilation in the lungs with a particular emphasis on the role of gravity. At the end of this chapter, the reader should be able to:

- Identify the major volumes and capacities in a spirogram
- Describe differences in the helium dilution and plethysmography methods of measuring lung volumes
- Calculate minute ventilation
- Predict changes in arterial P_{CO_2} based on changes in alveolar ventilation and carbon dioxide production
- Describe the differences between anatomic and physiologic dead space
- Predict the effect of changes in body position on the regional distribution of ventilation

VOLUMES   **FLOWS**

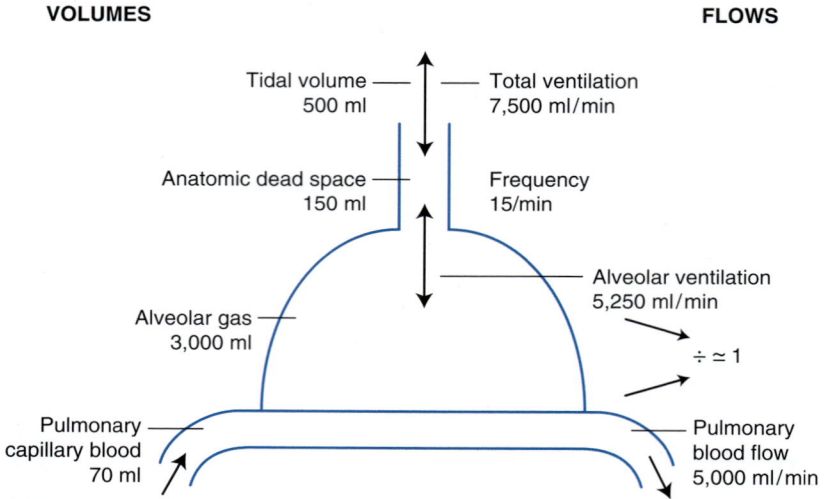

Tidal volume —— Total ventilation
500 ml   7,500 ml/min

Anatomic dead space —— Frequency
150 ml   15/min

Alveolar ventilation
5,250 ml/min

Alveolar gas
3,000 ml $\div \simeq 1$

Pulmonary —— Pulmonary
capillary blood   blood flow
70 ml   5,000 ml/min

Figure 2.1. Diagram of a lung showing typical volumes and flows. There is considerable variation around these values depending on the size and sex of the patient. (Modified with permission of John Wiley & Sons from West JB. *Ventilation/Blood Flow and Gas Exchange*. 5th ed. Oxford, UK: Blackwell; 1990:3; permission conveyed through Copyright Clearance Center, Inc.)

The next three chapters discuss how inspired air gets to the alveoli, how oxygen and carbon dioxide cross the blood-gas interface, and how they are moved to and from the lung by the blood. These functions are carried out by ventilation, diffusion, and blood flow, respectively.

Figure 2.1 is a highly simplified diagram of a lung that is used throughout the book. The various bronchi that make up the conducting airways (see Figures 1.3 and 1.4) are now represented by a single tube labeled "anatomic dead space." This leads into the gas-exchanging region of the lung, which is bounded by the blood-gas interface and the pulmonary capillary blood. With each inspiration, about 500 ml of air enters the lung (*tidal volume*) and about the same volume leaves. Note how small a proportion of the total lung volume is represented by the anatomic dead space. The larger the volume of the dead space, the smaller the volume of fresh gas entering the alveoli. Also note the very small volume of capillary blood compared with that of alveolar gas (compare with Figure 1.7).

LUNG VOLUMES

Before looking at the movement of gas into the lung, a brief glance at the static volumes of the lung is helpful. Some of these can be measured with a water-bell spirometer (**Figure 2.2**), although electronic devices have now

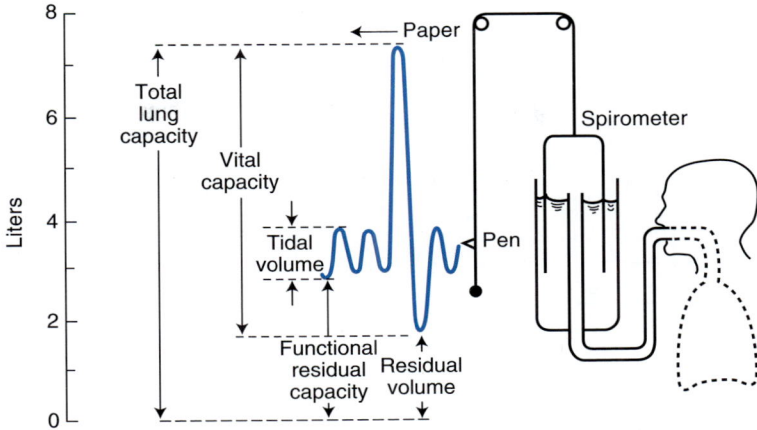

Figure 2.2. Lung volumes. Note that the total lung capacity, functional residual capacity, and residual volume cannot be measured with the spirometer.

replaced the classic water spirometer shown in this figure. During exhalation, the bell goes up and the pen down, marking a moving chart. First, normal breathing can be seen (*tidal volume*). The volume of gas in the lung after a normal (or tidal) expiration is the *functional residual capacity (FRC)*. Next, the individual took a maximal inspiration and followed this by a maximal expiration. The exhaled volume is called the *vital capacity*. Some gas does remain in the lung after a maximal expiration and is referred to as the *residual volume*.

Neither the FRC, residual volume, nor total lung capacity can be measured with a simple spirometer, and instead, can only be measured using other methods. One such method—a gas dilution technique—is shown in **Figure 2.3**. The subject is connected to a spirometer containing a known concentration of helium, which is virtually insoluble in blood. After some breaths, the helium concentrations in the spirometer and lung become the same.

The amount of helium present before equilibration (concentration times volume) is represented as follows:

$$C_1 \times V_1$$

Because no helium is lost, this must equal the amount of helium after equilibration:

$$C_2 \times (V_1 + V_2)$$

We can rearrange these equations and calculate the volume of the lung (V_2) as follows:

$$V_2 = V_1 \times \frac{C_1 - C_2}{C_2}$$

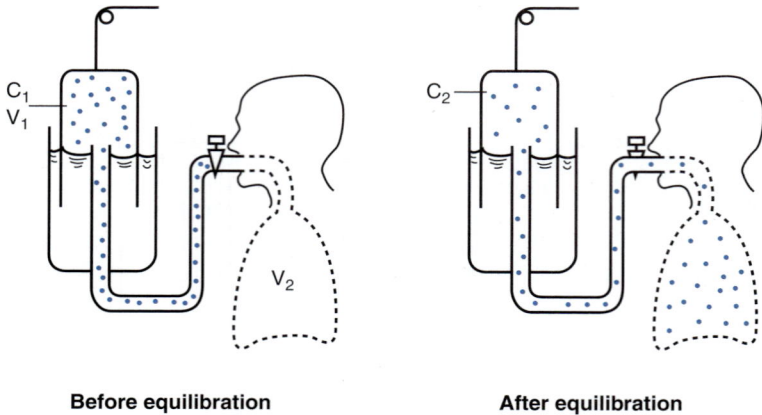

Before equilibration   **After equilibration**

$$C_1 \times V_1 = C_2 \times (V_1 + V_2)$$

Figure 2.3. Measurement of the functional residual capacity by helium dilution.

In practice, oxygen is added to the spirometer during equilibration to make up for that consumed by the subject, and also carbon dioxide is absorbed.

Another way of measuring the FRC is with a body plethysmograph (**Figure 2.4**). This is a large airtight box, like an old telephone booth, in which the subject sits. At the end of a normal expiration, a shutter closes the mouthpiece, and the subject is asked to make respiratory efforts. As the subject tries to inhale, he or she expands the gas in the lungs; lung volume increases, and, based on the principles of Boyle's law, which states that pressure × volume is constant at a constant temperature, the box pressure rises because its gas volume decreases.

If the pressures in the box before and after the inspiratory effort are P_1 and P_2, respectively, V_1 is the preinspiratory box volume, and ΔV is the change in volume of the box (or lung), we can therefore write:

$$P_1 V_1 = P_2(V_1 - \Delta V)$$

Thus, ΔV can be obtained.

Next, we apply Boyle's law to the gas in the lung and see that:

$$P_3 V_2 = P_4(V_2 + \Delta V)$$

where P_3 and P_4 are the mouth pressures before and after the inspiratory effort, and V_2 is the FRC. Thus, FRC can be obtained.

The body plethysmograph measures the total volume of gas in the lung, including any that is trapped behind closed airways and, therefore, does not communicate with the mouth (an example is shown in Figure 7.9). By

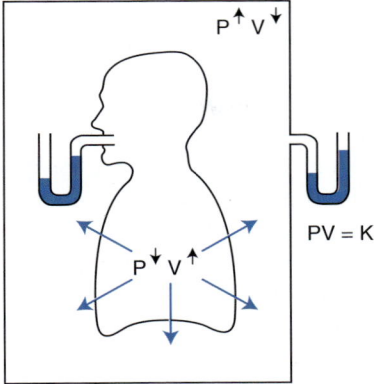

Figure 2.4. Measurement of FRC with a body plethysmograph. When the subject makes an inspiratory effort against a closed airway, he or she slightly increases the volume of his lung, airway pressure decreases, and box pressure increases. From Boyle's law, lung volume is obtained (see text).

contrast, the helium dilution method measures only communicating gas or ventilated lung volume. In healthy individuals, these volumes are virtually the same, but in patients with lung disease, the ventilated volume may be considerably less than the total volume because of gas trapped behind obstructed airways.

Lung Volumes

- Tidal volume and vital capacity can be measured with a simple spirometer.
- Total lung capacity, functional residual capacity, and residual volume are measured using helium dilution or body plethysmography.
- Helium is used because of its very low solubility in blood.
- The use of the body plethysmograph depends on Boyle's law, PV = K, at constant temperature.

VENTILATION

If the volume exhaled with each breath is 500 ml (Figure 2.1) and there are 12 breaths·min^{-1}, the total volume leaving the lung each minute is 500 × 12 = 6,000 ml·min^{-1}. This is known as the *total ventilation* or the *minute ventilation*. The volume of air entering the lung is very slightly greater because more oxygen is taken in than carbon dioxide is given out. Total ventilation is typically 5,000 to 6,000 ml·min^{-1} at rest in healthy adults and can rise to much higher levels with exercise or in response to a variety of other stimuli.

However, not all the air that passes the lips reaches the alveolar gas compartment where gas exchange occurs. Of each 500 ml inhaled in Figure 2.1, 150 ml remains behind in the anatomic dead space. Thus, the volume of fresh gas entering the respiratory zone each minute is $(500 - 150) \times 12$ or 4,200 ml·min^{-1}. This is called the *alveolar ventilation* and is of key importance because it represents the amount of fresh inspired air available for gas exchange (strictly, the alveolar ventilation is also measured on expiration, but the volume is almost the same). Note that even though only 350 ml of fresh gas enters the alveoli with each breath, the alveolar volume still expands by the full size of the tidal volume as 150 ml of gas left over in the anatomic dead space at the end of the previous exhalation is drawn into the alveoli with each breath before the fresh gas enters.

The total (or minute) ventilation can be measured easily by having the subject breathe through a valve box that separates the inspired from the expired gas, and collecting all the expired gas in a bag. The alveolar ventilation is more difficult to determine. One way is to measure the volume of the anatomic dead space (see below) and calculate the dead space ventilation (dead space volume × respiratory frequency). This is then subtracted from the total ventilation.

We can summarize this conveniently with symbols (**Figure 2.5**). Using V to denote volume, and the subscripts T, D, and A to denote tidal, dead space, and alveolar, respectively, we see that:

$$V_T = V_D + V_A$$

Taking into account the respiratory frequency n, we get:

$$V_T \cdot n = V_D \cdot n + V_A \cdot n$$

We see therefore that:

$$\dot{V}_E = \dot{V}_D + \dot{V}_A$$

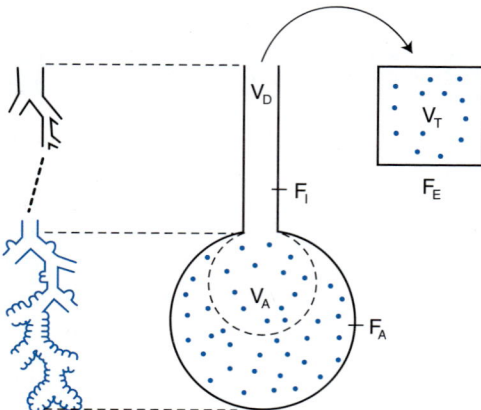

Figure 2.5. The tidal volume (V_T) is a mixture of gas from the anatomic dead space (V_D) and a contribution from the alveolar gas (V_A). The concentrations of CO_2 are shown by the *dots*. F, fractional concentration; I, inspired; E, expired. Compare Figure 1.4.

where $\dot{V}$ means volume per unit time, $\dot{V}_E$ is expired total (or minute) ventilation, and $\dot{V}_D$ and $\dot{V}_A$ are the dead space and alveolar ventilations, respectively (see Appendix A for a summary of symbols).

Rearranging this equation, we see that alveolar ventilation—that portion of ventilation which participates in gas exchanges—is determined by the balance between total and dead space ventilation:

$$\dot{V}_A = \dot{V}_E - \dot{V}_D$$

A difficulty with this method is that the anatomic dead space is not easy to measure, although a value for it can be assumed with little error. Note that alveolar ventilation can be increased by raising either tidal volume or respiratory frequency (or both). Increasing tidal volume is often more effective because this reduces the fraction of each breath occupied by the anatomic dead space, which is referred to as the dead space fraction.

Another way of measuring alveolar ventilation in normal subjects is from the concentration of CO_2 in expired gas (Figure 2.5). A small portion of each inhaled breath, which contains essentially no CO_2, is left behind in the conducting airways. Because no gas exchange occurs in the anatomic dead space, there is no CO_2 there at the end of inspiration, all of the expired CO_2 comes from the alveolar gas.

$$\dot{V}_{CO_2} = \dot{V}_A \times \frac{\%CO_2}{100}$$

$\dot{V}_{CO_2}$ refers to the CO_2 output or production, while the $\%CO_2/100$ is often called the fractional concentration and is denoted by F_{CO_2}.

Therefore,

$$\dot{V}_{CO_2} = \dot{V}_A \times F_{CO_2}$$

which can be rearranged to give:

$$\dot{V}_A = \frac{\dot{V}_{CO_2}}{F_{CO_2}}$$

Thus, the alveolar ventilation can be obtained by dividing the CO_2 output by the alveolar fractional concentration of this gas.

Note that the partial pressure of CO_2 (denoted P_{CO_2}) is proportional to the fractional concentration of the gas in the alveoli, or $P_{CO_2} = F_{CO_2} \times K$, where K is a constant which is the total pressure.

Therefore,

$$\dot{V}_A = \frac{\dot{V}_{CO_2}}{P_{CO_2}} \times K$$

This is called the alveolar ventilation equation.

Because in healthy individuals, the P_{CO_2} of alveolar gas and arterial blood are virtually identical, the arterial P_{CO_2} can be used to determine alveolar ventilation. This relationship between alveolar ventilation and P_{CO_2} is of crucial importance. If the alveolar ventilation is halved (and CO_2 production remains unchanged), for example, the alveolar and arterial P_{CO_2} will double. CO_2 production at rest is usually constant, but it is affected by metabolic activity. It is increased by factors such as exercise, fever, infection, nutritional intake, and seizures and decreased by hypothermia and fasting.

ANATOMIC DEAD SPACE

This is the volume of the conducting airways (Figures 1.3 and 1.4). The normal value is about 150 ml, and it increases with large inspirations because of the traction or pull exerted on the bronchi by the surrounding lung parenchyma. The dead space also depends on the size and posture of the subject.

The volume of the anatomic dead space can be measured by *Fowler's method* (**Figure 2.6**). The subject breathes through a valve box, and the sampling tube of a rapid nitrogen analyzer continuously samples gas at the lips (Figure 2.6A). Following a single inspiration of 100% O_2, the N_2 concentration rises as the dead space gas is increasingly washed out by alveolar gas. Finally, an almost uniform gas concentration is seen, representing pure alveolar gas. This phase is often called the alveolar "plateau," although in healthy individuals, it is not quite flat, and in patients with lung disease, it may rise steeply. Expired volume is also recorded. Carbon dioxide is sometimes substituted for nitrogen, but the measurements in such cases become much more complicated in patients with lung disease because of inequality of blood flow and ventilation in the lung.

The dead space is found by plotting N_2 concentration against expired volume and drawing a vertical line such that area A is equal to area B in Figure 2.6B. The dead space is the volume expired up to the vertical line. In effect, this method measures the volume of the conducting airways down to the midpoint of the transition from dead space to alveolar gas.

PHYSIOLOGIC DEAD SPACE

Another way of measuring dead space is *Bohr's method*. Figure 2.5 shows that all the expired CO_2 comes from the alveolar gas and none from the dead space. Therefore, we can write:

$$V_T \cdot F_{ECO_2} = V_A \cdot F_{ACO_2}$$

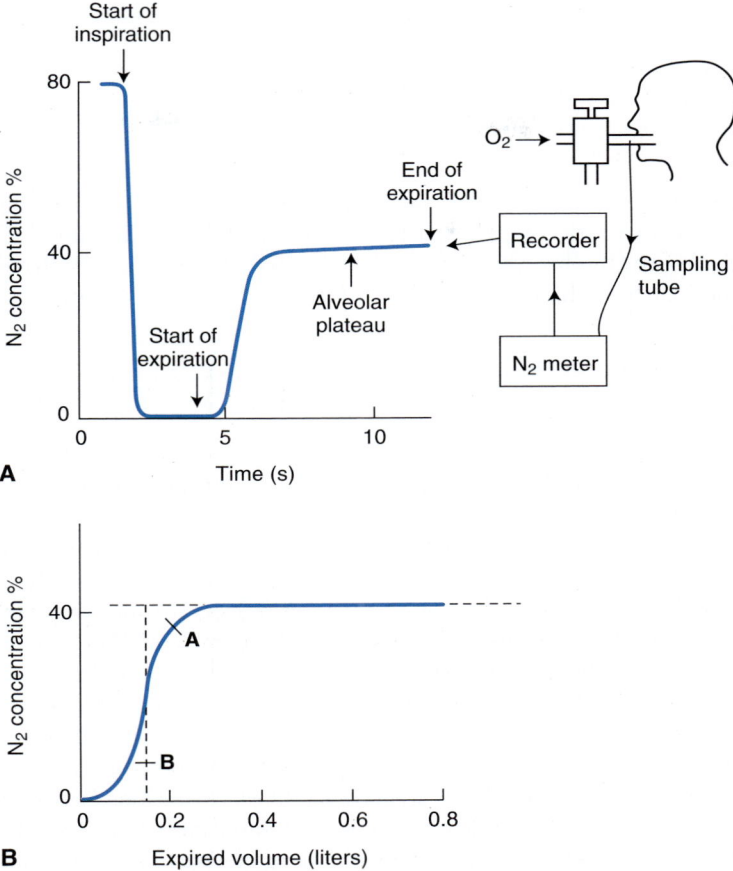

Figure 2.6. Fowler method of measuring the anatomic dead space with a rapid N_2 analyzer. **A.** Shows that following a test inspiration of 100% O_2, the N_2 concentration rises during expiration to an almost level "plateau" representing pure alveolar gas. In **(B)**, N_2 concentration is plotted against expired volume, and the dead space is the volume up to the *vertical dashed line*, which makes the areas *A* and *B* equal.

Recall that tidal volume is composed of the alveolar volume and dead space volume:

$$V_T = V_A + V_D$$

Rearranging this, we see:

$$V_A = V_T - V_D$$

Substituting the term on the right into the first equation above, we see that

$$V_T \cdot F_{ECO_2} = (V_T - V_D) \cdot F_{ACO_2}$$

We can therefore calculate the ratio of the dead space volume to the tidal volume as:

$$\frac{V_D}{V_T} = \frac{P_{A_{CO_2}} - P_{E_{CO_2}}}{P_{A_{CO_2}}} \quad \text{(Bohr equation)}$$

where A and E refer to alveolar and mixed expired, respectively (see Appendix A). The normal ratio of dead space to tidal volume is in the range of 0.2 to 0.35 during resting breathing. In healthy individuals, the P_{CO_2} in alveolar gas and that in arterial blood are virtually identical so that the equation is therefore often written:

$$\frac{V_D}{V_T} = \frac{P_{a_{CO_2}} - P_{E_{CO_2}}}{P_{a_{CO_2}}}$$

It should be noted that the Fowler's and Bohr's methods measure somewhat different things. Fowler's method measures the volume of the conducting airways down to the level where the rapid dilution of inspired gas occurs with gas already in the lung. This volume is determined by the geometry of the rapidly expanding airways (Figure 1.5), and because it reflects the morphology of the lung, it is called the *anatomic dead space*. Bohr's method measures the volume of the lung that does not eliminate CO_2. Because this is a functional measurement, the volume is called the *physiologic dead space*. In normal subjects, the volumes are very nearly the same. However, in patients with either acute or chronic lung disease, the physiologic dead space may be considerably larger because of inequality of blood flow and ventilation within the lung (see Chapter 5). The size of the physiologic dead space is very important. The larger it is, the greater the total ventilation an individual must generate to ensure an adequate amount of air enters the alveoli to participate in gas exchange.

Ventilation

- Total ventilation is tidal volume × respiratory frequency.
- Alveolar ventilation is the amount of fresh gas getting to the alveoli, or $(V_T - V_D) \times n$.
- Anatomic dead space is the volume of the conducting airways, about 150 ml in adults.
- Physiologic dead space is the volume of gas that does not eliminate CO_2.
- The two dead spaces are almost the same in healthy individuals, but the physiologic dead space is increased in both acute and chronic lung diseases.

REGIONAL DIFFERENCES IN VENTILATION

So far, we have been assuming that all regions of the normal lung have the same ventilation. However, it has been shown that the lower regions of the lung ventilate better than the upper zones. This can be demonstrated if a subject inhales radioactive xenon gas (**Figure 2.7**). When the xenon-133 enters the counting field, its radiation penetrates the chest wall and can be recorded by a bank of counters or a radiation camera. In this way, the volume of the inhaled xenon going to various regions can be determined.

Figure 2.7 shows the results obtained in a series of normal volunteers using this method. It can be seen that ventilation per unit volume is greatest near the bottom of the lung and becomes progressively smaller toward the top. Other measurements show that when the subject is in the supine position, this difference disappears, with the result that apical and basal ventilations become the same. However, in that posture, the ventilation of the lowermost (posterior) lung exceeds that of the uppermost (anterior) lung. Again, in the lateral position (subject on his or her side), the dependent lung is best ventilated. The cause of these regional differences in ventilation is discussed in Chapter 7.

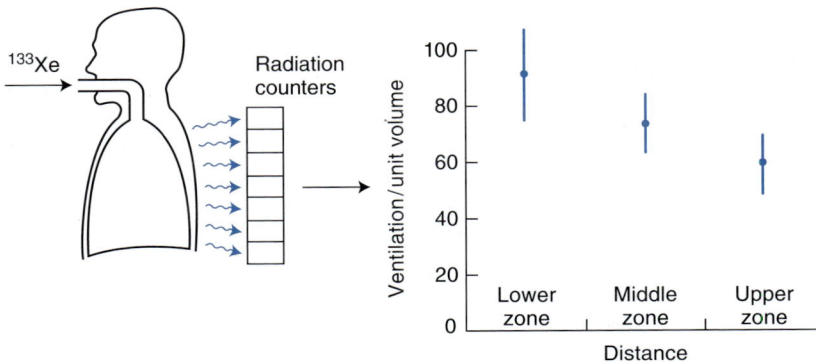

Figure 2.7. Measurement of regional differences in ventilation with radioactive xenon. When the gas is inhaled, its radiation can be detected by counters outside the chest. Note that the ventilation decreases from the lower to upper regions of the upright lung.

KEY CONCEPTS

1. Lung volumes that cannot be measured with a simple spirometer include the total lung capacity, the functional residual capacity, and the residual volume. These can be determined by helium dilution or the body plethysmograph.

2. Alveolar ventilation is the volume of fresh (non–dead space) gas entering the respiratory zone per minute. It can be determined from the alveolar ventilation equation, that is, the CO_2 output divided by the fractional concentration of CO_2 in the expired gas.

3. The concentration of CO_2 (and therefore its partial pressure) in alveolar gas and arterial blood is inversely related to the alveolar ventilation.

4. The anatomic dead space is the volume of the conducting airways and can be measured from the nitrogen concentration following a single inspiration of 100% oxygen (Fowler's method).

5. The physiologic dead space is the volume of lung that does not eliminate CO_2. It is measured by Bohr's method using arterial and expired CO_2.

6. The lower regions of the lung are better ventilated than the upper regions because of the effects of gravity on the lung.

CLINICAL VIGNETTE

A 20-year-old college student is brought into the emergency department at 1:00 AM where she is noted to be confused and barely able to speak, and her breath smells strongly of alcohol. Her friends who brought her in left before any information could be obtained about her. Concerned about her ability to protect her airway and the fact that she may swallow oral secretions into her lungs (aspiration), the emergency physician intubates the patient. This involves passing a tube through her mouth into her trachea so that she can be attached to a ventilator. The ventilator is placed on a mode that allows her to set her own respiratory rate and tidal volume. The respiratory therapist reviews the information on the ventilator's display and notes that her respiratory rate is 8 breaths per minute and her tidal volume is 300 ml.

- How does her total ventilation compare to what you would expect for a healthy individual of this age? What could account for this change?
- What is her dead space as a fraction of her tidal volume compared to prior to her illness?
- What change would you expect to see in her arterial P_{CO_2} compared to before her illness?

QUESTIONS

For each question, choose the one best answer.

1. A healthy individual with no underlying lung disease is laying on a table in the position depicted in the figure below. Which of the labeled regions of the lung (A–C) would you expect to receive the greatest ventilation per unit volume?

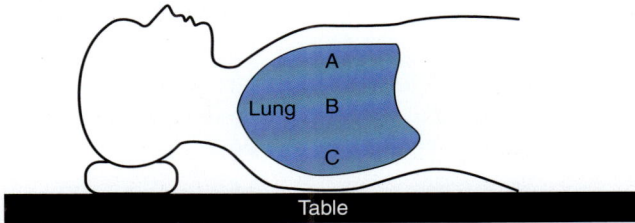

A. A
B. B
C. C

2. An otherwise healthy patient is intubated and started on mechanical ventilation because he was comatose and not making any breathing efforts after a drug overdose. The ventilator settings include a tidal volume of 450 ml and a respiratory rate of 12 breaths·min⁻¹. Using data obtained from the ventilator and an arterial blood gas, the respiratory therapist estimates that the patient's dead space fraction $\left(\dfrac{V_D}{V_T}\right)$ is 0.3. Based on these data, what is the patient's approximate alveolar ventilation?
   A. 1 liter·min⁻¹
   B. 1.6 liter·min⁻¹
   C. 3.8 liter·min⁻¹
   D. 5.4 liter·min⁻¹
   E. 7.0 liter·min⁻¹

3. In a measurement of FRC by helium dilution, the original and final helium concentrations were 10% and 6%, and the spirometer volume was kept at 5 liters. What is the volume of the FRC in liters?
   A. 2.5
   B. 3.0
   C. 3.3
   D. 3.8
   E. 5.0

4. A patient sits in a body plethysmograph (body box) and makes an expiratory effort against his closed glottis. What happens to the following: pressure in the lung airways, lung volume, box pressure, box volume?

	Airway Pressure	Lung Volume	Box Pressure	Box Volume
A.	↓	↑	↑	↓
B.	↓	↑	↓	↑
C.	↑	↓	↑	↓
D.	↑	↓	↓	↑
E.	↑	↑	↓	↓

5. If CO_2 production remains constant and alveolar ventilation is increased threefold, the alveolar P_{CO_2}, after a steady state is reached, will be what percentage of its former value?
   A. 25
   B. 33
   C. 50
   D. 100
   E. 300

6. A 56-year-old woman is started on mechanical ventilation after presenting to the emergency department with acute respiratory failure. The ventilator is set to deliver a tidal volume of 750 ml 10 times per minute. After transfer to the ICU, the physician decreases her tidal volume to 500 ml and raises her respiratory rate to 15 breaths·min^{-1}. She is heavily sedated and does not initiate any breaths beyond what the ventilator gives to her (in other words, total ventilation is fixed). She is not having fevers or seizures and is not receiving nutrition. Which of the following changes would you expect to occur as a result of the physician's intervention?
   A. Decreased airway resistance
   B. Decreased arterial P_{CO_2}
   C. Increased alveolar ventilation
   D. Increased CO_2 production
   E. Increased dead space fraction

7. A 40-year-old man is receiving mechanical ventilation in the ICU after an admission for severe respiratory failure. The ventilator settings include a tidal volume of 600 ml and respiratory rate of 15 breaths·min^{-1}.

The patient is in a deep coma and cannot increase his total ventilation beyond what the ventilator is set to deliver. On his 5th hospital day, he develops high fevers and is determined to have a new blood stream infection. Which of the following changes would be expected as a result of this change in the patient's condition?

A. Decreased anatomic dead space

B. Decreased physiologic dead space

C. Increased arterial P_{CO_2}

D. Increased ventilation to the dependent regions of the lung

E. Increased volume of gas delivered to the alveoli with each breath

8. In the figure below, the blue line depicts changes in lung volume as a function of time in an individual performing spirometry. Which of the labeled volumes or capacities in the spirogram can actually be measured with the spirometer?

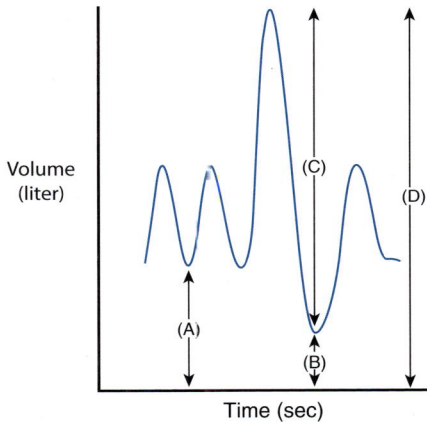

A. A

B. B

C. C

D. D

9. A 62-year-old man is receiving invasive mechanical ventilation after suffering a cardiac arrest with anoxic brain injury. While rounding on the patient on the 2nd day in the hospital, you note the following data:

Parameter	Day 1	Day 2
Arterial P_{CO_2} (mm Hg)	45	35
Dead space fraction (%)	32	32

The patient remains in a coma and does not take any breaths beyond those provided by the ventilator. If there were no changes made in the set respiratory rate or tidal volume between day 1 and 2, which of the following could account for the observed change in his $Paco_2$?

A. A new infection
B. Increase in his minute ventilation
C. Initiation of a protocol to lower his body temperature
D. Initiation of nutritional intake through a feeding tube
E. Recurrent seizures

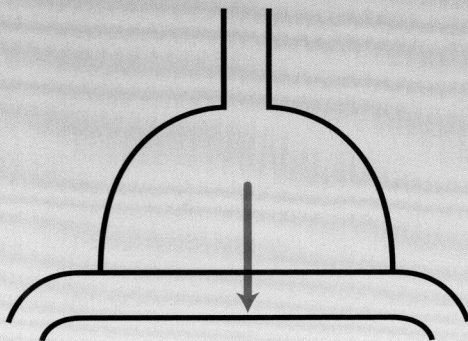

Diffusion

How Gas Gets Across
the Blood-Gas Barrier

3

This chapter considers how gases move across the blood-gas barrier. After describing the basic laws of diffusion, we distinguish between diffusion- and perfusion-limited gases. We then analyze oxygen uptake along the pulmonary capillary and how this varies under different conditions. The chapter then examines how diffusion capacity is measured using carbon monoxide and how to account for the finite reaction rate of oxygen with hemoglobin. The chapter concludes with a brief description of the interpretation of diffusion capacity measurements and the diffusion properties of carbon dioxide. At the end of this chapter, the reader should be able to:

- List the variables that determine the rate of transfer of a gas through a sheet of tissue
- Describe the difference between perfusion-limited and diffusion-limited gases
- Predict the effect of exercise, thickening of the alveolar-capillary barrier, and decreased alveolar P_{O_2} on oxygen uptake along the pulmonary capillary
- Calculate the diffusing capacity of the lung for carbon monoxide
- Explain the significance of reductions in the measured diffusing capacity for carbon monoxide

In the last chapter, we looked at how gas is moved from the atmosphere to the alveoli, or in the reverse direction. We now come to the transfer of gas across the blood-gas barrier. This process occurs by *diffusion*. Only 80 years ago, some physiologists believed that the lung secreted oxygen into the capillaries, that is, the oxygen was moved in an energy-dependent manner from a region of lower to one of higher partial pressure. Such a process was thought to occur in the swim bladder of fish, and it requires energy. But more accurate measurements showed that this does not occur in the lung and that all gases move across the alveolar wall by passive diffusion.

LAWS OF DIFFUSION

Diffusion through tissues is described by Fick's law (**Figure 3.1**). This states that the rate of transfer of a gas through a sheet of tissue like a postage stamp is proportional to the tissue area and the difference in gas partial pressure between the two sides, and inversely proportional to the tissue thickness. As we have seen, the area of the blood-gas barrier in the lung is enormous (50 to 100 m^2), and the thickness is only 0.3 μm in many places (Figure 1.1), so the dimensions of the barrier are ideal for diffusion. The rate of transfer is also proportional to a diffusion constant, which depends on the properties of the tissue and the particular gas. The constant is proportional to the solubility of the gas and inversely proportional to the square root of the molecular weight (Figure 3.1). This explains why CO_2 diffuses through tissue sheets about 20 times more rapidly than does O_2, as it has a much higher solubility but a relatively similar molecular weight.

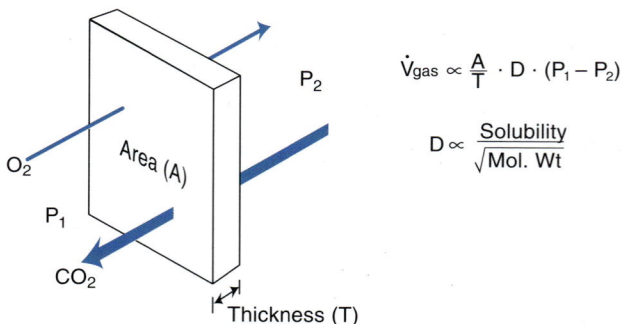

$$\dot{V}_{gas} \propto \frac{A}{T} \cdot D \cdot (P_1 - P_2)$$

$$D \propto \frac{Solubility}{\sqrt{Mol.\ Wt}}$$

Figure 3.1. Diffusion through a tissue sheet. The amount of gas transferred is proportional to the area (A), a diffusion constant (D), and the difference in partial pressure $(P_1 - P_2)$ and is inversely proportional to the thickness (T). The constant is proportional to the gas solubility but inversely proportional to the square root of its molecular weight. As a result, carbon dioxide diffuses more rapidly than does oxygen.

Fick's Law of Diffusion

- The rate of diffusion of a gas through a tissue slice is proportional to the surface area and the partial pressure difference.
- Diffusion rate is inversely proportional to the thickness of the tissue slice.
- Diffusion rate is proportional to the solubility of the gas in the tissue but inversely proportional to the square root of the molecular weight.

DIFFUSION AND PERFUSION LIMITATIONS

Suppose a red blood cell enters a pulmonary capillary of an alveolus that contains a foreign gas such as carbon monoxide or nitrous oxide. How rapidly will the partial pressure in the blood rise? **Figure 3.2** shows the time courses of several gases as the red blood cell moves through the capillary, a process that takes about 0.75 s. Look first at carbon monoxide. When

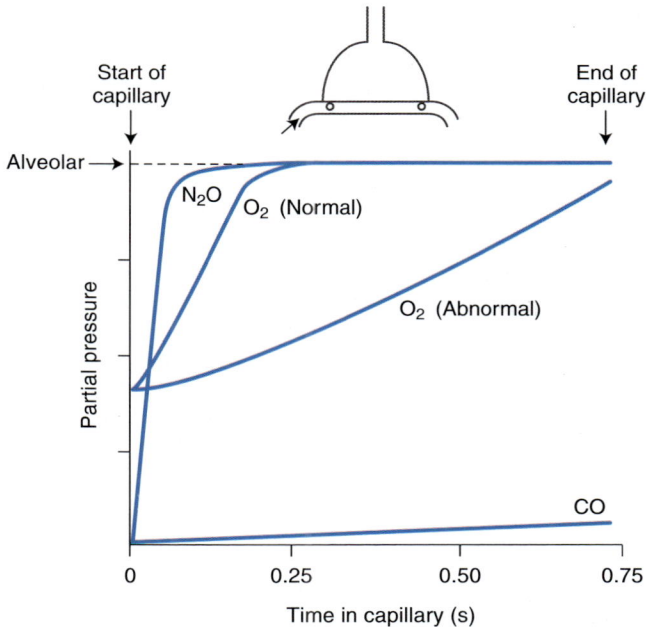

Figure 3.2. Uptake of carbon monoxide, nitrous oxide, and O_2 along the pulmonary capillary. Note that the blood partial pressure of nitrous oxide virtually reaches that of alveolar gas very early in the capillary, so the transfer of this gas is perfusion limited. By contrast, the partial pressure of carbon monoxide in the blood is almost unchanged, so its transfer is diffusion limited. O_2 transfer can be perfusion limited or partly diffusion limited, depending on the conditions.

the red cell enters the capillary, carbon monoxide moves rapidly across the extremely thin blood-gas barrier from the alveolar gas into the red blood cell. As a result, the content of carbon monoxide in the cell rises. However, because of the tight bond that forms between carbon monoxide and hemoglobin within the cell, a large amount of carbon monoxide can be taken up by the cell with almost no increase in partial pressure. Thus, as the cell moves through the capillary, the carbon monoxide partial pressure in the blood hardly changes, so that no appreciable back pressure develops, and the gas continues to move rapidly across the alveolar wall. It is clear, therefore, that the amount of carbon monoxide that gets into the blood is limited by the diffusion properties of the blood-gas barrier and not by the amount of blood available.* The transfer of carbon monoxide is therefore said to be *diffusion limited*.

This can be contrasted with the time course of nitrous oxide. When this gas moves across the alveolar wall into the blood, no combination with hemoglobin takes place. As a result, the blood has nothing like the avidity for nitrous oxide that it has for carbon monoxide, and the partial pressure rises rapidly. Indeed, Figure 3.2 shows that the partial pressure of nitrous oxide in the blood has virtually reached that of the alveolar gas by the time the red cell is only one-tenth of the way along the capillary. After this point, almost no nitrous oxide is transferred. Thus, the amount of this gas taken up by the blood depends entirely on the amount of available blood flow and not at all on the diffusion properties of the blood-gas barrier. The transfer of nitrous oxide is therefore *perfusion limited*.

What of O_2? Its time course lies between those of carbon monoxide and nitrous oxide. O_2 combines with hemoglobin (unlike nitrous oxide) but with nothing like the avidity of carbon monoxide. In other words, the rise in partial pressure when O_2 enters a red blood cell is much greater than is the case for the same number of molecules of carbon monoxide. Figure 3.2 shows that the Po_2 of the red blood cell as it enters the capillary is already about four-tenths of the alveolar value because of the O_2 in mixed venous blood. Under typical resting conditions, the capillary Po_2 virtually reaches that of alveolar gas when the red cell is about one-third of the way along the capillary. Under these conditions, O_2 transfer is perfusion limited like nitrous oxide. However, in some abnormal circumstances when the diffusion properties of the lung are impaired, for example, because of thickening of the blood-gas barrier, the blood Po_2 does not reach the alveolar value by the end of the capillary, and now there is some diffusion limitation as well.

A more detailed analysis shows that whether a gas is diffusion limited or not depends essentially on its solubility in the blood-gas barrier compared

---

*This introductory description of carbon monoxide transfer is not completely accurate because of the rate of reaction of carbon monoxide with hemoglobin (see later).

with its "solubility" in blood (actually the slope of the dissociation curve; see Chapter 6). For a gas like carbon monoxide, these are very different, whereas for a gas like nitrous oxide, they are the same. An analogy is the rate at which sheep can enter a field through a gate. If the gate is narrow but the field is large, the number of sheep that can enter in a given time is limited by the size of the gate (diffusion limited). However, if both the gate and the field are small (or both are big), the number of sheep is limited by the size of the field (perfusion limited).

OXYGEN UPTAKE ALONG THE PULMONARY CAPILLARY

Let us take a closer look at the uptake of O_2 by blood as it moves through a pulmonary capillary. **Figure 3.3A** shows that the Po_2 in a red blood cell entering the capillary, referred to as the mixed venous Po_2, is normally about 40 mm Hg. Across the blood-gas barrier, only 0.3 μm away, the alveolar Po_2 is 100 mm Hg. Oxygen floods down this large pressure gradient, and the Po_2 in the red cell rapidly rises; indeed, as we have seen, it very nearly reaches the Po_2 of alveolar gas by the time the red cell is only one-third of its way along the capillary or about 0.25 s. Thus, under normal circumstances, the difference in Po_2 between alveolar gas and end-capillary blood is immeasurably small—a mere fraction of a mm Hg. Because nearly complete equilibration occurs in only a fraction of the time the red cell spends in the pulmonary capillary, there is a considerable reserve capacity for diffusion, which is useful in the face of various conditions that thicken the blood-gas barrier or the reduce the pressure gradient across the barrier.

With heavy exercise, the pulmonary blood flow is greatly increased, and the time normally spent by the red cell in the capillary, about 0.75 s, may be reduced to as little as one-third of this. Although the time for diffusion is decreased, in healthy individuals breathing air, there is generally still no measurable fall in end-capillary Po_2. However, if the blood-gas barrier is markedly thickened by disease so that oxygen diffusion is impeded, the rate of rise of Po_2 in the red blood cells is correspondingly slow, and the Po_2 may not reach that of alveolar gas before the red blood cell leaves the pulmonary capillary. In this case, a measurable difference between alveolar gas and end-capillary blood for Po_2 may occur.

Another way of stressing the diffusion properties of the lung is to lower the alveolar Po_2 (**Figure 3.3B**). Suppose that this has been reduced to 50 mm Hg, by the individual either going to high altitude or inhaling a low O_2 mixture. Now, although the Po_2 in the red cell at the start of the capillary may only be about 20 mm Hg, the partial pressure difference responsible for driving the O_2 across the blood-gas barrier has been reduced from 60 mm Hg

A

B

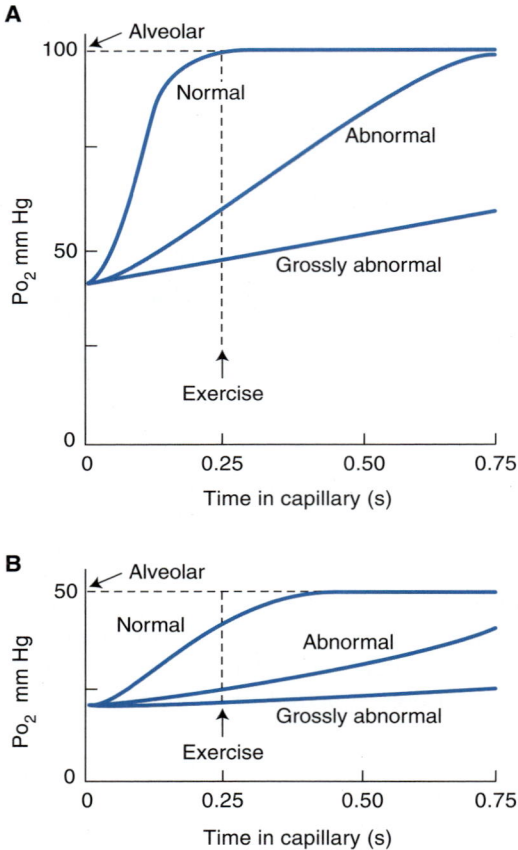

Figure 3.3. Oxygen time courses in the pulmonary capillary when diffusion is normal and abnormal (e.g., because of thickening of the blood-gas barrier by disease). **A.** Shows time courses when the alveolar P_{O_2} is normal. **B.** Shows slower oxygenation when the alveolar P_{O_2} is abnormally low. Note that in both cases, severe exercise reduces the time available for oxygenation.

(Figure 3.3A) to only 30 mm Hg, thereby slowing movement of O_2 across the blood gas barrier. In addition, the rate of rise of P_{O_2} for a given increase in O_2 concentration in the blood is less than it was because of the steep slope of the O_2 dissociation curve when the P_{O_2} is low (see Chapter 6). For both of these reasons, therefore, the rise in P_{O_2} along the capillary is relatively slow, and failure to reach the alveolar P_{O_2} is more likely. Thus, severe exercise at very high altitude is one of the few situations in which diffusion impairment of O_2 transfer in healthy individuals can be convincingly demonstrated. By the same token, patients with a thickened blood-gas barrier may show evidence of diffusion impairment if they breathe a low oxygen mixture, especially if they exercise as well.

Diffusion of Oxygen Across the Blood-Gas Barrier

- Red blood cells spend only about 0.75 s in the pulmonary capillary at rest.
- At rest, the Po_2 of the blood virtually reaches that of the alveolar gas after about one-third of its time in the capillary.
- There is considerable reserve capacity for diffusion across the blood gas barrier.
- Exercise reduces the time red blood cells spend in the pulmonary capillary.
- The diffusion process is challenged by exercise, alveolar hypoxia, and thickening of the blood-gas barrier.

MEASUREMENT OF DIFFUSING CAPACITY

For both clinical and research purposes, it can be helpful to measure the diffusing capacity of the lung. Because the transfer of carbon monoxide is limited solely by diffusion, it is the gas of choice for this measurement. At one time, O_2, which can be diffusion limited under certain circumstances, was employed under hypoxic conditions (Figure 3.3B), but this technique is no longer used.

The laws of diffusion (Figure 3.1) state that the amount of gas transferred across a sheet of tissue is proportional to the area (A), a diffusion constant (D, determined by the solubility and molecular weight of the gas), and the difference in partial pressure, and inversely proportional to the thickness (T), or

$$\dot{V}_{gas} = \frac{A}{T} \cdot D \cdot (P_1 - P_2)$$

Now, for a complex structure like the blood-gas barrier of the lung, it is not possible to measure the area and thickness during life. Instead, the equation is rewritten as:

$$\dot{V}_{gas} = D_L \cdot (P_1 - P_2)$$

where D_L is called the *diffusing capacity of the lung* and includes the area, thickness, and diffusion properties of the sheet and the gas concerned. Thus, the diffusing capacity for carbon monoxide is given by:

$$D_L = \frac{\dot{V}_{CO}}{P_1 - P_2}$$

where P_1 and P_2 are the partial pressures of alveolar gas and capillary blood, respectively. But as we have seen (Figure 3.2), the partial pressure of carbon monoxide in capillary blood is extremely small and can generally be neglected. Thus, the equation can be rewritten as:

$$D_L = \frac{\dot{V}_{CO}}{P_{A_{CO}}}$$

or, in words, the diffusing capacity of the lung for carbon monoxide is the volume of carbon monoxide transferred in milliliters per minute per mm Hg of alveolar partial pressure.

A frequently used test is the *single-breath method*, in which a single inspiration of a dilute mixture of carbon monoxide is made and the rate of disappearance of carbon monoxide from the alveolar gas during a 10-s breath-hold is calculated. This is usually done by measuring the inspired and expired concentrations of carbon monoxide with an infrared analyzer. The alveolar concentration of carbon monoxide is not constant during the breath-holding period, but allowance can be made for that. Helium is also added to the inspired gas to give a measurement of lung volume by dilution.

The normal value of the diffusing capacity for carbon monoxide at rest is about 25 ml·min^{-1}·mm Hg^{-1}, and it increases to two or three times this value on exercise because of recruitment and distension of pulmonary capillaries (see Chapter 4), which increases the volume of blood in the pulmonary capillaries capable of taking up carbon monoxide.

Measurement of Diffusing Capacity

- Carbon monoxide is used because the uptake of this gas is diffusion limited.
- Normal diffusing capacity is about 25 ml·min^{-1}·mm Hg^{-1}.
- Diffusing capacity increases on exercise.

REACTION RATES WITH HEMOGLOBIN

So far we have assumed that all the resistance to the movement of O_2 and CO resides in the blood-gas barrier. However, Figure 1.1 shows that the path length from the alveolar wall to the center of a red blood cell exceeds that in the wall itself, so that some of the diffusion resistance is located within the capillary. In addition, there is another type of resistance to gas transfer that is most conveniently discussed with diffusion, that is, the resistance caused by the finite rate of reaction of O_2 or CO with hemoglobin inside the red blood cell.

When O_2 (or CO) is added to blood, its combination with hemoglobin is quite fast, being well on the way to completion in 0.2 s. However, oxygenation occurs so rapidly in the pulmonary capillary (Figure 3.3) that even this rapid

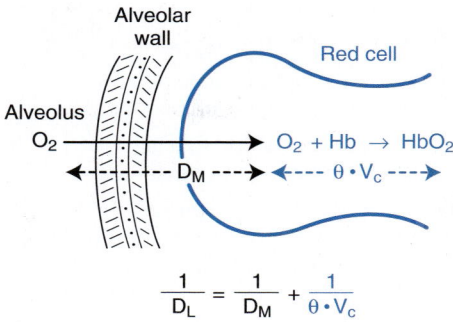

Figure 3.4. The diffusing capacity of the lung (D_L) is made up of two components: that due to the diffusion process itself and that attributable to the time taken for O_2 (or CO) to react with hemoglobin.

reaction significantly delays the loading of O_2 by the red cell. Thus, the uptake of O_2 (or CO) can be regarded as occurring in two stages: (1) diffusion of O_2 through the blood-gas barrier (including the plasma and red cell interior) and (2) reaction of O_2 with hemoglobin (**Figure 3.4**). In fact, it is possible to sum the two resultant resistances to produce an overall "diffusion" resistance.

We saw that the diffusing capacity of the lung (D_L) is defined as $D_L = \dot{V}_{gas} / (P_1 - P_2)$, that is, as the flow of gas divided by a pressure difference. Thus, the inverse of D_L is pressure difference divided by flow, which is analogous to electrical resistance. The resistance of the blood-gas barrier in Figure 3.4 is shown as $1/D_M$, where M means membrane. Now, the rate of reaction of O_2 (or CO) with hemoglobin can be described by θ, which gives the rate in milliliters per minute of O_2 (or CO) that combine with 1 ml of blood per mm Hg partial pressure of O_2 (or CO). This is analogous to the "diffusing capacity" of 1 ml of blood and, when multiplied by the volume of capillary blood (V_c), gives the effective "diffusing capacity" of the rate of reaction of O_2 with hemoglobin. Again its inverse, $1/(\theta \cdot V_c)$, describes the resistance of this reaction. Because the processes of moving across the blood-gas barrier and combing with hemoglobin are essentially in series with each other, the total diffusion resistance can be determined by adding the resistances offered by the membrane and the blood to obtain the total diffusion resistance. Thus, the complete equation is:

$$\frac{1}{D_L} = \frac{1}{D_M} + \frac{1}{\theta \cdot V_c}$$

In practice, the resistances offered by the membrane and blood components are approximately equal, so that a reduction of capillary blood volume or concentration of hemoglobin by disease can reduce the measured diffusing capacity of the lung. θ for CO is reduced if a subject breathes a high O_2 mixture, because the O_2 competes with the CO for hemoglobin. As a result, the measured diffusing capacity is reduced by O_2 breathing. In fact, it is possible to separately determine D_M and V_c by measuring the diffusing capacity for CO at different alveolar Po_2 values.

Reaction Rates of O_2 and CO with Hemoglobin

- The reaction rate of O_2 with hemoglobin is fast, but because so little time is available in the capillary, this rate can become a limiting factor.
- The resistance to the uptake of O_2 attributable to reaction rate is probably about the same as that due to diffusion across the blood-gas barrier.
- The reaction rate of CO can be altered by changing the alveolar P_{O_2}. In this way, the separate contributions of the diffusion properties of the blood-gas barrier and the volume of capillary blood can be derived.

INTERPRETATION OF DIFFUSING CAPACITY FOR CO

It is clear that the measured diffusing capacity of the lung for CO depends not only on the area and thickness of the blood-gas barrier but also on the volume of blood and concentration of hemoglobin in the pulmonary capillaries. Furthermore, in the diseased lung, the measurement is affected by the distribution of diffusion properties, alveolar volume, and capillary blood. For these reasons, the term *transfer factor* is sometimes used (particularly in Europe) to emphasize that the measurement does not solely reflect the diffusion properties of the lung. To obtain more specific information about the blood-gas barrier itself in clinical practice, the measured diffusion capacity is adjusted for the hemoglobin concentration and alveolar volume.

CO_2 TRANSFER ACROSS THE PULMONARY CAPILLARY

We have seen that diffusion of CO_2 through tissue is about 20 times faster than that of O_2 because of the much higher solubility of CO_2 (Figure 3.1). At first sight, therefore, it seems unlikely that CO_2 elimination could be affected by diffusion difficulties, and indeed, this has been the general belief. However, the reaction of CO_2 with blood is complex (see Chapter 6), and although there is some uncertainty about the rates of the various reactions, it is possible that a difference between end-capillary blood and alveolar gas can develop if the blood-gas barrier is diseased.

KEY CONCEPTS

1. Fick's law states that the rate of diffusion of a gas through a tissue sheet is proportional to the area of the sheet and the partial pressure difference across it, and inversely proportional to the thickness of the sheet.

2. Examples of diffusion- and perfusion-limited gases are carbon monoxide and nitrous oxide, respectively. Oxygen transfer is normally perfusion limited, but some diffusion limitation may occur with intense exercise, thickening of the blood-gas barrier, and alveolar hypoxia.

3. The diffusing capacity of the lung is measured using inhaled carbon monoxide. The value increases markedly on exercise.

4. The finite reaction rate of oxygen with hemoglobin can reduce its transfer rate into the blood, and the effect is similar to that of reducing the diffusion rate.

5. Carbon dioxide transfer across the blood-gas barrier is probably not diffusion limited.

CLINICAL VIGNETTE

A 40-year-old woman who is a lifelong nonsmoker presents for evaluation of worsening shortness of breath (dyspnea) over a 6-month period. On examination, she had a high respiratory rate and limited chest excursion when asked to take a maximal inhalation. On auscultation, she had fine inspiratory crackles in the posterior lower lung fields bilaterally. A chest radiograph showed low lung volumes with "reticular" or netlike opacities in the lower lung zones. On pulmonary function testing, she had a decreased lung volume and a diffusing capacity for carbon monoxide that was less than half the normal value. Arterial blood gases were measured while she was at rest and following a vigorous walk around the clinic. She had a normal arterial P_{O_2} at rest, but it fell significantly with exercise. She was referred for surgical lung biopsy, which revealed areas of dense fibrosis with collagen deposition and thickening of the alveolar walls.

- Why is the diffusing capacity for carbon monoxide decreased?
- Why did the arterial P_{O_2} decrease with exercise?
- How could you improve the transfer of oxygen across the blood-gas barrier?
- What would you expect her arterial P_{CO_2} to be?

QUESTIONS

For each question, choose the one best answer.

1. Using Fick's law of diffusion of gases through a tissue slice, if gas X is 4 times as soluble and has 4 times the molecular weight as gas Y, what is the ratio of the diffusion rates of X to Y?

A. 0.25
B. 0.5
C. 2
D. 4
E. 8

2. An exercising subject breathes a low concentration of CO in a steady state. If the alveolar Pco is 0.5 mm Hg and the CO uptake is 30 ml·min⁻¹, what is the diffusing capacity of the lung for CO in ml·min⁻¹·mm Hg⁻¹?
   A. 20
   B. 30
   C. 40
   D. 50
   E. 60

3. In a normal person, doubling the diffusing capacity of the lung would be expected to:
   A. Decrease arterial P_{CO_2} during resting breathing
   B. Increase resting oxygen uptake when the subject breathes 10% oxygen
   C. Increase the uptake of nitrous oxide during anesthesia
   D. Increase the arterial P_{O_2} during resting breathing
   E. Increase maximal oxygen uptake at extreme altitude

4. The figure below depicts the time course of changes in the partial pressure of two gases (Gas A and Gas B) as blood moves through the pulmonary capillaries. Which of these two gases is diffusion limited?

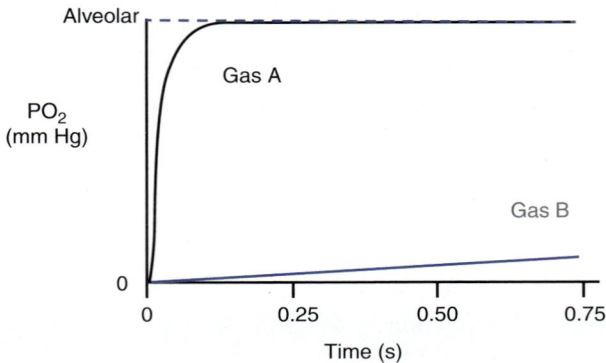

A. Gas A
B. Gas B

5. The figure below depicts the charges in the P_{O_2} as blood traverses the pulmonary capillaries under two conditions, A and B. Which of the following could account for the time course of the change in P_{O_2} observed under condition B compared to condition A?

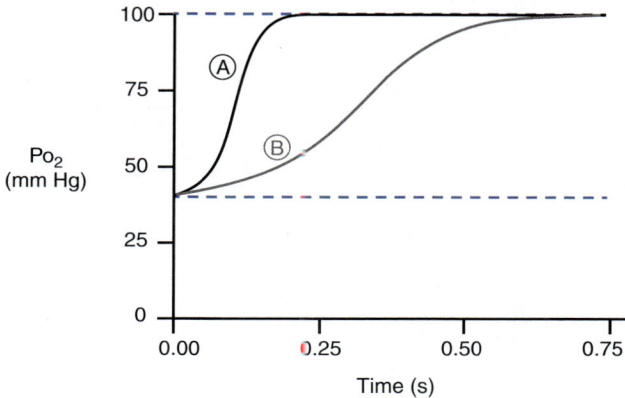

A. Ascent to high altitude
B. Decreased minute ventilation
C. Exercise
D. Increased inspired oxygen fraction
E. Thickening of the blood-gas barrier

6. A 48-year-old patient undergoes pulmonary function testing as part of an evaluation for increasing dyspnea and is found to have a measured diffusing capacity for carbon monoxide of 32 ml·min^{-1}·mm Hg^{-1}, which is 10% higher than the predicted value for this individual. Which of the following conditions could account for this observation?
A. Diffuse alveolar hemorrhage, in which red blood cells leak into the alveolar space
B. Emphysema, which causes loss of pulmonary capillaries
C. Pulmonary embolism, which cuts off the blood supply to part of the lung
D. Pulmonary fibrosis, which causes thickening of the blood-gas barrier
E. Severe anemia

7. A 63-year-old man with pulmonary fibrosis of unknown cause is referred for a cardiopulmonary exercise test in preparation for lung transplantation. He earlier underwent a lung biopsy, which revealed that the thin part of the blood-gas barrier in the involved areas was 0.9 μm in thickness. The diffusing capacity for carbon monoxide was only 40% of the predicted value. Compared to a healthy individual, which of the

following findings would you expect to see on the exercise test in this patient?
A. Decreased anatomic dead space volume
B. Decreased alveolar P_{O_2}
C. Decreased arterial P_{O_2}
D. Decreased inspired P_{O_2}
E. Increased rate of diffusion across the blood-gas barrier

8. A 58-year-old woman with long-standing use of ibuprofen for osteoarthritis presents to her doctor because of excessive tiredness. Laboratory studies reveal a hemoglobin concentration of 9 g·dl^{-1} (normal 13 to 15 g·dl^{-1}). Which of the following abnormalities would you most likely observe?
A. Decreased diffusing capacity for carbon monoxide
B. Decreased functional residual capacity
C. Decreased residual volume
D. Increased physiologic dead space
E. Increased ventilation to the upper lung zones

9. The figure below shows histopathologic specimens from a normal lung and that of a patient with a diffuse parenchymal lung disease. The pulmonary capillaries are located in the walls of the alveoli in each image. Which of the following would you expect to find in the patient compared to the normal lung?

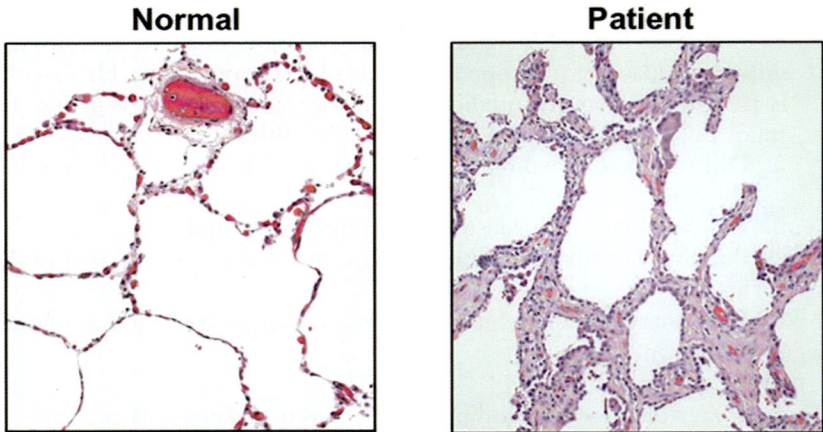

Normal   **Patient**

A. Difference between alveolar and end capillary P_{O_2} during exercise
B. Increased alveolar P_{O_2}
C. Increased diffusion capacity for carbon monoxide
D. Increased rate of transfer of oxygen across the blood-gas barrier
E. Increased reaction rate of oxygen with hemoglobin

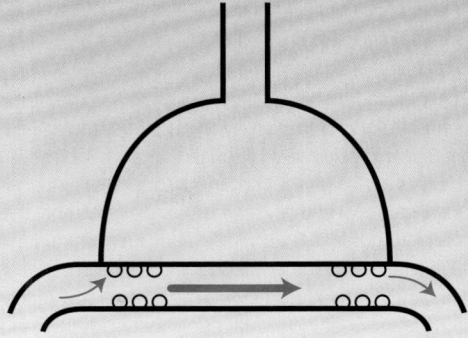

Blood Flow and Metabolism

4

How the Pulmonary Circulation Removes Gas from the Lung and Alters Some Metabolites

- Pressures Within Pulmonary Blood Vessels
- Pressures Around Pulmonary Blood Vessels
- Pulmonary Vascular Resistance
- Measurement of Pulmonary Blood Flow
- Distribution of Blood Flow
- Active Control of the Circulation
- Water Balance in the Lung
- Other Functions of the Pulmonary Circulation
- Metabolic Functions of the Lung

We now turn to how the respiratory gases are removed from the lung. First the pressures inside and outside the pulmonary blood vessels are considered and then pulmonary vascular resistance is introduced. Next, we look at the measurement of total pulmonary blood flow and its uneven distribution caused by gravity. Active control of the circulation is then addressed, followed by fluid balance in the lung. Finally, other functions of the pulmonary circulation are dealt with, particularly the metabolic functions of the lung. At the end of this chapter, the reader should be able to:

- Predict the effects of changes in lung volume, pulmonary vascular pressures, and alveolar oxygen tensions on pulmonary vascular resistance
- Calculate pulmonary vascular resistance, cardiac output and net capillary filtration pressure
- Describe how the balance of alveolar pressure and pulmonary artery and venous pressure affects blood flow in different regions of the lung
- Explain the mechanism and physiologic role of hypoxic pulmonary vasoconstriction
- Describe the fate of various substances as they cross the pulmonary circulation

The pulmonary circulation begins at the main pulmonary artery, which receives the mixed venous blood pumped by the right ventricle. This artery then branches successively like the system of airways (Figure 1.3) and, indeed, the pulmonary arteries accompany the airways as far as the terminal bronchioles in what is often called the bronchovascular bundle. Beyond that, they break up to supply the capillary bed that lies in the walls of the alveoli (Figures 1.6 and 1.7). The pulmonary capillaries form a dense network in the alveolar wall that makes an exceedingly efficient arrangement for gas exchange (Figures 1.1, 1.6, and 1.7). So rich is the mesh that some physiologists feel that it is misleading to talk of a network of individual capillary segments and prefer to regard the capillary bed as a sheet of flowing blood interrupted in places by posts (Figure 1.6), rather like an underground parking garage. The oxygenated blood is then collected from the capillary bed by the small pulmonary veins that run between the lobules and eventually unite to form the four large veins, which drain into the left atrium.

At first sight, this circulation appears to be simply a small version of the systemic circulation, which begins at the aorta and ends in the right atrium. However, there are important differences between the two circulations in terms of both structure and function.

PRESSURES WITHIN PULMONARY BLOOD VESSELS

The pressures in the pulmonary circulation are remarkably low. The systolic and diastolic pressures in the main pulmonary artery are about 25 and 8 mm Hg, respectively, while the mean pressure is only about 15 mm Hg (**Figure 4.1**), roughly one-sixth of the typical mean pressure in the aorta (100 mm Hg). The pressures in the right and left atriums are not very dissimilar—about 2 and 5 mm Hg, respectively. Thus, the pressure differences from inlet to outlet of the pulmonary and systemic systems are about $(15 - 5) = 10$ and $(100 - 2) = 98$ mm Hg, respectively—a factor of 10.

In keeping with these low pressures, the walls of the pulmonary artery and its branches are remarkably thin and contain relatively little smooth muscle (they are easily mistaken for veins). This is in striking contrast to the systemic circulation, where the arteries generally have thick walls and the arterioles in particular have abundant smooth muscle.

The reasons for these differences become clear when the functions of the two circulations are compared. The systemic circulation regulates the supply of blood to various organs, including those which may be far above the level of the heart (e.g., the brain). By contrast, the lung is required to accept the whole of the cardiac output at all times and is rarely concerned with directing blood from one region to another, except in response to localized alveolar hypoxia (see below). As a result, its arterial pressure is as low as necessary to lift blood to the top of the lung. This keeps the work of the right heart as small as is feasible for efficient gas exchange to occur in the lung.

The pressure within the pulmonary capillaries is uncertain. The best evidence suggests that it lies about halfway between pulmonary arterial and

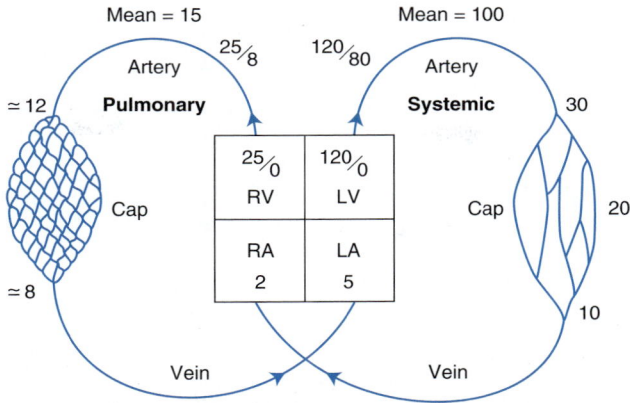

Figure 4.1. Comparison of pressures (mm Hg) in the pulmonary and systemic circulations. Hydrostatic differences modify these.

venous pressure and that probably much of the pressure drop occurs within the capillary bed itself. Certainly, the distribution of pressures along the pulmonary circulation is far more symmetrical than in its systemic counterpart, where most of the pressure drop is just upstream of the capillaries (Figure 4.1). In addition, the pressure within the pulmonary capillaries varies considerably throughout the lung because of hydrostatic effects (see below).

PRESSURES AROUND PULMONARY BLOOD VESSELS

The pulmonary capillaries are unique in that they are virtually surrounded by gas (Figures 1.1 and 1.7). It is true that there is a very thin layer of epithelial cells lining the alveoli, but the capillaries receive little support from this and, consequently, are liable to collapse or distend, depending on the pressures within and around them. The latter is very close to alveolar pressure. (The pressure in the alveoli is usually close to atmospheric pressure; indeed, during breath-holding with the glottis open, the two pressures are identical.) Under some special conditions, the effective pressure around the capillaries is reduced by the surface tension of the fluid lining the alveoli. But usually, the effective pressure is alveolar pressure, and when this rises above the pressure inside the capillaries, they collapse. The pressure difference between the inside and outside of the capillaries is often called the *transmural pressure*.

What is the pressure around the pulmonary arteries and veins? This can be considerably less than alveolar pressure. As the lung expands, these larger blood vessels are pulled open by the radial traction of the elastic lung

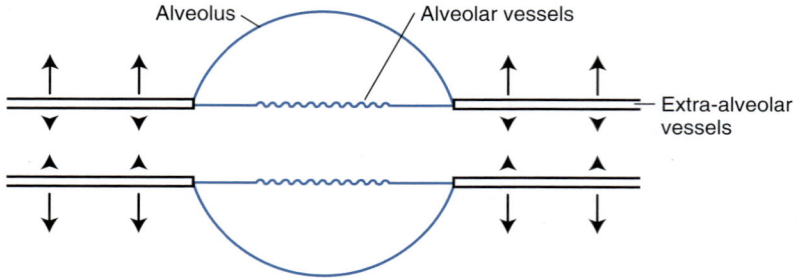

Figure 4.2. "Alveolar" and "extra-alveolar" vessels. The first are mainly the capillaries and are exposed to alveolar pressure. The second are pulled open by the radial traction of the surrounding lung parenchyma, and the effective pressure around them is therefore lower than alveolar pressure. (Reprinted from Hughes JMB, Glazier JB, Maloney JE, et al. Effect of lung volume on the distribution of pulmonary blood flow in man. *Respir Physiol.* 1968;4(1):58-72. Copyright © 1968 Elsevier. With permission.)

parenchyma that surrounds them (**Figures 4.2 and 4.3**). Consequently, the effective pressure around them is low; in fact, there is some evidence that this pressure is even less than the pressure around the whole lung (intrapleural pressure). This paradox can be explained by the mechanical advantage that develops when a relatively rigid structure such as a blood vessel or bronchus is surrounded by a rapidly expanding elastic material such as lung parenchyma. In any event, both the arteries and veins increase their caliber as the lung expands.

The behavior of the capillaries and the larger blood vessels is so different they are often referred to as alveolar and extra-alveolar vessels, respectively (Figure 4.2). Alveolar vessels are exposed to alveolar pressure and include the capillaries and the slightly larger vessels in the corners of the alveolar walls. Their caliber is determined by the relationship between alveolar pressure and

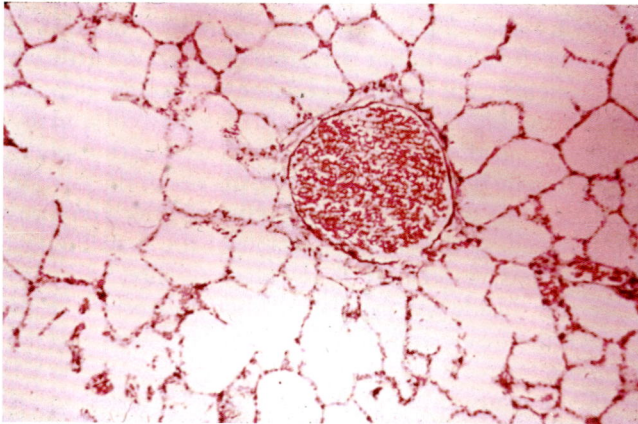

Figure 4.3. Section of lung showing many alveoli and an extra-alveolar vessel (in this case, a small vein) with its perivascular sheath.

the pressure within them. Extra-alveolar vessels include all the arteries and veins that run through the lung parenchyma. Their caliber is greatly affected by lung volume because this determines the expanding pull, or radial traction, of the parenchyma on their walls. The very large vessels near the hilum are outside the lung substance and are exposed to intrapleural pressure.

Alveolar and Extra-alveolar Vessels

- Alveolar vessels are exposed to alveolar pressure and are compressed if this increases.
- Extra-alveolar vessels are exposed to a pressure less than alveolar and are pulled open by the radial traction of the surrounding parenchyma.

PULMONARY VASCULAR RESISTANCE

It is useful to describe the resistance of a system of blood vessels as follows:

$$\text{Vascular resistance} = \frac{\text{input pressure} - \text{output pressure}}{\text{blood flow}}$$

This is analogous to electrical resistance, which is the difference in voltage divided by current. The number for vascular resistance is certainly not a complete description of the pressure-flow properties of the system. For example, the number usually depends on the magnitude of the blood flow. Nevertheless, it often allows a helpful comparison of different circulations or the same circulation under different conditions.

We have seen that the total pressure drop from the pulmonary artery to left atrium in the pulmonary circulation is only some 10 mm Hg, compared to about 100 mm Hg for the systemic circulation. Because the blood flows through the two circulations are virtually identical, it follows that the pulmonary vascular resistance is only one-tenth that of the systemic circulation. The pulmonary blood flow is about 6 liters·min^{-1}, so that, in numbers, the pulmonary vascular resistance is (15 − 5)/6 or about 1.7 mm Hg·liter^{-1}·min.* The high resistance of the systemic circulation is largely caused by very muscular arterioles that allow the regulation of blood flow to various organs of the body. The pulmonary circulation has no such vessels and appears to have as low a resistance as is compatible with distributing the blood in a thin film over a vast area in the alveolar walls.

---

*Pulmonary vascular resistance is sometimes expressed in the units dyne·s·cm^{-5}. The normal value is then in the region of 100.

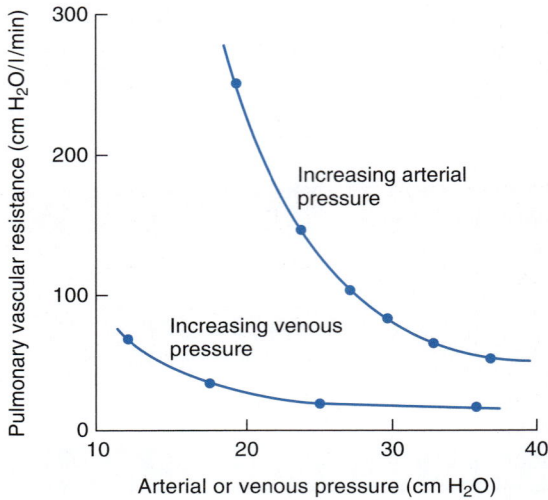

Figure 4.4. Fall in pulmonary vascular resistance as the pulmonary arterial or venous pressure is raised. When the arterial pressure was changed, the venous pressure was held constant at 12 cm water, and when the venous pressure was changed, the arterial pressure was held at 37 cm water. (Data from an excised animal lung preparation.)

Although the normal pulmonary vascular resistance is extraordinarily small, it has a remarkable facility for becoming even smaller as the pressure within the vessels rises. **Figure 4.4** shows that an increase in either pulmonary arterial or venous pressure causes pulmonary vascular resistance to fall. Two mechanisms are responsible for this. Under normal conditions, some capillaries are either closed or open but with no blood flow. As the pressure rises, these vessels begin to conduct blood, thus lowering the overall resistance. This is termed *recruitment* (**Figure 4.5**) and is apparently the chief mechanism for the fall in pulmonary vascular resistance that occurs as the pulmonary artery pressure is raised from low levels. The reason some vessels are unperfused at low perfusing pressures is not fully understood but perhaps is caused by random differences in the geometry of the complex network (Figure 1.6), which result in preferential channels for flow.

At higher vascular pressures, widening of individual capillary segments occurs. This increase in caliber, or *distension*, is hardly surprising in view of the

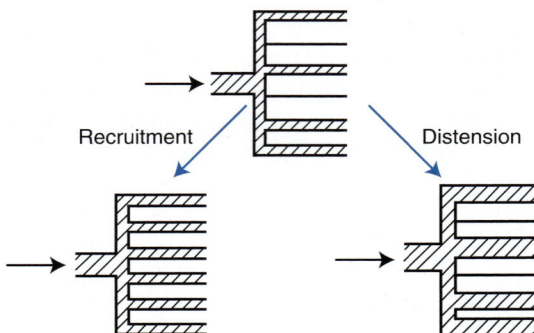

Figure 4.5. Recruitment (opening of previously closed vessels) and distension (increase in caliber of vessels). These are the two mechanisms for the decrease in pulmonary vascular resistance that occurs as vascular pressures are raised.

very thin membrane that separates the capillary from the alveolar space (see Figure 1.1). Distension is probably chiefly a change in shape of the capillaries from near flattened to more circular. There is evidence that the capillary wall strongly resists stretching. Distension is apparently the predominant mechanism for the fall in pulmonary vascular resistance at relatively high vascular pressures. However, recruitment and distension often occur together and are the major reason pulmonary vascular resistance decreases with exercise.

Another important determinant of pulmonary vascular resistance is *lung volume*. The caliber of the extra-alveolar vessels (Figure 4.2) is determined by a balance between various forces. As we have seen, they are pulled open as the lung expands. As a result, their vascular resistance is low at large lung volumes. On the other hand, resistance is high when lung volume is low because their walls contain smooth muscle and elastic tissue, which resist distension and tend to reduce the caliber of the vessels (**Figure 4.6**). Indeed, if the lung is completely collapsed, the smooth muscle tone of these vessels is so effective that the pulmonary artery pressure has to be raised several centimeters of water above downstream pressure before any flow at all occurs. This is called a *critical opening pressure*.

Is the vascular resistance of the capillaries influenced by lung volume? This depends on whether alveolar pressure changes with respect to the pressure inside the capillaries, that is, whether their transmural pressure alters. If alveolar pressure rises with respect to capillary pressure, the vessels tend to be squashed, and their resistance rises. This usually occurs when a normal subject takes a deep inspiration, because the vascular pressures fall since the heart is surrounded by intrapleural pressure, which falls on inspiration. However, the pressures in the pulmonary circulation do not remain steady after such a maneuver. An additional factor is that the caliber of the capillaries is reduced at large lung volumes

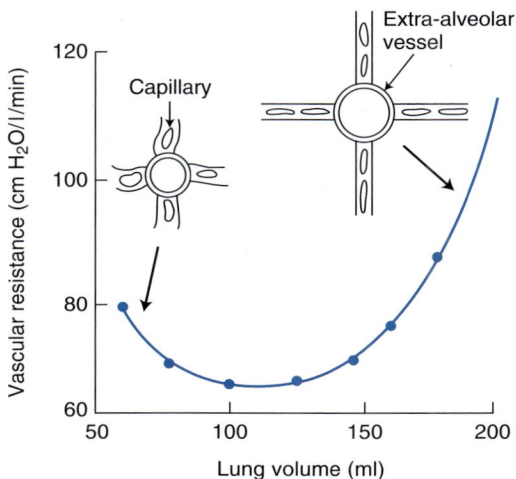

Figure 4.6. Effect of lung volume on pulmonary vascular resistance when the transmural pressure of the capillaries is held constant. At low lung volumes, resistance is high because the extra-alveolar vessels become narrow. At high volumes, the capillaries are stretched, and their caliber is reduced. Note that the resistance is least at normal breathing volumes.

because of stretching across the walls. An analogy is a piece of thin-walled rubber tubing that is stretched across its diameter. The caliber is then greatly reduced. Thus, even if the transmural pressure of the capillaries is not changed with large lung inflations, their vascular resistance increases (Figure 4.6).

Because of the role of smooth muscle in determining the caliber of the extra-alveolar vessels, substances that cause smooth muscle contraction increase pulmonary vascular resistance. These include serotonin, histamine, norepinephrine, and endothelin. The important role of hypoxia is discussed later. These drugs are particularly effective vasoconstrictors when the lung volume is low and the expanding forces on the vessels are weak. Substances that can relax smooth muscle in the pulmonary circulation include acetylcholine, calcium channel blockers, nitric oxide, phosphodiesterase-5 inhibitors, and prostacyclin (PGI_2).

Pulmonary Vascular Resistance

- Is normally very small
- Decreases on exercise because of recruitment and distension of capillaries
- Increases at high and low lung volumes
- Increases due to alveolar hypoxia, as well as endothelin, histamine, serotonin, thromboxane A2
- Decreases due to acetylcholine, calcium channel blockers, nitric oxide, phosphodiesterase inhibitors, prostacyclin (PGI_2)

MEASUREMENT OF PULMONARY BLOOD FLOW

The volume of blood passing through the lungs each minute ($\dot{Q}$) can be calculated using the *Fick principle*. This states that the O_2 consumption per minute ($\dot{V}O_2$) measured at the mouth is equal to the amount of O_2 taken up by the blood in the lungs per minute. Because the O_2 concentration in the blood entering the lungs is $C\bar{v}_{O_2}$ and that in the blood leaving is Ca_{O_2}, we have

$$\dot{V}O_2 = \dot{Q}(Ca_{O_2} - C\bar{v}_{O_2})$$

which can be arranged to give

$$\dot{Q} = \frac{\dot{V}O_2}{Ca_{O_2} - C\bar{v}_{O_2}}$$

$\dot{V}O_2$ can be measured by collecting the expired gas in a large spirometer and measuring its O_2 concentration. More modern systems estimate this variable using flow sensors and oxygen analyzers connected to a mouthpiece that measure the amount of oxygen consumed per breath and sum over the total breaths taken each minute. Mixed venous blood is obtained from a catheter in the pulmonary artery and arterial blood by puncture of the radial artery. Pulmonary blood flow can also be measured by one of several dilution techniques, in which a dye or other indicator is injected into the venous circulation, and its concentration in arterial blood is recorded or cold saline is infused and the downstream change in temperature of the blood is measured. The Fick principle and dilution techniques are of great importance, but they will not be considered in more detail here because they fall within the province of cardiovascular physiology.

DISTRIBUTION OF BLOOD FLOW

So far, we have been assuming that all parts of the pulmonary circulation behave identically. However, considerable inequality of blood flow exists within the upright human lung. This can be shown by a modification of the radioactive xenon method used to measure the distribution of ventilation (Figure 2.7). To measure blood flow, the xenon is dissolved in saline and injected into a peripheral vein (**Figure 4.7**). When it reaches the pulmonary

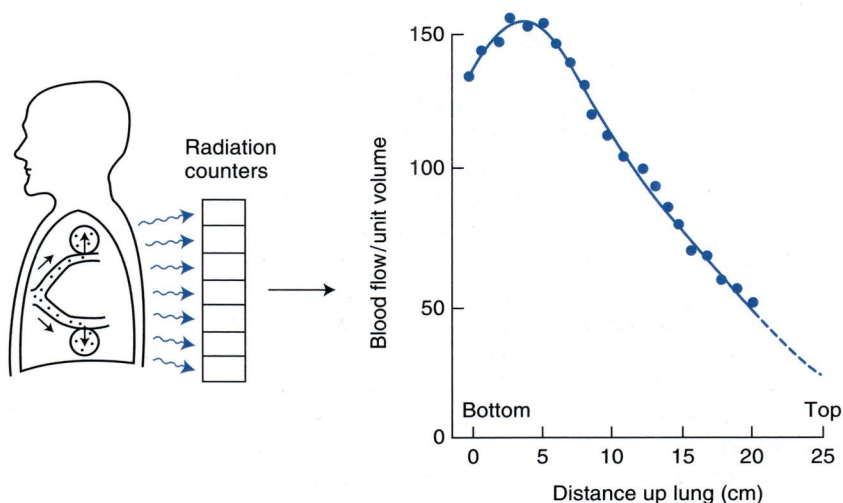

Figure 4.7. Measurement of the distribution of blood flow in the upright human lung, using radioactive xenon. The dissolved xenon is evolved into alveolar gas from the pulmonary capillaries. The units of blood flow are such that if flow were uniform, all values would be 100. Note the small flow at the apex. (Redrawn from Hughes JMB, Glazier JB, Maloney JE, et al. Effect of lung volume on the distribution of pulmonary blood flow in man. *Respir Physiol*. 1968;4(1):58-72. Copyright © 1968 Elsevier. With permission.)

capillaries, it is evolved into alveolar gas because of its low solubility, and the distribution of radioactivity can be measured by counters over the chest during breath-holding.

In the upright human lung, blood flow decreases almost linearly from bottom to top, reaching very low values at the apex (Figure 4.7). This distribution is affected by change of posture and exercise. When the subject lies supine, the apical zone blood flow increases, but the basal zone flow remains virtually unchanged, with the result that the distribution from apex to base becomes almost uniform. However, in this posture, blood flow in the posterior (lower or dependent) regions of the lung exceeds flow in the anterior parts. Measurements on subjects suspended upside down show that apical blood flow may exceed basal flow in this position. On mild exercise, both upper and lower zone blood flows increase, and the regional differences become less.

The uneven distribution of blood flow can be explained by the hydrostatic pressure differences within the blood vessels. If we consider the pulmonary arterial system as a continuous column of blood, the difference in pressure between the top and bottom of a lung 30 cm high will be about 30 cm water, or 23 mm Hg. This is a large pressure difference for such a low-pressure system as the pulmonary circulation (Figure 4.1), and its effects on regional blood flow are shown in **Figure 4.8**.

There may be a region at the top of the lung (*zone 1*), where pulmonary arterial pressure falls below alveolar pressure (normally close to atmospheric

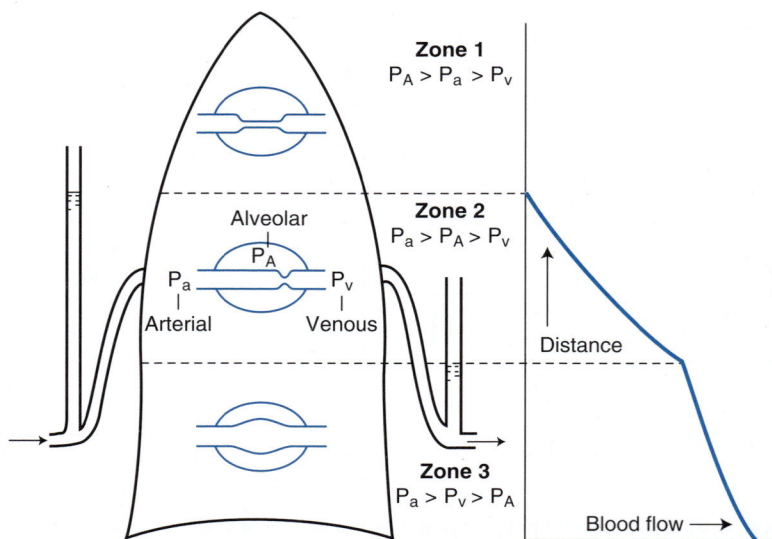

Figure 4.8. Explanation of the uneven distribution of blood flow in the lung, based on the pressures affecting the capillaries. See text for details. (Reproduced with permission from West JB, Dollery CT, Naimark A. Distribution of blood flow in isolated lung; relation to vascular and alveolar pressures. *J Appl Physiol*. 1964; 19(4):713-724. Copyright © 1964 the American Physiological Society. All rights reserved.)

pressure). If this occurs, the capillaries are squashed flat, and no flow is possible. Zone 1 does *not* occur under normal conditions, because the pulmonary arterial pressure is just sufficient to raise blood to the top of the lung, but may be present if the arterial pressure is reduced (e.g., with septic shock or hemorrhage) or if alveolar pressure is raised, as occurs during positive pressure ventilation. This ventilated but unperfused lung is useless for gas exchange and is called *alveolar dead space*.

Farther down the lung (*zone 2*), pulmonary arterial pressure increases because of the hydrostatic effect and now exceeds alveolar pressure. However, venous pressure is still very low and is less than alveolar pressure, which leads to remarkable pressure-flow characteristics. Under these conditions, blood flow is determined by the difference between arterial and alveolar pressures (not the usual arterial-venous pressure difference). Indeed, venous pressure has no influence on flow unless it exceeds alveolar pressure.

This behavior can be modeled with a flexible rubber tube inside a glass chamber (**Figure 4.9**). When chamber pressure is greater than downstream pressure, the rubber tube collapses at its downstream end, and the pressure inside the tube at this point limits flow. The pulmonary capillary bed is clearly very different from a rubber tube. Nevertheless, the overall behavior is similar and is often called the Starling resistor, sluice, or waterfall effect. Because arterial pressure is increasing down the zone but alveolar pressure is the same throughout the lung, the pressure difference responsible for flow increases. In addition, increasing recruitment of capillaries occurs down this zone.

In *zone 3*, venous pressure now exceeds alveolar pressure, and flow is determined in the usual way by the arterial-venous pressure difference. The increase in blood flow down this region of the lung is apparently caused chiefly by distension of the capillaries. The pressure within them (lying between arterial and venous) increases down the zone, while the pressure outside (alveolar) remains constant. Thus, their transmural pressure rises and, indeed, measurements show that their mean width increases. Recruitment of previously

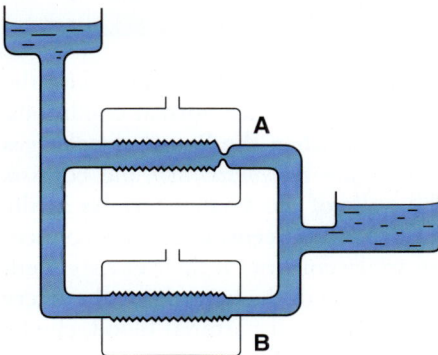

Figure 4.9. Two Starling resistors, each consisting of a thin rubber tube inside a container. When chamber pressure exceeds downstream pressure as in **A**, flow is independent of downstream pressure. However, when downstream pressure exceeds chamber pressure as in **B**, flow is determined by the upstream-downstream difference.

closed vessels may also play some part in the increase in blood flow down this zone.

The scheme shown in Figure 4.8 summarizes the role played by the capillaries in determining the distribution of blood flow. At low lung volumes, the resistance of the extra-alveolar vessels becomes important, and a reduction of regional blood flow is seen, starting first at the base of the lung, where the parenchyma is least expanded (see Figure 7.8). This region of reduced blood flow is sometimes called *zone 4* and can be explained by the narrowing of the extra-alveolar vessels, which occurs when the lung around them is poorly inflated (Figure 4.6).

Distribution of Blood Flow

- Gravity causes large differences down the lung.
- In zone 1, there is no flow because pulmonary artery pressure is less than alveolar pressure. This is not seen under normal conditions.
- In zone 2, flow is determined by the difference between arterial and alveolar pressures.
- In zone 3, flow is determined by the difference between arterial and venous pressures.
- In zones 2 and 3, flow increases down each zone.

There are other factors causing uneven blood flow in the lung. The complex, partly random arrangement of blood vessels and capillaries (Figure 1.6) causes some inequality of blood flow at any given level in the lung. There is also evidence that blood flow decreases along the acinus, with peripheral parts less well supplied with blood. Some measurements suggest that the peripheral regions of the whole lung receive less blood flow than the central regions.

ACTIVE CONTROL OF THE CIRCULATION

We have seen that passive factors dominate the vascular resistance and the distribution of flow in the pulmonary circulation under normal conditions. However, a remarkable active response occurs when the P_{O_2} of alveolar gas is reduced. This is known as *hypoxic pulmonary vasoconstriction* and consists of contraction of smooth muscle in the walls of the small arterioles in the hypoxic region. This response does not depend on central nervous connections, as excised segments of pulmonary artery constrict if their environment is made hypoxic, indicating there is a local action of the hypoxia on the artery itself. The P_{O_2} of the alveolar gas, not the pulmonary arterial blood, chiefly determines the response. This can be proved by perfusing a lung with blood of a high Po_2 while keeping the alveolar Po_2 low. Under these conditions, the response still occurs.

The vessel wall becomes hypoxic as a result of diffusion of oxygen over the very short distance from the wall to the surrounding alveoli. Recall that a small pulmonary artery is very closely surrounded by alveoli (compare the proximity of alveoli to the small pulmonary vein in Figure 4.3). The stimulus-response curve of this constriction is very nonlinear (**Figure 4.10**). When the alveolar Po_2 is altered in the region above 100 mm Hg, little change in vascular resistance is seen. However, when the alveolar Po_2 is reduced below approximately 70 mm Hg, marked vasoconstriction may occur, and at a very low Po_2, the local blood flow may be almost abolished.

The mechanism of hypoxic pulmonary vasoconstriction remains a subject of much research. An increase in cytoplasmic calcium ion concentration is the major trigger for smooth muscle contraction and occurs as a result of a variety of factors. Research has shown, for example, that inhibition of voltage-gated potassium channels and membrane depolarization are involved, leading to increased cytoplasmic calcium ion concentrations.

Endothelium-derived vasoactive substances also play a large role in regulating vascular tone. One such factor is nitric oxide (NO), which is formed from L-arginine via catalysis by endothelial NO synthase (eNOS) (**Figure 4.11**). NO activates soluble guanylate cyclase and increases the synthesis of guanosine $3',5'$-cyclic monophosphate (cyclic GMP). cGMP subsequently inhibits

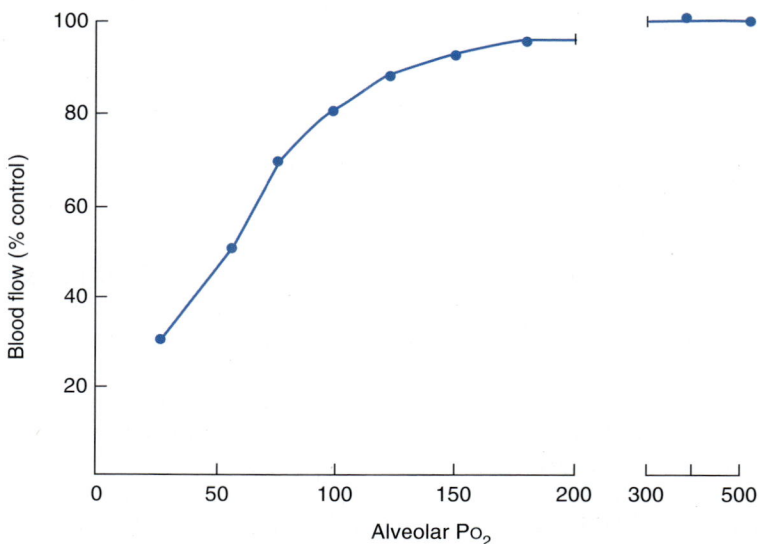

Figure 4.10. Effect of reducing alveolar Po_2 on pulmonary blood flow. (Data from anesthetized cat.) (From Barer GR, et al. *J Physiol*. 1970;211:139.)

Airspaces

(1) Inhalation from sinuses

Smooth muscle

GTP   cGMP → Myosin light chain
dephosphorylation

NO→ Guanylate Cyclase

Endothelium

O_2 NO

NADPH → eNOS → NADP

L-Arginine

Vascular space

Ca^{2+}
(2) Shear forces

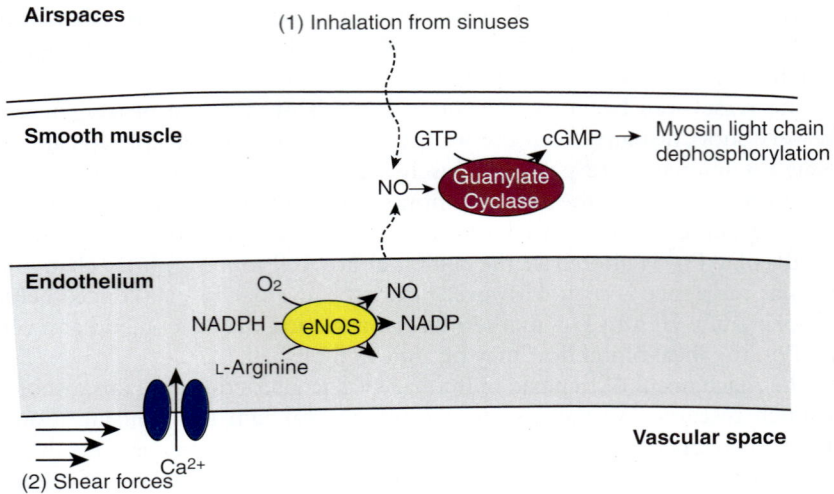

Figure 4.11. Mechanism of action of nitric oxide (NO) on pulmonary vascular smooth muscle. Nitric oxide is delivered through two mechanisms: (1) inhalation of NO produced in the sinuses and (2) endogenous production in response to shear forces, which trigger an influx of calcium that combines with endothelial nitric oxide synthetase (eNOS) to produce NO from oxygen, NADHP, and L-arginine. NO from either source diffuses into smooth muscle where it catalyzes conversion of GTP to cGMP. Increased concentration cGMP causes myosin light chain dephosphorylation, decoupling, and subsequent smooth muscle relaxation.

calcium channels, preventing a rise in intracellular calcium concentrations and promoting vasodilation. NO synthase inhibitors augment hypoxic pulmonary vasoconstriction in animal preparations, while administration of NO in low concentrations (10 to 40 ppm) by the inhalational route reduces hypoxic pulmonary vasoconstriction in humans. Disruption of the eNOS gene has been shown to cause pulmonary hypertension in animal models.

Pulmonary vascular endothelial cells also release potent vasoconstrictors such as endothelin-1 (ET-1) and thromboxane A_2 (TXA_2), which play a role in normal physiology and disease. Endothelin receptor antagonists are now part of treatment regimens for many patients with pulmonary hypertension.

Hypoxic vasoconstriction has the effect of directing blood flow away from hypoxic regions of lung. These regions may result from bronchial obstruction or alveolar filling, and by diverting blood flow, the deleterious effects on gas exchange are reduced. At high altitude, the Po_2 is reduced throughout the lung with the result that generalized pulmonary vasoconstriction occurs, leading to a rise in pulmonary arterial pressure. But probably, the most important situation in which this mechanism operates is at birth. During fetal life, the pulmonary vascular resistance is very high, partly because of hypoxic vasoconstriction, and only some 15% of the cardiac output goes through the lungs (see Figure 9.5). When the first breath oxygenates the alveoli, the vascular resistance falls dramatically because of relaxation of vascular smooth muscle, and the pulmonary blood flow increases enormously.

Other active responses of the pulmonary circulation have been described. A low blood pH (acidemia) causes vasoconstriction, especially when alveolar hypoxia is present, while severe hypothermia attenuates this response.

Hypoxic Pulmonary Vasoconstriction

- Alveolar hypoxia constricts small pulmonary arteries.
- Probably a direct effect of the low P_{O_2} on vascular smooth muscle.
- Its release is critical at birth in the transition from placental to air breathing.
- Directs blood flow away from poorly ventilated areas of the diseased lung in the adult.

The autonomic nervous system exerts a weak control, with an increase in sympathetic outflow causing stiffening of the walls of the pulmonary arteries and vasoconstriction. Iron deficiency causes increased vasoconstriction in response to alveolar hypoxia.

WATER BALANCE IN THE LUNG

Because only 0.3 μm of tissue separates the capillary blood from the air in the lung (Figure 1.1), the problem of keeping the alveoli free of fluid is critical. Fluid exchange across the capillary endothelium obeys Starling's law. The force tending to push fluid *out* of the capillary is the capillary hydrostatic pressure minus the hydrostatic pressure in the interstitial fluid, or $P_c - P_i$. The force tending to pull fluid in is the colloid osmotic pressure of the proteins of the blood minus that of the proteins of the interstitial fluid, or $\pi_c - \pi_i$. This force depends on the reflection coefficient σ, which is a measure of the effectiveness of the capillary wall in preventing the passage of proteins across it. Thus,

$$\text{net fluid out} = K[(P_c - P_i) - \sigma(\pi_c - \pi_i)]$$

where K is a constant called the filtration coefficient. This is called Starling's equation.

Net fluid out is not typically calculated in practice due to our ignorance of many of the values. Nevertheless, the principles encapsulated in the equation help us understand various physiological and clinical situations. The colloid osmotic pressure within the capillary is about 25 to 28 mm Hg. The capillary hydrostatic pressure is probably about halfway between arterial and venous pressure and is much higher at the bottom of the lung than at the top. The colloid osmotic pressure of the interstitial fluid is not known but is about

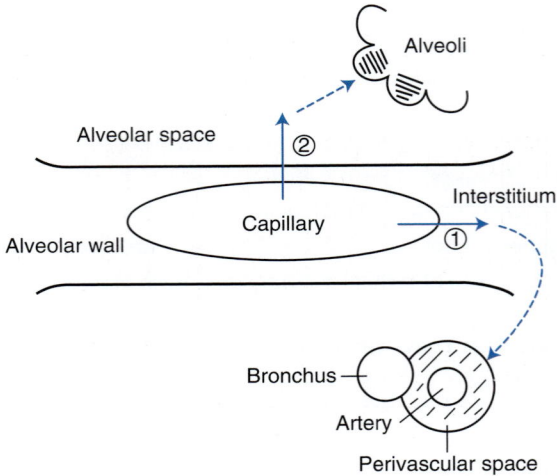

Figure 4.12. Two possible paths for fluid that moves out of the pulmonary capillaries. Fluid that enters the interstitium initially finds its way into the perivascular space (*1*). Later, fluid may cross the alveolar wall (*2*).

20 mm Hg in lung lymph. However, this value may be higher than that in the interstitial fluid around the capillaries. The interstitial hydrostatic pressure is unknown, but some measurements show it is substantially below atmospheric pressure. It is probable that the net pressure of the Starling equation is outward, causing a small lymph flow of perhaps 20 ml·h^{-1} in humans under normal conditions.

Where does fluid go when it leaves the capillaries? **Figure 4.12** shows that fluid that leaks out into the interstitium of the alveolar wall tracks through the interstitial space to the perivascular and peribronchial space within the lung. Numerous lymphatics run in the perivascular spaces, and these help to transport the fluid to the hilar lymph nodes. In addition, the pressure in these perivascular spaces is low, thus forming a natural sump for the drainage of fluid. The earliest form of pulmonary edema[†] is characterized by engorgement of these peribronchial and perivascular spaces and is known as interstitial edema. The rate of lymph flow from the lung increases considerably if the capillary pressure is raised over a long period.

In a later stage of pulmonary edema, fluid may cross the alveolar epithelium into the alveolar spaces (Figure 4.12). When this occurs, the alveoli fill with fluid one by one, and because they are then unventilated, no oxygenation of the blood passing through them is possible. What prompts fluid to start moving across into the alveolar spaces is not known, but it may occur when

---

[†]For a more extensive discussion of pulmonary edema, see the companion volume, West JB, Luks AM. *West's Pulmonary Pathophysiology: The Essentials.* 9th ed. Philadelphia, PA: Wolters Kluwer; 2017.

the maximal drainage rate through the interstitial space is exceeded and the pressure there rises too high. Fluid that reaches the alveolar spaces is actively pumped out by a sodium-potassium ATPase pump in epithelial cells. Alveolar edema is much more serious than interstitial edema because of the interference with pulmonary gas exchange.

OTHER FUNCTIONS OF THE PULMONARY CIRCULATION

The chief function of the pulmonary circulation is to move blood to and from the blood-gas barrier so that gas exchange can occur. However, it has other important functions. One is to act as a reservoir for blood. We saw that the lung has a remarkable ability to reduce its pulmonary vascular resistance as its vascular pressures are raised through the mechanisms of recruitment and distension (Figure 4.5). The same mechanisms allow the lung to increase its blood volume with relatively small rises in pulmonary arterial or venous pressures. This occurs, for example, when a subject lies down after standing and blood drains from the legs into the lung.

Another function of the lung is to filter blood. Small blood thrombi are removed from the circulation before they can reach the brain or other vital organs. Many white blood cells are trapped by the lung and later released, although the value of this is not clear.

METABOLIC FUNCTIONS OF THE LUNG

The lung has important metabolic functions in addition to gas exchange. Because the lung is the only organ except the heart that receives the whole circulation, it is uniquely suited to modifying bloodborne substances, including a number of vasoactive substances (**Table 4.1**). A substantial fraction of all the vascular endothelial cells in the body are located in the lung. The metabolic functions of the vascular endothelium are only briefly dealt with here because many fall within the province of pharmacology.

The only known example of biological activation by passage through the pulmonary circulation is the conversion of the relatively inactive polypeptide angiotensin I to the potent vasoconstrictor angiotensin II. The latter, which is up to 50 times more active than its precursor, is unaffected by passage through the lung. The conversion of angiotensin I is catalyzed by angiotensin-converting enzyme, or ACE, which is located in small pits in the surface of the capillary endothelial cells.

Many vasoactive substances are completely or partially inactivated during passage through the lung. ACE inactivates up to 80% of bradykinin. The lung

Table 4.1	Fate of Substances in the Pulmonary Circulation
Substance	**Fate**
Peptides	
Angiotensin I	Converted to angiotensin II by ACE
Angiotensin II	Not Affected
Vasopressin	Not Affected
Bradykinin	Up to 80% inactivated
Amines	
Serotonin	Almost completely removed
Norepinephrine	Up to 30% removed
Histamine	Not affected
Dopamine	Not affected
Arachidonic acid metabolites	
Prostaglandins E_2 and $F_{2\alpha}$	Almost completely removed
Prostaglandins A_1 and A_2	Not affected
Prostacyclin (PGI_2)	Not affected
Leukotrienes	Almost completely removed

is the major site of inactivation of serotonin (5-hydroxytryptamine), but this is not by enzymatic degradation but by an uptake and storage process (Table 4.1). Some of the serotonin may be transferred to platelets in the lung or stored in some other way and released during anaphylaxis. The prostaglandins E_1, E_2, and $F_{2\alpha}$ are also inactivated in the lung, which is a rich source of the responsible enzymes. Norepinephrine is also taken up by the lung to some extent (up to 30%). Histamine appears not to be affected by the intact lung but is readily inactivated by slices.

Some vasoactive materials pass through the lung without significant gain or loss of activity. These include epinephrine, prostaglandins A_1 and A_2, angiotensin II, and vasopressin (ADH).

Several vasoactive and bronchoactive substances are metabolized in the lung and may be released into the circulation under certain conditions. Important among these are the arachidonic acid metabolites. Arachidonic acid is formed through the action of the enzyme phospholipase A_2 on phospholipid bound to cell membranes. There are two major synthetic pathways, the initial reactions being catalyzed by the enzymes lipoxygenase and cyclooxygenase, respectively. The first produces the leukotrienes, which include the mediator originally described as slow-reacting substance of anaphylaxis (SRS-A). These compounds cause airway constriction and may have an important role in asthma. Other leukotrienes are involved in inflammatory responses.

The prostaglandins are potent vasoconstrictors or vasodilators. Prostaglandin E_2 plays an important role in the fetus because it helps to relax the patent ductus arteriosus, while prostaglandin I_2 is a potent pulmonary vasodilator that is used in the treatment of patients with increased pulmonary artery pressure. Prostaglandins also affect platelet aggregation, are active in other systems, such as the kallikrein-kinin clotting cascade, and may have a role in the bronchoconstriction of asthma. There is also evidence that the lung plays a role in the clotting mechanism of blood under normal and abnormal conditions. For example, there are a large number of mast cells containing heparin in the interstitium. In addition, the lung is able to secrete special immunoglobulins, particularly IgA, in the bronchial mucus that contribute to its defenses against infection.

Synthetic functions of the lung include the synthesis of phospholipids such as dipalmitoyl phosphatidylcholine, which is a component of pulmonary surfactant (see Chapter 7). Protein synthesis is also clearly important because collagen and elastin form the structural framework of the lung. Under some conditions, proteases are apparently liberated from leukocytes in the lung, causing breakdown of collagen and elastin, and this may result in emphysema. Another significant area is carbohydrate metabolism, especially the elaboration of mucopolysaccharides of bronchial mucus.

KEY CONCEPTS

1. The pressures within the pulmonary circulation are much lower than in the systemic circulation. Also the capillaries are exposed to alveolar pressure, whereas the pressures around the extra-alveolar vessels are lower.

2. Pulmonary vascular resistance is low and falls even more when cardiac output increases because of recruitment and distension of the capillaries. Pulmonary vascular resistance increases at very low or high lung volumes.

3. Blood flow is unevenly distributed in the upright lung. There is a higher flow at the base than at the apex as a result of gravity. If capillary pressure is less than alveolar pressure at the top of the lung, the capillaries collapse, and there is no blood flow (zone 1). There is also uneven blood flow at any given level in the lung because of random variations of the blood vessels.

4. Hypoxic pulmonary vasoconstriction reduces the blood flow to poorly ventilated regions of the lung. Release of this mechanism is largely responsible for a large increase in blood flow to the lung at birth.

5. Fluid movement across the capillary endothelium is governed by the Starling equilibrium.

6. The pulmonary circulation has many metabolic functions, notably the conversion of angiotensin I to angiotensin II by angiotensin-converting enzyme.

CLINICAL VIGNETTE

A 24-year-old man is admitted to the hospital after suffering pelvic and femur fractures in a high-speed motor vehicle collision. While recovering on the wards after surgical repair of his fractures, he had sudden onset of left-sided chest pain and severe difficulty breathing. He noted that the pain was stabbing in nature and increased with movement, coughing or deep breathing, a phenomenon referred to as "pleuritic" pain. He had an elevated heart rate and respiratory rate but a normal blood pressure and no abnormal findings on lung auscultation. A chest radiograph showed decreased vascular markings in the left lower lung field. A CT scan with intravenous contrast showed a lack of blood flow to the entire left lower lobe, consistent with a pulmonary embolism (a blood clot in the pulmonary artery). He then underwent echocardiography, which showed normal right ventricular function and only a small increase in his pulmonary artery systolic pressure above the normal range.

- If the circulation to the entire left lower lobe was occluded, why did the pulmonary artery pressure only rise a small amount above normal?
- What would be expected to happen to the blood flow to the apex of the right lung?
- What would happen to dead-space ventilation and alveolar ventilation?

QUESTIONS

For each question, choose the one best answer.

1. The figure below depicts changes in pulmonary vascular resistance as a function of lung volume. Which of the following best accounts for the observed change in resistance as lung volume changes from Point A to Point B?

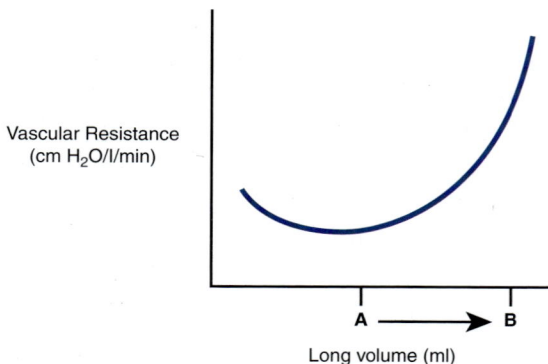

Vascular Resistance
(cm H_2O/l/min)

A ⟶ B

Long volume (ml)

A. Decreased endothelin-1 concentration in the pulmonary vasculature
B. Increased nitric oxide concentration in the pulmonary vasculature
C. Increased radial traction on extra-alveolar vessels
D. Recruitment and distention due to increased blood flow
E. Stretching of intra-alveolar vessels

2. As part of a research project, a healthy individual performs a cardiopulmonary exercise test with a right heart catheter in place to monitor pulmonary vascular resistance with progressive exercise.

Time Point	Pulmonary Vascular Resistance (mm Hg·liter^{-1}·min)
Pre-exercise	2.5
Mid-exercise	2.2
Maximal exercise	1.7

Which of the following accounts for the observed change in pulmonary vascular resistance with progressive exercise?
A. Decreased blood pH
B. Increased endothelin-1 concentration in the pulmonary vasculature
C. Increased zone 1 blood flow conditions
D. Increased sympathetic nervous system outflow
E. Recruitment and distention of the pulmonary capillaries

3. A patient with pulmonary vascular disease has mean pulmonary arterial and venous pressures of 55 and 5 mm Hg, respectively, while the cardiac output is 3 liters·min^{-1}. What is his or her pulmonary vascular resistance in mm Hg·liters^{-1}·min?
A. 0.5
B. 1.7
C. 2.5
D. 5
E. 17

4. A patient with a long history of tobacco use presents to the emergency department with acute onset of dyspnea. After a chest radiograph shows a dense left lower lobe opacity, a CT scan of the chest is obtained and shows collapse of the left lower lobe due to a mass lesion obstructing the left lower lobe bronchus. Which of the following changes would you expect to see in the left lower lobe as a result of this finding?
A. Decreased conversion of angiotensin I to angiotensin II
B. Distention of extra-alveolar vessels
C. Increased pulmonary venous pressure
D. Smooth muscle constriction in the pulmonary arterioles
E. Smooth muscle relaxation in the pulmonary venules

5. A patient undergoes placement of a right heart catheter and radial arterial catheter during an evaluation for valvular heart disease. The O_2 concentrations of mixed venous and arterial blood are found to be 16 and 20 ml per 100 ml, respectively, while the O_2 consumption is estimated to be 300 ml·min^{-1}. Which of the following is the patient's pulmonary blood flow in liters·min^{-1}?

   A. 2.5
   B. 5
   C. 7.5
   D. 10
   E. 75

6. You are conducting an experiment involving an isolated, perfused, and mechanically ventilated lung. Catheters and pressure gauges are placed that allow you to measure the pulmonary arterial and venous and alveolar pressure in a specific region of the lung. Based on the displayed values, what will happen to blood flow in this region as a result of the intervention?

Time Point	$P_{arterial}$ (mm Hg)	$P_{alveolar}$ (mm Hg)	P_{venous} (mm Hg)
Pre-intervention	12	4	7
Post-intervention	12	9	5

   A. Decrease in flow because the driving pressure becomes arterial minus venous pressure
   B. Decrease in flow because the driving pressure becomes arterial minus alveolar pressure
   C. Increase in flow because the driving pressure becomes alveolar minus venous pressure
   D. Increase in flow because the driving pressure becomes arterial minus venous pressure
   E. No change in blood flow

7. A healthy individual is participating in a research experiment and undergoes placement of a pulmonary artery catheter. Measurements are made before and after an intervention. Based on the data shown in the table, which of the following is the most likely intervention performed on this individual?

Time Point	Pulmonary Vascular Resistance (mm Hg·liter^{-1}·min)	Mean Pulmonary Artery Pressure (mm Hg)	Cardiac Output (liter·min^{-1})
Pre-intervention	3.2	23	5.6
Post-intervention	2.5	21	6.4

A. Intravenous administration of endothelin
B. Intravenous administration of histamine
C. Intravenous administration of prostacyclin
D. Intravenous administration of serotonin
E. Inhalation of a gas mixture with an F_IO_2 of 0.12

8. If the pressures in the capillaries and interstitial space at the top of the lung are 3 and 0 mm Hg, respectively, and the colloid osmotic pressures of the blood and interstitial fluid are 25 and 5 mm Hg, respectively, what is the net pressure in mm Hg moving fluid into the capillaries?
A. 17
B. 20
C. 23
D. 27
E. 33

9. A 45-year-old man is admitted with severe right lower lobe pneumonia. On the second hospital day, his hypoxemia worsens and a repeat chest radiograph shows increased opacities in both lungs. A blood gas reveals a pH of 7.47 and an arterial Po_2 of 55 mm Hg, while an echocardiogram demonstrates normal left ventricular function and left atrial size but significantly increased systolic pulmonary artery pressure. Which of the following factors likely accounts for the findings on his echocardiogram?
A. Decreased alveolar Po_2
B. Decreased arterial Po_2
C. Decreased sympathetic nervous system activity
D. Increased blood pH
E. Increased pulmonary venous pressure

10. Following admission for a severe myocardial infarction, a 62-year-old woman has increasing difficulty breathing. Laboratory studies reveal a serum albumin of 4.1 mg·dl^{-1} (normal >4.0 mg·dl^{-1}) and an arterial Po_2 of 55 mm Hg, while a chest radiograph demonstrates a large heart and diffuse bilateral opacities, consistent with pulmonary edema. An echocardiogram demonstrates a dilated left ventricle with decreased systolic function, an enlarged left atrium, and mildly increased systolic pulmonary artery pressure. Which of the following factors most likely accounts for the findings on chest radiography in this patient?
A. Decreased arterial Po_2
B. Decreased colloid osmotic pressure
C. Increased lymphatic drainage from the pulmonary interstitium
D. Increased pulmonary capillary hydrostatic pressure
E. Recruitment and distention of the pulmonary vasculature

11. Administration of an angiotensin converting enzyme (ACE) inhibitor would be expected to have which of the following effects in the lung?
   A. Decreased inactivation of bradykinin
   B. Decreased uptake and storage of serotonin
   C. Increased conversion of arachidonic acid to prostaglandin
   D. Increased enzymatic degradation of angiotensin II
   E. Increased lung uptake of norepinephrine

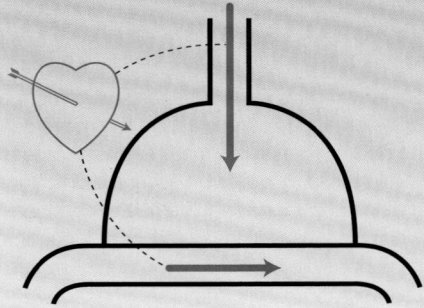

Ventilation-Perfusion Relationships

5

How Matching of Gas and Blood Determines Gas Exchange

- **Oxygen Transport from Air to Tissues**
- **Hypoventilation**
- **Diffusion Limitation**
- **Shunt**
- **The Ventilation-Perfusion Ratio**
- **Effect of Altering the Ventilation-Perfusion Ratio of a Lung Unit**
- **Regional Gas Exchange in the Lung**
- **Effect of Ventilation-Perfusion Inequality on Overall Gas Exchange**
- **Distributions of Ventilation-Perfusion Ratios**
- **Ventilation-Perfusion Inequality as a Cause of CO_2 Retention**
- **Measurement of Ventilation-Perfusion Inequality**

This chapter is devoted to the primary function of the lung, that is, gas exchange. First, a theoretical ideal lung is considered. Then we review three mechanisms of hypoxemia: hypoventilation, diffusion limitation, and shunt. The difficult concept of ventilation-perfusion inequality is then introduced, and to illustrate this, the regional differences of gas exchange in the upright human lung are described. Then we examine how ventilation-perfusion inequality impairs overall gas exchange, including not only the effects on oxygen but also the effects on carbon dioxide. Methods of measuring ventilation-perfusion inequality are then briefly discussed. At the end of this chapter, the reader should be able to:

- Calculate the shunt fraction and the alveolar-arterial P_{O_2} difference
- Predict changes in the P_{O_2} and P_{CO_2} for a given lung unit based on changes in the ventilation-perfusion ratio
- Describe regional differences in blood flow and ventilation in the upright lung and their effects on ventilation-perfusion ratios and oxygenation
- Use clinical and laboratory data to identify the cause of hypoxemia
- Compare the effect of increased ventilation on CO_2 elimination and oxygenation in the setting of ventilation-perfusion inequality

69

So far we have considered the movement of air to and from the blood-gas interface, the diffusion of gas across it, and the movement of blood to and from the barrier. It would be natural to assume that if all these processes were adequate, normal gas exchange within the lung would be assured. Unfortunately, this is not so because of another factor that is critical for adequate gas exchange—the matching of ventilation and blood flow within various regions of the lung. Indeed, mismatching of ventilation and blood flow is responsible for most of the defective gas exchange in acute and chronic pulmonary diseases.

After taking a preliminary look at normal O_2 transfer, we will examine the primary reasons that individuals develop an abnormally low Po_2 in arterial blood, referred to as hypoxemia. We shall then consider three relatively simple causes of hypoxemia—hypoventilation, diffusion limitation, and shunt—and then look more closely at the final and very important cause, ventilation-perfusion inequality.

OXYGEN TRANSPORT FROM AIR TO TISSUES

Figure 5.1 shows how the Po_2 falls as the gas moves from the atmosphere in which we live to the mitochondria where it is utilized. The Po_2 of air is 20.93% of the total dry gas pressure (i.e., excluding water vapor). At sea level, the barometric pressure is 760 mm Hg, and at the body temperature of 37°C, the water vapor pressure of moist inspired gas (which is fully saturated with water vapor) is 47 mm Hg. Thus, the Po_2 of inspired air is $(20.93/100) \times (760 - 47)$, or 149 mm Hg (say 150).

Figure 5.1 is drawn for a hypothetical perfect lung, and it shows that by the time the O_2 has reached the alveoli, the Po_2 has fallen to about 100 mm Hg, that is, by one-third. This is because the Po_2 of alveolar gas is determined by a balance between two processes: the removal of O_2 by pulmonary capillary blood on the one hand and its continual replenishment by alveolar ventilation on the other. (Strictly, alveolar ventilation is not continuous but is breath by breath. However, the fluctuation in alveolar Po_2 with each breath is only about 3 mm Hg, because the tidal volume is small compared with the volume of gas in the lung, so the process can be regarded as continuous.) The rate of removal of O_2 from the lung is governed by the O_2 consumption of the tissues and varies little under resting conditions. In practice, therefore, the alveolar Po_2 is largely determined by the level of alveolar ventilation. The same applies to the alveolar Pco_2, which is normally about 40 mm Hg.

When the systemic arterial blood reaches the tissue capillaries, O_2 diffuses to the mitochondria, where the Po_2 is much lower. The "tissue" Po_2 probably differs considerably throughout the body, and in some cells at least, the Po_2 is as low as 1 mm Hg. However, the lung is an essential link in the chain of O_2 transport, and any decrease of Po_2 in arterial blood must result in a lower

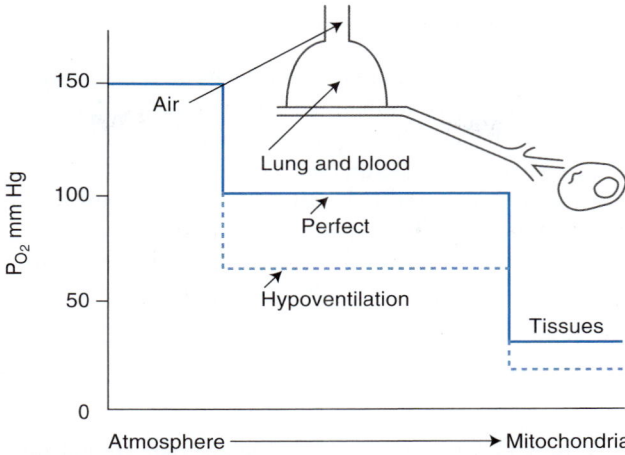

Figure 5.1. Scheme of the O_2 partial pressures from air to tissues. The *solid line* shows a hypothetical perfect situation, and the *broken line* depicts hypoventilation. Hypoventilation depresses the P_{O_2} in the alveolar gas and, therefore, in the tissues.

tissue P_{O_2} other things being equal. For the same reasons, impaired pulmonary gas exchange causes a rise in tissue P_{CO_2}.

While this is how normal gas exchange takes place, in some situations, these processes go awry and patients develop hypoxemia. This can happen for one of several reasons, referred to as hypoventilation, shunt, diffusion abnormality, and ventilation-perfusion inequality.

Four Causes of Hypoxemia

- Hypoventilation
- Diffusion limitation
- Shunt
- Ventilation-perfusion inequality

HYPOVENTILATION

We have seen that the alveolar P_{O_2} is determined by a balance between the rate of removal of O_2 by the blood, which is set by the metabolic demands of the tissues, and the rate of replenishment of O_2 by alveolar ventilation. Thus, if the alveolar ventilation is abnormally low, the alveolar P_{O_2}

falls. For similar reasons, the P_{CO_2} rises. This is known as hypoventilation (Figure 5.1).

Causes of hypoventilation include such drugs as opiates and barbiturates that depress the central drive to the respiratory muscles, damage to the chest wall, weakness or paralysis of the respiratory muscles, and a high resistance to breathing (e.g., a very severe asthma attack). Some diseases, such as morbid obesity, may cause hypoventilation by affecting both central respiratory drive and respiratory mechanics. Hypoventilation always causes an increased alveolar and, therefore, arterial P_{CO_2}. The relationship between alveolar ventilation and P_{CO_2} was derived on p. 21 in the alveolar ventilation equation:

$$P_{CO_2} = \frac{\dot{V}_{CO_2}}{\dot{V}_A} \times K$$

where $\dot{V}_{CO_2}$ is the CO_2 production, $\dot{V}_A$ is the alveolar ventilation, and K is a constant. This means that if the alveolar ventilation is halved, the P_{CO_2} is doubled, once a steady state has been established.

The relationship between the fall in P_{O_2} and the rise in P_{CO_2} that occurs in hypoventilation can be calculated from the *alveolar gas equation* if we know the composition of inspired gas and the respiratory exchange ratio R. The latter is given by the CO_2 production/O_2 consumption, is determined by the metabolism of the tissues in a steady state, and varies based on the balance of fuels consumed by a given individual (i.e., carbohydrate, fat, and protein). It is sometimes known as the respiratory quotient. A simplified form of the alveolar gas equation is

$$P_{A_{O_2}} = P_{I_{O_2}} - \frac{P_{A_{CO_2}}}{R} + F$$

where F is a small correction factor (typically about 2 mm Hg for air breathing), which we can ignore. This equation shows that if R has its normal value of 0.8, the fall in alveolar P_{O_2} is slightly greater than is the rise in P_{CO_2} during hypoventilation. The full version of the equation is given in Appendix A.

Hypoventilation always reduces the alveolar and arterial P_{O_2} except when the subject breathes an enriched O_2 mixture. In this case, the added amount of O_2 per breath can easily make up for the reduced flow of inspired gas (try question 3 at the end of the chapter). If alveolar ventilation is suddenly increased (e.g., by voluntary hyperventilation), it may take several minutes for the alveolar P_{O_2} and P_{CO_2} to assume their new steady-state values. This is because of the different O_2 and CO_2 stores in the body. The CO_2 stores are much greater than the O_2 stores because of the large amount of CO_2 in the form of bicarbonate in the blood and interstitial fluid (see Chapter 6). Therefore, the alveolar P_{CO_2} takes longer to come to equilibrium, and during the nonsteady state, the R value of expired gas is high as the CO_2 stores are washed out. Opposite changes occur with the onset of hypoventilation.

Hypoventilation

- Always increases the alveolar and arterial P_{CO_2}
- Decreases the P_{O_2} unless additional O_2 is inspired
- Hypoxemia is easily reversed by adding O_2 to the inspired gas

DIFFUSION LIMITATION

Figure 5.1 shows that in a perfect lung, the P_{O_2} of arterial blood would be the same as that in alveolar gas. In real life, this is not so. One reason is that although the P_{O_2} of the blood rises closer and closer to that of alveolar gas as the blood traverses the pulmonary capillary (Figure 3.3), it never quite reaches it. Under normal conditions, the P_{O_2} difference between alveolar gas and end-capillary blood resulting from incomplete diffusion is immeasurably small but is shown schematically in **Figure 5.2.** As we have seen, the difference can become larger during exercise (due to decreases in the capillary transit time of red blood cells), or when the blood-gas barrier is thickened, or if a low O_2 mixture is inhaled (Figure 3.3B). However, diffusion limitation rarely causes hypoxemia at rest at sea level even when lung disease affects the blood-gas barrier because the red blood cells spend enough time in the pulmonary capillary to allow nearly complete equilibration.

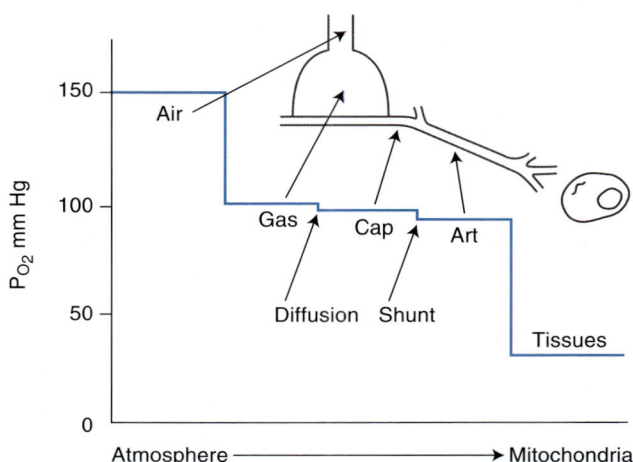

Figure 5.2. Scheme of O_2 transfer from air to tissues showing the depression of arterial P_{O_2} caused by diffusion and shunt. (Modified with permission of John Wiley & Sons from West JB. *Ventilation/Blood Flow and Gas Exchange*. 5th ed. Oxford, UK: Blackwell; 1990:3; permission conveyed through Copyright Clearance Center, Inc.)

SHUNT

Another reason why the P_{O_2} of arterial blood is less than that in alveolar gas is shunted blood. *Shunt* refers to blood that enters the arterial system without going through ventilated areas of the lung. In the normal lung, some of the bronchial artery blood is collected by the pulmonary veins after it has perfused the bronchi and its O_2 has been partly depleted. Another source is a small amount of coronary venous blood that drains directly into the cavity of the left ventricle through the thebesian veins. The effect of the addition of this poorly oxygenated blood is to depress the arterial P_{O_2}. Some individuals have an abnormal vascular connection between a small pulmonary artery and vein (pulmonary arteriovenous malformation). Some forms of cardiac disease cause direct addition of venous blood to arterial blood across a defect between the right and left sides of the heart.

When the shunt is caused by the addition of mixed venous blood to blood draining from the capillaries, it is possible to calculate the amount of the shunt flow (**Figure 5.3**). The total amount of O_2 leaving the system is the total blood flow $\dot{Q}_T$ multiplied by the O_2 concentration in the arterial blood, Ca_{O_2}, or $\dot{Q}_T \times Ca_{O_2}$. This must equal the sum of the amounts of O_2 in the shunted blood, and end-capillary blood, $(\dot{Q}_T - \dot{Q}_S) \times Cc'_{O_2}$. Thus,

$$\dot{Q}_T \times Ca_{O_2} = \dot{Q}_S \times C\bar{v}_{O_2} + (\dot{Q}_T - \dot{Q}_S) \times Cc'_{O_2}$$

Rearranging gives:

$$\frac{\dot{Q}_S}{\dot{Q}_T} = \frac{Cc'_{O_2} - Ca_{O_2}}{Cc'_{O_2} - C\bar{v}_{O_2}}$$

The O_2 concentration of end-capillary blood is usually calculated from the alveolar P_{O_2} and the oxygen dissociation curve (see Chapter 6). The ratio of shunt flow to total flow is called the shunt fraction.

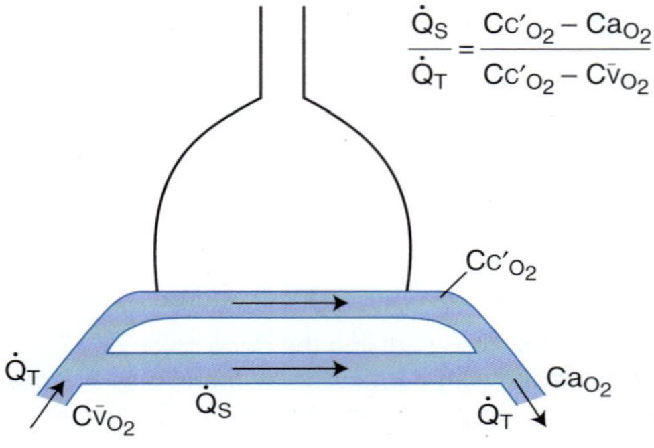

Figure 5.3. Measurement of shunt flow. The oxygen carried in the arterial blood equals the sum of the oxygen carried in the capillary blood and that in the shunted blood (see text).

When the shunt is caused by blood that does not have the same O_2 concentration as mixed venous blood (e.g., bronchial vein blood), it is generally not possible to calculate its true magnitude. However, it is often useful to calculate an "as if" shunt, that is, what the shunt *would* be if the observed depression of arterial O_2 concentration were caused by the addition of mixed venous blood. In healthy individuals, the normal shunt fraction resulting from bronchial and thebesian vein flow is about 5%, whereas in certain forms of lung disease, it can rise to much higher values.

An important feature of a shunt is that the hypoxemia cannot be abolished by giving an individual 100% O_2 to breathe. This is because the shunted blood that bypasses ventilated alveoli is never exposed to the higher alveolar Po_2, so it continues to depress the arterial Po_2. However, some elevation of the arterial Po_2 occurs because of the O_2 added to the capillary blood of ventilated lung, which can be valuable in some patients. Most of the added O_2 is in the dissolved form, rather than attached to hemoglobin, because the blood that is perfusing ventilated alveoli is nearly fully saturated (see Chapter 6). The response to supplemental oxygen administration when shunt is present varies based on the shunt fraction (**Figure 5.4**). Giving the subject 100% O_2 to breathe is a very sensitive measurement of shunt because when the Po_2 is high, a small depression of arterial O_2 concentration causes a relatively large fall in Po_2 due to the almost flat slope of the O_2 dissociation curve in this region (**Figure 5.5**).

A shunt usually does not result in a raised Pco_2 in arterial blood, even though the shunted blood is rich in CO_2. The reason is that the chemoreceptors sense any elevation of arterial Pco_2 and respond by increasing ventilation. This reduces the Pco_2 of the unshunted blood until the arterial Pco_2 is normal. Indeed, in some patients with a shunt, the arterial Pco_2 is low because the hypoxemia increases respiratory drive (see Chapter 8).

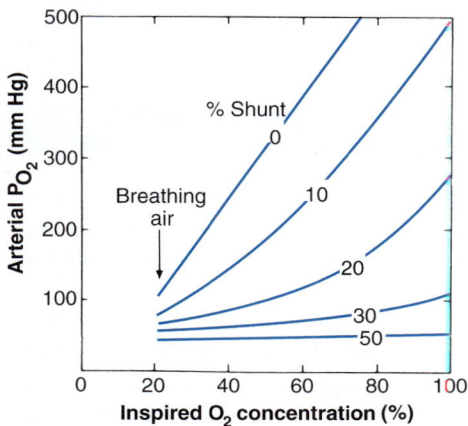

Figure 5.4. Response of the arterial Po_2 to increased inspired oxygen concentrations in a lung with various amounts of shunt. Note that the Po_2 remains far below the normal level for 100% oxygen. Nevertheless, useful gains in oxygenation occur even with severe degrees of shunting. (This diagram shows typical values only; changes in cardiac output, oxygen uptake, etc., affect the position of the lines.) (From West JB. *Pulmonary Pathophysiology: The Essentials.* 8th ed. Philadelphia, PA: Lippincott Williams & Wilkins; 2003:Figure 9-3.)

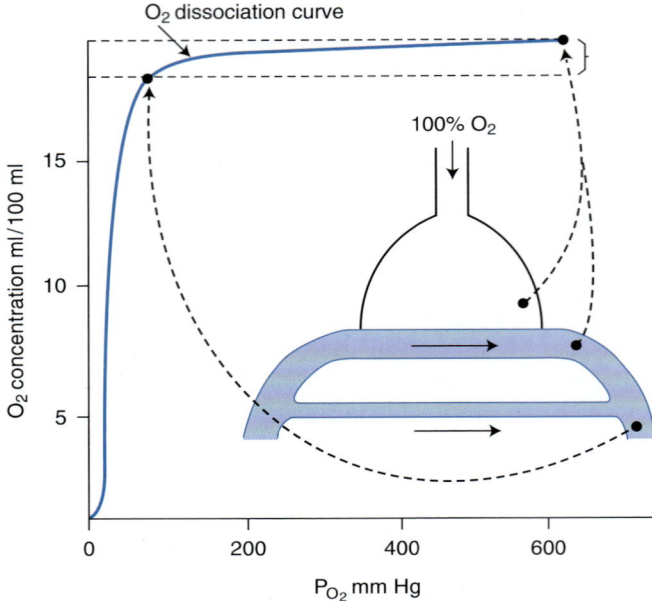

Figure 5.5. Depression of arterial P_{O_2} by shunt during 100% O_2 breathing. The addition of a small amount of shunted blood with its low O_2 concentration greatly reduces the P_{O_2} of arterial blood. This is because the O_2 dissociation curve is nearly flat when the P_{O_2} is very high.

Shunt

- Hypoxemia responds poorly to added inspired O_2.
- When 100% O_2 is inspired, the arterial P_{O_2} does not rise to the expected level—a useful diagnostic test.
- If the shunt is caused by mixed venous blood, its size can be calculated from the shunt equation.

THE VENTILATION-PERFUSION RATIO

So far, we have considered three of the four causes of hypoxemia: hypoventilation, diffusion, and shunt. We now come to the last cause, which is both the most common and the most difficult to understand, namely, ventilation-perfusion inequality.

A critical factor in maintaining efficient gas exchange and preventing hypoxemia is ensuring that lung units receive a balanced mix of ventilation and perfusion; if ventilation and blood flow are mismatched in various regions of the lung, impaired transfer of both O_2 and CO_2 results. The key to understanding how this happens is the ventilation-perfusion ratio.

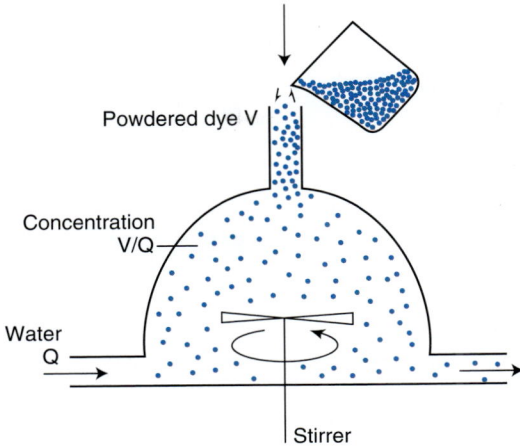

Figure 5.6. Model to illustrate how the ventilation-perfusion ratio determines the P_{O_2} in a lung unit. Powdered dye is added by ventilation at the rate V and removed by blood flow Q to represent the factors controlling alveolar P_{O_2}. The concentration of dye is given by V/Q. (Republished with permission of John Wiley & Sons from West JB. *Ventilation/Blood Flow and Gas Exchange.* 5th ed. Oxford, UK: Blackwell; 1990; permission conveyed through Copyright Clearance Center, Inc.)

Consider a model of a lung unit (Figure 2.1) in which the uptake of O_2 is being mimicked using dye and water (**Figure 5.6**). Powdered dye is continuously poured into the unit to represent the addition of O_2 by alveolar ventilation. Water is pumped continuously through the unit to represent the blood flow that removes the O_2. A stirrer mixes the alveolar contents, a process normally accomplished by gaseous diffusion. The key question is: What determines the concentration of dye (or O_2) in the alveolar compartment and, therefore, in the effluent water (or blood)?

It is clear that both the rate at which the dye is added (ventilation) and the rate at which water is pumped (blood flow) will affect the concentration of dye in the model. What may not be intuitively clear is that the concentration of dye is determined by the ratio of these rates. In other words, if dye is added at the rate of V g·min^{-1} and water is pumped through at Q liters·min^{-1}, the concentration of dye in the alveolar compartment and effluent water is V/Q g·liter^{-1}.

In exactly the same way, the concentration of O_2 (or, better, P_{O_2}) in any lung unit is determined by the ratio of ventilation to blood flow. This is true not only for O_2 but also for CO_2, N_2, and any other gas that is present under steady-state conditions. This is why the ventilation-perfusion ratio plays such a key role in pulmonary gas exchange.

EFFECT OF ALTERING THE VENTILATION-PERFUSION RATIO OF A LUNG UNIT

Let us take a closer look at the way alterations in the ventilation-perfusion ratio of a lung unit affect its gas exchange. **Figure 5.7A** shows the P_{O_2} and P_{CO_2} in a unit with a normal ventilation-perfusion ratio (about 1, see

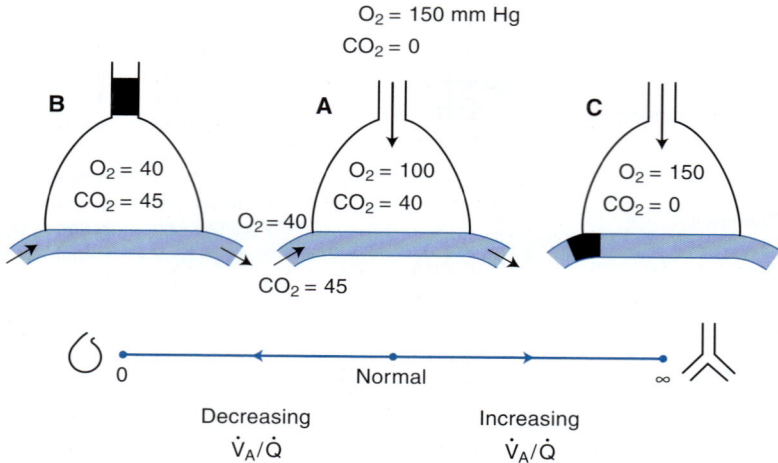

Figure 5.7. Effect of altering the ventilation-perfusion ratio on the P_{O_2} and P_{CO_2} in a lung unit. (Republished with permission of John Wiley & Sons from West JB. *Ventilation/ Blood Flow and Gas Exchange*. 5th ed. Oxford, UK: Blackwell; 1990; permission conveyed through Copyright Clearance Center, Inc.)

Figure 2.1). The inspired air has a P_{O_2} of 150 mm Hg (Figure 5.1) and a P_{CO_2} of 0. The mixed venous blood entering the unit has a P_{O_2} of 40 mm Hg and a P_{CO_2} of 45 mm Hg. The alveolar P_{O_2} of 100 mm Hg is determined by a balance between the addition of O_2 by ventilation and its removal by blood flow. The normal alveolar P_{CO_2} of 40 mm Hg is set similarly.

Now suppose that the ventilation-perfusion ratio of the unit is gradually reduced by obstructing its ventilation, leaving its blood flow unchanged (**Figure 5.7B**). This could occur, for example, due to mucous or a tumor obstructing the airway. It is clear that the O_2 in the unit will fall and the CO_2 will rise, although the relative changes of these two are not immediately obvious.* However, we can easily predict what will eventually happen when the ventilation is completely abolished (ventilation-perfusion ratio of 0). Now the O_2 and CO_2 of alveolar gas and end-capillary blood must be the same as those of mixed venous blood. (In practice, completely obstructed units eventually collapse, but we can neglect such long-term effects at the moment.) Note that we are assuming that what happens in one lung unit out of a very large number does not affect the composition of the mixed venous blood.

---

*The alveolar gas equation is not applicable here because the respiratory exchange ratio is not constant. The appropriate equation is

$$\frac{\dot{V}_A}{\dot{Q}} = 8.63 \ R \ \frac{Ca_{O_2} - C\bar{v}_{O_2}}{Pa_{CO_2}}$$

This is called the ventilation-perfusion ratio equation. See Appendix B for more details.

Suppose instead that the ventilation-perfusion ratio is increased by decreasing blood flow (**Figure 5.7C**). This could occur, for example, due to a blood clot partially obstructing a blood vessel, a problem known as a pulmonary embolism. Now the O_2 rises and the CO_2 falls, eventually reaching the composition of inspired gas when blood flow is abolished (ventilation-perfusion ratio of infinity). Thus, as the ventilation-perfusion ratio of the unit is altered, its gas composition approaches that of mixed venous blood or inspired gas.

A convenient way of depicting these changes is to use the O_2-CO_2 diagram (**Figure 5.8**). In this, P_{O_2} is plotted on the x axis, and P_{CO_2} is plotted on the y axis. First, locate the normal alveolar gas composition, point A (P_{O_2} = 100, P_{CO_2} = 40). If we assume that blood equilibrates with alveolar gas at the end of the capillary (Figure 3.3), this point can equally well represent the end-capillary blood. Next find the mixed venous point $\bar{v}$ (P_{O_2} = 40, P_{CO_2} = 45). The bar above v means "mixed" or "mean." Finally, find the inspired point I (P_{O_2} = 150, P_{CO_2} = 0). Also, note the similarities between Figures 5.7 and 5.8.

The line joining $\bar{v}$ to I passing through A shows the changes in alveolar gas (and end-capillary blood) composition that can occur when the ventilation-perfusion ratio is either decreased below normal (A → $\bar{v}$) or increased above normal (A → I). Indeed, this line indicates *all* the possible alveolar gas compositions in a lung that is supplied with gas of composition I and blood of composition $\bar{v}$. For example, such a lung could not contain an alveolus with a P_{O_2} of 70 and P_{CO_2} of 30 mm Hg, because this point does not lie on the ventilation-perfusion line. However, this alveolar composition *could* exist if the mixed venous blood or inspired gas were changed so that the line then passed through this point.

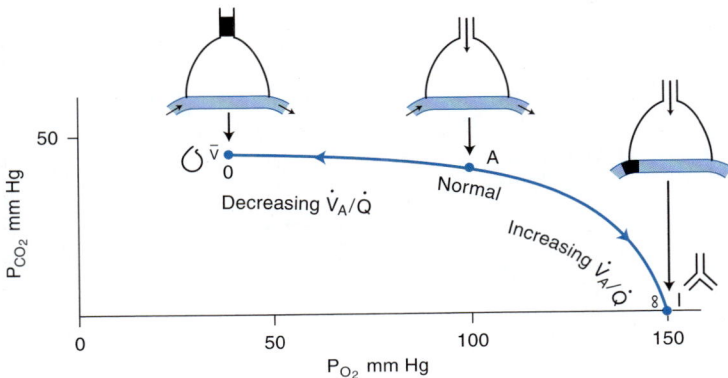

Figure 5.8. O_2-CO_2 diagram showing a ventilation-perfusion ratio line. The P_{O_2} and P_{CO_2} of a lung unit move along this line from the mixed venous point to the inspired gas point I as the ventilation-perfusion ratio is increased (compare Figure 5.7). (Republished with permission of John Wiley & Sons from West JB. *Ventilation/Blood Flow and Gas Exchange*. 5th ed. Oxford, UK: Blackwell; 1990; permission conveyed through Copyright Clearance Center, Inc.)

REGIONAL GAS EXCHANGE IN THE LUNG

Ventilation and perfusion are not constant throughout the lung, and, instead vary from top to bottom due to the effects of gravity and other factors. This has implications for ventilation-perfusion ratios across the lung which affects the exchange of gases in the different regions. We saw in Figures 2.7 and 4.7 that ventilation increases slowly from top to bottom of the lung and blood flow increases more rapidly (**Figure 5.9**). As a consequence, the ventilation-perfusion ratio is abnormally high at the top of the lung (where the blood flow is minimal) and much lower at the bottom. We can now use these regional differences in ventilation-perfusion ratio on an O_2-CO_2 diagram (Figure 5.8) to depict the resulting differences in gas exchange.

Figure 5.10 shows the upright lung divided into imaginary horizontal "slices," each of which is located on the ventilation-perfusion line by its own ventilation-perfusion ratio. This ratio is high at the apex, so this point is found toward the right end of the line, whereas the base of the lung is to the left of normal (compare Figure 5.8). It is clear that the Po_2 of the alveoli (horizontal axis) decreases markedly down the lung, whereas the Pco_2 (vertical axis) increases much less.

Figure 5.11 illustrates the values that can be read off a diagram like Figure 5.10. (Of course, there will be variations between individuals; the chief aim of this approach is to describe the principles underlying gas exchange

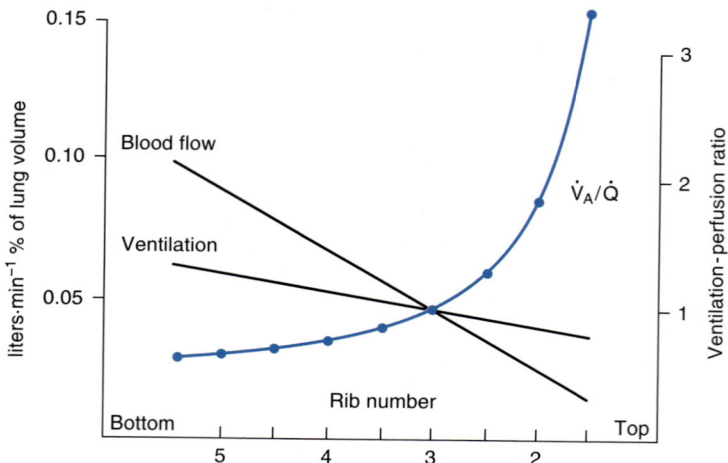

Figure 5.9. Distribution of ventilation and blood flow down the upright lung (compare Figures 2.7 and 4.7). Note that the ventilation-perfusion ratio decreases down the lung. (From West JB. *Ventilation/Blood Flow and Gas Exchange*. 5th ed. Oxford, UK: Blackwell; 1990.)

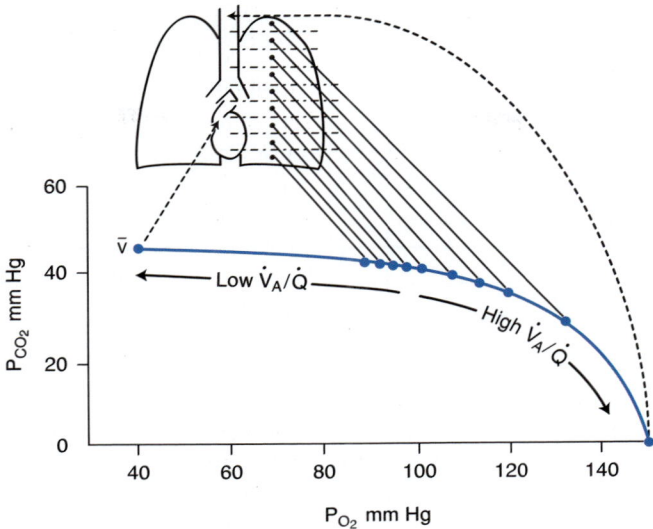

Figure 5.10. Result of combining the pattern of ventilation-perfusion ratio inequality shown in Figure 5.9 with the effects of this on gas exchange as shown in Figure 5.8. Note that the high ventilation-perfusion ratio at the apex results in a high P_{O_2} and low P_{CO_2} there. The opposite is seen at the base. (From West JB. *Ventilation/Blood Flow and Gas Exchange*. 5th ed. Oxford, UK: Blackwell; 1990.)

rather than determine specific values.) Note first that the volume of the lung in the slices is less near the apex than the base. Ventilation is less at the top than the bottom, but the differences in blood flow are more marked. Consequently, the ventilation-perfusion ratio decreases down the lung, and all the differences in gas exchange follow from this. Note that the P_{O_2} changes by over 40 mm Hg, whereas the difference in P_{CO_2} between apex and base is much less. The variation in P_{N_2} is, in effect, by default because the total pressure in the alveolar gas is the same throughout the lung.

The regional differences in P_{O_2} and P_{CO_2} imply differences in the end-capillary concentrations of these gases, which can be obtained from the appropriate dissociation curves (Chapter 6). Note the surprisingly large difference in pH down the lung, which reflects the considerable variation in P_{CO_2} of the blood. The minimal contribution to overall O_2 uptake made by the apex can be mainly attributed to the very low blood flow there. The difference in CO_2 output between apex and base is much less because this can be shown to be more closely related to ventilation. As a result, the respiratory exchange ratio (CO_2 output/O_2 uptake) is higher at the apex than at the base. On exercise, when the distribution of blood flow becomes more uniform, the apex assumes a larger share of the O_2 uptake.

Vol (%)	V̇A (l/min)	Q̇ (l/min)	V̇A/Q̇	P_{O_2} (mm Hg)	P_{CO_2} (mm Hg)	P_{N_2} (mm Hg)	O_2 conc. (ml/100 ml)	CO_2 conc. (ml/100 ml)	pH	O_2 in (ml/min)	CO_2 out (ml/min)
7	0.24	0.07	3.3	132	28	553	20.0	42	7.51	4	8
13	0.82	1.29	0.63	89	42	582	19.2	49	7.39	60	39

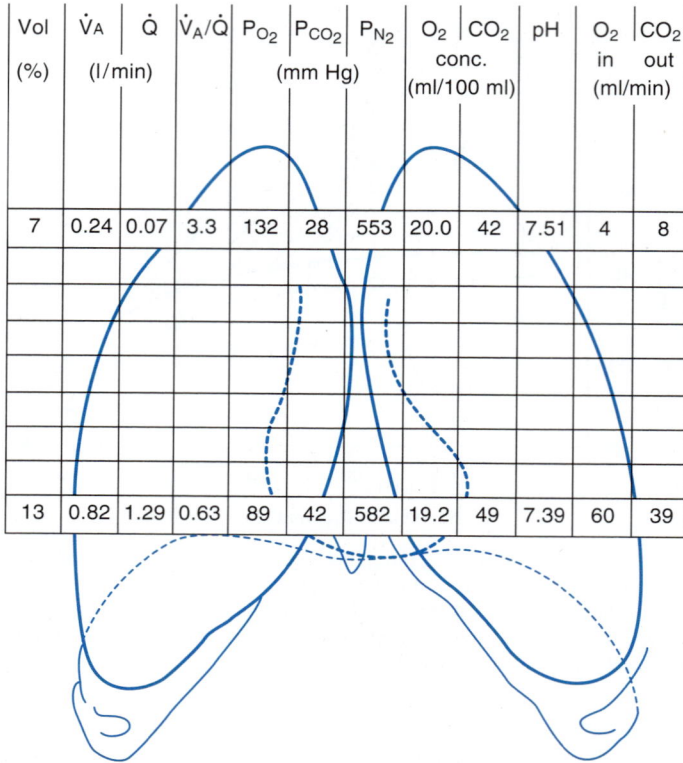

Figure 5.11. Regional differences in gas exchange down the normal lung. Only the apical and basal values are shown for clarity.

EFFECT OF VENTILATION-PERFUSION INEQUALITY ON OVERALL GAS EXCHANGE

Although the regional differences in gas exchange discussed above are of interest, more important to the body as a whole is whether uneven ventilation and blood flow affect the overall gas exchange of the lung, that is, its ability to take up O_2 and put out CO_2. It turns out that a lung with ventilation-perfusion inequality is not able to transfer as much O_2 and CO_2 as a lung that is uniformly ventilated and perfused, other things being equal. Or if the same amounts of gas are being transferred (because these are set by the metabolic demands of the body), the lung with ventilation-perfusion inequality cannot maintain as high an arterial P_{O_2} or as low an arterial P_{CO_2} as a homogeneous lung with good ventilation-perfusion matching throughout, again other things being equal.

The reason why a lung with uneven ventilation and blood flow has difficulty oxygenating arterial blood can be illustrated by looking at the differ-

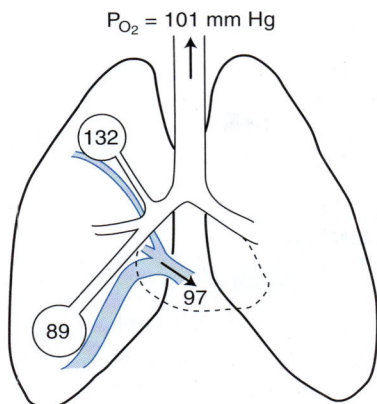

P_{O_2} = 101 mm Hg

132

97

89

Figure 5.12. Depression of the arterial P_{O_2} by ventilation-perfusion inequality. In this diagram of the upright lung, only two groups of alveoli are shown, one at the apex and another at the base. The relative sizes of the airways and blood vessels indicate their relative ventilations and blood flows. Because most of the blood comes from the poorly oxygenated base, depression of the blood P_{O_2} is inevitable. (Reprinted from West JB. Blood-flow, ventilation, and gas exchange in the lung. *The Lancet.* 1963;282(7316):1055-1058. Copyright © 1963 Elsevier. With permission.)

ences down the upright lung (**Figure 5.12**). Here, the P_{O_2} at the apex is some 40 mm Hg higher than at the base of the lung. However, the major share of the blood leaving the lung comes from the lower zones, where the P_{O_2} is low. This has the result of depressing the arterial P_{O_2}. By contrast, the expired alveolar gas comes more uniformly from apex and base because the differences of ventilation are much less than those for blood flow (Figure 5.9). By the same reasoning, the arterial P_{CO_2} will be elevated because it is higher at the base of the lung than at the apex (Figure 5.11).

An additional reason that uneven ventilation and blood flow depress the arterial P_{O_2} is shown in **Figure 5.13**. This depicts three groups of alveoli with low, normal, and high ventilation-perfusion ratios. The O_2 concentrations of the effluent blood are 16, 19.5, and 20 ml per 100 ml, respectively. Even though there is an equal number of low and high ventilation-perfusion ratio alveoli, the high ventilation-perfusion ratio alveoli cannot compensate for the problems caused by the low ventilation-perfusion units. Due to the nonlinear shape of the oxygen dissociation curve, units with a high ventilation-perfusion ratio do not increase the oxygen concentration of their blood very much despite the relatively high P_{O_2}. As a result, they add relatively little oxygen to the blood, compared with the decrement caused by the alveoli with the low ventilation-perfusion ratio. Thus, mixed capillary blood has a lower O_2 concentration than that from units with a normal ventilation-perfusion ratio. This explanation for the depression of P_{O_2} does not apply to the elevation of the P_{CO_2} because the CO_2 dissociation curve is almost linear in the working range (discussed below).

The net result of these mechanisms is a depression of the arterial P_{O_2} below that of the mixed alveolar P_{O_2}—the so-called alveolar-arterial P_{O_2} difference. In the healthy upright lung, this difference is of trivial magnitude, being only about 4 mm Hg due to ventilation-perfusion inequality. Its development is described here only to illustrate how uneven ventilation and blood flow must

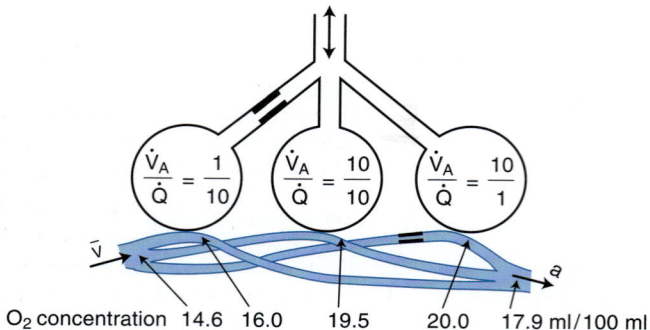

Figure 5.13. Additional reason for the depression of arterial Po$_2$ by mismatching of ventilation and blood flow. The lung units with a high ventilation-perfusion ratio add relatively little oxygen to the blood, compared with the decrement caused by alveoli with a low ventilation-perfusion ratio. (Modified with permission of John Wiley & Sons from West JB. *Ventilation/Blood Flow and Gas Exchange*. 5th ed. Oxford, UK: Blackwell; 1990; permission conveyed through Copyright Clearance Center, Inc.)

result in depression of the arterial Po$_2$. In acute and chronic lung disease, the lowering of arterial Po$_2$ by this mechanism can be extreme.

DISTRIBUTIONS OF VENTILATION-PERFUSION RATIOS

It is possible to obtain information about the distribution of ventilation-perfusion ratios in patients with lung disease by infusing into a peripheral vein a mixture of dissolved inert gases having a range of solubilities and then measuring the concentrations of the gases in arterial blood and expired gas. The details of this technique are too complex to be described here, and it is used for research purposes rather than in a clinical pulmonary function laboratory. The technique returns a distribution of ventilation and blood flow plotted against ventilation-perfusion ratio with 50 compartments equally spaced on a log scale.

Figure 5.14 shows a typical result from a young healthy individual. Note that all the ventilation and blood flow goes to compartments close to the normal ventilation-perfusion ratio of about 1.0, and, in particular, there is no blood flow to the unventilated compartment (shunt). The distributions in patients with lung disease are often very different. An example from a patient with chronic bronchitis and emphysema is shown in **Figure 5.15**. Note that although much of the ventilation and blood flow goes to compartments with ventilation-perfusion ratios near normal, considerable blood flow is going to compartments with ventilation-perfusion ratios of between 0.03 and 0.3. Blood from these units will be poorly oxygenated and will depress the arterial

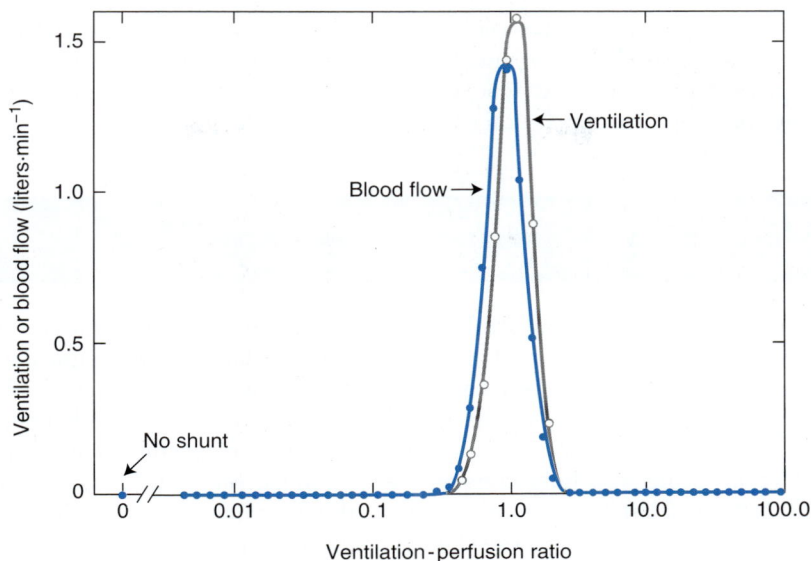

Figure 5.14. Distribution of ventilation-perfusion ratios in a young normal subject. Note the narrow dispersion and absence of shunt. (Redrawn from Wagner, et al. *J Clin Invest*. 1974;54:54.)

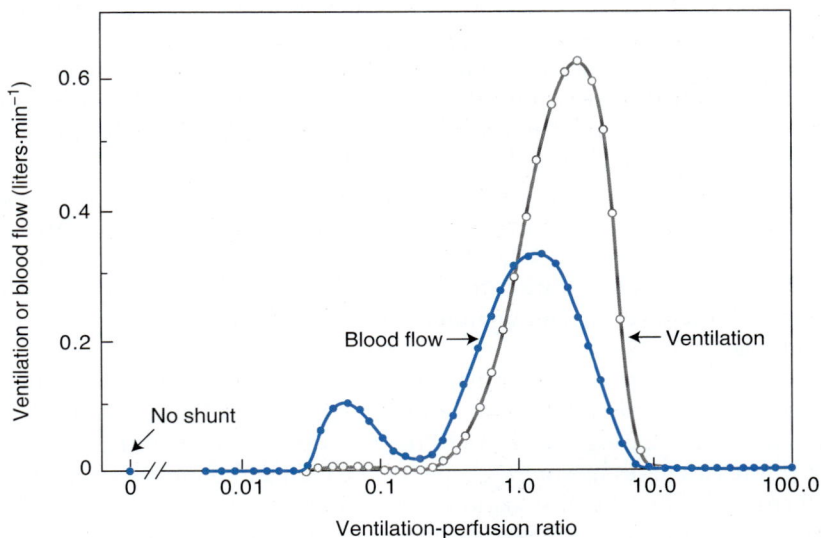

Figure 5.15. Distribution of ventilation-perfusion ratios in a patient with chronic bronchitis and emphysema. Note particularly the blood flow to lung units with very low ventilation-perfusion ratios. Compare Figure 5.14. (Redrawn from Wagner, et al. *J Clin Invest*. 1974;54:54.)

P_{O_2}. There is also excessive ventilation to lung units with ventilation-perfusion ratios up to 10. These units are inefficient at eliminating CO_2. This particular patient had arterial hypoxemia but a normal arterial P_{CO_2} (see below). Other patterns are seen in other types of lung disease.

VENTILATION-PERFUSION INEQUALITY AS A CAUSE OF CO_2 RETENTION

Imagine a lung that is uniformly ventilated and perfused and that is transferring normal amounts of O_2 and CO_2. Suppose that in some magical way, the matching of ventilation and blood flow is suddenly disturbed while everything else remains unchanged. What happens to gas exchange? It transpires that the effect of this "pure" ventilation-perfusion inequality (i.e., everything else held constant) is to reduce *both* the O_2 uptake and CO_2 output of the lung. In other words, the lung becomes less efficient as a gas exchanger for both gases. Hence, mismatching ventilation and blood flow must cause both hypoxemia and hypercapnia (CO_2 retention), other things being equal.

However, in practice, patients with undoubted ventilation-perfusion inequality, such as those with chronic obstructive lung disease or pneumonia, often have a normal arterial P_{CO_2}. The reason for this is that whenever the chemoreceptors sense a rising P_{CO_2}, there is an increase in ventilatory drive (Chapter 8). The consequent increase in ventilation to the alveoli is usually effective in returning the arterial P_{CO_2} to normal. However, such patients can only maintain a normal P_{CO_2} at the expense of this increased ventilation to their alveoli; the ventilation in excess of what they would normally require is sometimes referred to as *wasted ventilation* and is necessary because the lung units with abnormally high ventilation-perfusion ratios are inefficient at eliminating CO_2. Such units are said to constitute an *alveolar dead space*. This is in addition to the anatomic dead space discussed earlier. Together, the alveolar and anatomic dead space comprise the physiologic dead space.

While the increase in ventilation to a lung with ventilation-perfusion inequality is usually effective at reducing the arterial P_{CO_2}, it is much less effective at increasing the arterial P_{O_2}. The reason for the different behavior of the two gases lies in the shapes of the CO_2 and O_2 dissociation curves (Chapter 6). The CO_2 dissociation curve is almost straight in the physiological range, with the result that an increase in ventilation will raise the CO_2 output of lung units with both high and low ventilation-perfusion ratios. By contrast, the almost flat top of the O_2 dissociation curve means that only units with moderately low ventilation-perfusion ratios will benefit appreciably from the increased ventilation. Those units that are very high on the

Table 5.1 The Four Causes of Hypoxemia with Their Alveolar-Arterial P_{O_2} Difference and the Response of the Arterial P_{O_2} When 100% Oxygen Is Administered		
Cause of Hypoxemia	**A-a Difference**	**Response to O_2**
Hypoventilation	None	Good
Diffusion limitation	Increased	Good
Shunt	Increased	Small but often useful
$\dot{V}_A/\dot{Q}$ inequality	Increased	Good

dissociation curve (high ventilation-perfusion ratio) increase the O_2 concentration of their effluent blood very little (Figure 5.13). Those units that have a very low ventilation-perfusion ratio continue to put out blood with an O_2 concentration close to that of mixed venous blood. The net result is that the mixed arterial P_{O_2} rises only modestly, and some hypoxemia always remains (**Table 5.1**).

Ventilation-Perfusion Inequality

- The ventilation-perfusion ratio $\dot{V}_A/\dot{Q}$ determines the gas exchange in any single lung unit.
- Regional differences of $\dot{V}_A/\dot{Q}$ in the upright human lung cause a pattern of regional gas exchange.
- $\dot{V}_A/\dot{Q}$ inequality impairs the uptake or elimination of all gases by the lung.
- Although the elimination of CO_2 is impaired by $\dot{V}_A/\dot{Q}$ inequality, this can be corrected by increasing the ventilation to the alveoli.
- By contrast, the hypoxemia resulting from inequality cannot be eliminated by increases in ventilation.
- The different behavior of the two gases results from the different shapes of their dissociation curves.

MEASUREMENT OF VENTILATION-PERFUSION INEQUALITY

How can we assess the amount of ventilation-perfusion inequality in diseased lungs? Radioactive gases can be used to define topographical differences in ventilation and blood flow in the normal upright lung (Figures 2.7 and 4.7), but in most patients, large amounts of inequality exist between closely adjacent units, and this cannot be distinguished by counters over the chest. In practice, we turn to indices based on the resulting impairment of gas exchange.*

One useful measurement is the *alveolar-arterial* P_{O_2} *difference*, obtained by subtracting the arterial P_{O_2} from the so-called ideal alveolar P_{O_2}. The latter is the P_{O_2} that the lung *would* have if there were no ventilation-perfusion inequality, and it was exchanging gas at the same respiratory exchange ratio as the real lung. It is derived from the alveolar gas equation:

$$P_{A_{O_2}} = P_{I_{O_2}} - \frac{P_{A_{CO_2}}}{R} + F$$

The arterial P_{CO_2} is used for the alveolar value.

An example will clarify this. Suppose a patient who is breathing air at sea level has an arterial P_{O_2} of 50 mm Hg, an arterial P_{CO_2} of 60 mm Hg, and a respiratory exchange ratio of 0.8. The high P_{CO_2} indicates that hypoventilation is contributing to the patient's hypoxemia. The question is whether this is the only explanation or whether ventilation-perfusion inequality is also playing a role? This can be determined by calculating the alveolar-arterial P_{O_2} difference.

From the alveolar gas equation, the ideal alveolar P_{O_2} is given by:

$$P_{A_{O_2}} = 149 - \frac{60}{0.8} + F = 74 \, \text{mm Hg}$$

where the inspired P_{O_2} is 149 mm Hg and we ignore the small factor F. Thus, the alveolar-arterial P_{O_2} difference is approximately $(74 - 50) = 24$ mm Hg. The normal value is about 10 to 15 mm Hg, although it does increase with age. If hypoventilation was the sole cause of hypoxemia, the patient should have a value in this range. The fact that the patient's value is abnormally high and indicates that ventilation-perfusion inequality is an additional cause.

To use this equation, the inspired P_{O_2} must be accurately known, as is the case when a patient is breathing ambient air or receiving mechanical ventilation. However, the inspired P_{O_2} is variable in some forms of supplemental oxygen administration (nasal cannula, nonrebreather mask), which can make the equation difficult to use in clinical practice.

Additional information on the measurement of ventilation-perfusion inequality can be found in Chapter 10.

KEY CONCEPTS

1. The four causes of hypoxemia are hypoventilation, diffusion limitation, shunt, and ventilation-perfusion inequality

---

*For more details of this difficult subject, see West JB, Luks AM. *West's Pulmonary Pathophysiology.* 9th ed. Philadelphia, PA: Wolters Kluwer; 2017.

2. The two causes of hypercapnia, or CO_2 retention, are hypoventilation and ventilation-perfusion inequality.

3. Shunt is the only cause of hypoxemia in which the arterial Po_2 does not rise to the expected level when a patient is given 100% O_2 to breathe.

4. The ventilation-perfusion ratio determines the Po_2 and Pco_2 in any lung unit. Because the ratio is high at the top of the lung, Po_2 is high there and the Pco_2 is low.

5. Ventilation-perfusion inequality reduces the gas exchange efficiency of the lung for all gases. However, many patients with ventilation-perfusion inequality have a normal arterial Pco_2 because they increase the ventilation to their alveoli. By contrast, the arterial Po_2 is always low. The different behavior of the two gases is attributable to the different shapes of the two dissociation curves.

6. The alveolar-arterial Po_2 difference is a useful measure of ventilation-perfusion inequality. The alveolar Po_2 is calculated from the alveolar gas equation using the arterial Pco_2.

CLINICAL VIGNETTE

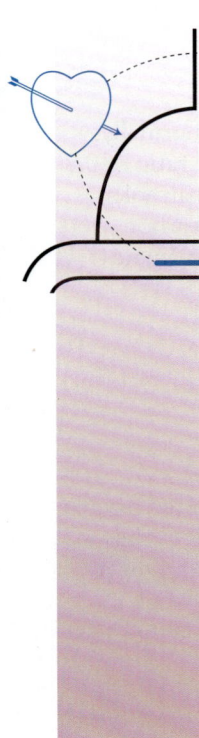

A 60-year-old man presents to the emergency department with a history of 2 days of worsening shortness of breath (dyspnea), cough, and sputum production following a viral upper respiratory tract infection. His outpatient clinic records state that he was a long-standing two-pack-per-day smoker who had been followed for several years in the pulmonary clinic for chronic dyspnea on exertion and daily cough productive of yellow sputum. Pulmonary function testing performed in clinic confirmed that he had chronic obstructive pulmonary disease (COPD). An arterial blood gas taken while breathing ambient air as an outpatient showed a pH of 7.38, Pco_2 of 45 mm Hg, and Po_2 of 73 mm Hg.

In the emergency department, he was visibly short of breath. His lips were slightly blue, and on lung auscultation, he had diffuse, high-pitched musical sounds on exhalation. A chest radiograph showed overinflated lungs with areas of abnormal lucency but no focal opacities. An arterial blood gas taken with him breathing ambient air showed pH 7.30, Pco_2 55 mm Hg, and Po_2 45 mm Hg. As part of his treatment, he was given oxygen by nasal cannula at a rate of 2 liter·min^{-1}. Arterial blood was taken 30 min later and showed that the Po_2 had increased to 90 mm Hg.

• Assuming a respiratory exchange ratio of 0.8, what was the alveolar-arterial oxygen difference in the outpatient clinic, and what does this tell you about the cause of hypoxemia at that time?

- What was the alveolar-arterial oxygen difference when the patient was seen in the emergency department? What does this tell you about the cause(s) of his hypoxemia at this time?
- Why was his Pco_2 higher in the emergency department than in clinic?
- What does the change in Po_2 following administration of supplemental oxygen tell you about the causes of his hypoxemia?

QUESTIONS

For each question, choose the one best answer.

1. An arterial blood gas is drawn on a climber shortly following ascent to an altitude of 4,500 m (14,800 ft) where the barometric pressure is 447 mm Hg. The arterial Po_2 is 55 mm Hg, while the arterial Pco_2 is 32 mm Hg. The Po_2 of moist inspired gas (in mm Hg) is:
   A. 44
   B. 63
   C. 75
   D. 84
   E. 98

2. An otherwise healthy individual who resides at sea level and normally has an arterial Pco_2 of 40 mm Hg and a respiratory exchange ratio of 0.8 takes an overdose of opiate pain medications, after which the alveolar ventilation decreases by 50%. If there is no change in either carbon dioxide production or oxygen consumption, what is the approximate alveolar Po_2 (in mm Hg) in this individual?
   A. 40
   B. 50
   C. 60
   D. 70
   E. 80

3. For this individual in Question 2, by how much does the inspired oxygen concentration (%) have to be raised to return the alveolar Po_2 to the preoverdose level?
   A. 7
   B. 11
   C. 15
   D. 19
   E. 23

4. A patient is receiving mechanical ventilation for severe respiratory failure due to pneumonia. Following a fall in the arterial Po_2 from 75 mm Hg to 55 mm Hg, the minute ventilation was noted to increase from 10 to 15 liter·min^{-1}. Which of the following would you expect to see as a result of this change in the patient's clinical condition?
   A. Decreased pulmonary vascular resistance
   B. Faster diffusion of carbon dioxide across the alveolar-capillary barrier
   C. Increased carbon dioxide elimination from units with high and low ventilation perfusion ratios
   D. Increased oxygen uptake from units with high ventilation perfusion ratios only
   E. Increased oxygen uptake from units with high and low ventilation perfusion ratios

5. If a climber on the summit of Mt. Everest (barometric pressure 253 mm Hg) maintains an alveolar Po_2 of 34 mm Hg and remains in a steady state with the respiratory exchange ratio (R) ≤ 1, his alveolar Pco_2 (in mm Hg) cannot be any higher than:
   A. 5
   B. 9
   C. 11
   D. 13
   E. 15

6. The distribution of ventilation-perfusion ($\dot{V}_A/\dot{Q}$) ratios in two patients, Patients 1 and 2, are displayed in the figure below. Each patient is breathing ambient air.

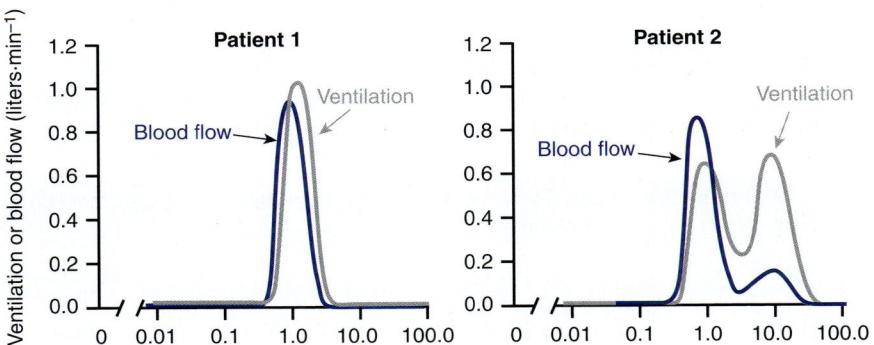

When compared to Patient 1, which of the following would you expect to find with Patient 2?
   A. Decreased rate of diffusion across the alveolar-capillary barrier
   B. Decreased shunt fraction
   C. Increased alveolar-arterial oxygen difference
   D. Increased arterial Po_2
   E. No change in arterial Po_2

7. In an experimental model, multiple variables are measured in blood taken from the end of the pulmonary capillaries at the base and apex of an upright lung. The results are displayed in the table below.

Location	P_{O_2} (mm Hg)	P_{CO_2} (mm Hg)	pH
Base	87	43	7.38
Apex	128	29	7.50

Which of the following best accounts for the observed changes in these parameters with movement from the base to the apex?
A. Decrease in the number of shunt units at the lung apex
B. Increase in blood flow with movement from base to apex
C. Increase in pulmonary arteriolar vasoconstriction at the lung apex
D. Increase in ventilation with movement from base to apex
E. Increase in the average ventilation-perfusion ratio at the lung apex

8. While hospitalized for injuries suffered in a motor vehicle collision, a previously healthy individual suffers a pulmonary embolism in which the left lower lobe pulmonary artery is occluded by a large thrombus. If alveolar ventilation remains constant throughout the lung, which of the following changes would you expect to see in the lung units served by this pulmonary artery?
A. Decreased pH of end-capillary blood
B. Hypoxic pulmonary vasoconstriction
C. Increased alveolar P_{CO_2}
D. Increased alveolar P_{O_2}
E. Increased CO_2 elimination

9. A patient with chronic lung disease undergoes a cardiopulmonary exercise test. An arterial blood gas is obtained while exhaled gases are monitored. Resting data are shown in the table below.

CO_2 Production (ml·min^{-1})	O_2 Consumption (ml·min^{-1})	Pa_{O_2} (mm Hg)	Pa_{CO_2} (mm Hg)
200	250	49	48

What is the approximate alveolar-arterial P_{O_2} difference (in mm Hg) at rest?
A. 10
B. 20
C. 30
D. 40
E. 50

10. A 52-year-old man with a history of heavy smoking presents to the emergency department with 2 days of dyspnea, fever, and a cough productive of rust-colored sputum. Arterial blood gases are performed upon arrival in the emergency department and after being placed on supplemental oxygen. The results are as follows:

F_{IO_2}	pH	Pa_{CO_2}	Pa_{CO_2}	HCO_3^-
0.21	7.48	32	51	23
0.80	7.47	33	55	23

What is the predominant mechanism(s) of his hypoxemia?
A. Diffusion limitation
B. Hypoventilation
C. Shunt
D. Ventilation-perfusion inequality
E. Hypoventilation and ventilation-perfusion inequality

11. A 60-year-old previously healthy woman is admitted with a severe left lower lobe pneumonia. Pulmonary artery and radial artery catheters are inserted for monitoring. The arterial and mixed venous oxygen contents are determined to be 17 ml per 100 ml and 12 ml per 100 ml, respectively, while the end-capillary oxygen content is estimated to be 20 ml per 100 ml. The arterial Po_2 is 55 mm Hg, and the arterial Pco_2 is 41 mm Hg. Which of the following would you expect to see as a result of this patient's clinical condition?
A. Decreased alveolar Po_2
B. Decreased ventilatory drive
C. Increased arterial Pco_2
D. Normal alveolar-arterial Po_2 difference
E. Suboptimal response to supplemental oxygen administration

12. A 35-year-old man is found to have a large arteriovenous malformation (fistula) in one of the lowest segments of his right lower lobe. Which of the following changes would you expect to see when the patient changes from the supine to the upright position?
A. Decreased alveolar Po_2
B. Decreased alveolar-arterial oxygen difference
C. Increased arterial Pco_2
D. Increased dead-space fraction
E. Increased shunt fraction

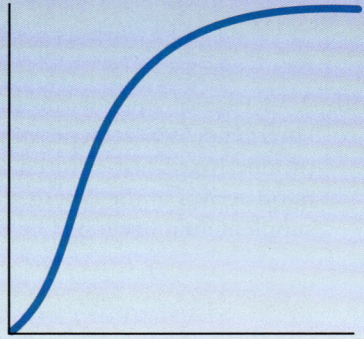

Gas Transport by the Blood

6

How Gases Are Moved to and from the Peripheral Tissues

- **Oxygen**
  Dissolved O_2
  Combination with Hemoglobin
  O_2 Dissociation Curve
- **Carbon Dioxide**
  CO_2 Carriage
  CO_2 Dissociation Curve
- **Acid-Base Status**
  Respiratory Acidosis
  Respiratory Alkalosis
  Metabolic Acidosis
  Metabolic Alkalosis
- **Blood-Tissue Gas Exchange**
  Diffusion
  Tissue P_{O_2}
  Mixed Venous P_{O_2}

We now consider the carriage of the respiratory gases, oxygen and carbon dioxide, by the blood. First, we look at the two means by which oxygen is transported, dissolved in blood, and bonded to hemoglobin, including the hemoglobin oxygen dissociation curve, and the factors affecting the oxygen affinity for hemoglobin. Then we look at the three ways that carbon dioxide is carried in the blood. Next, we consider the acid-base status of the blood and the four principal abnormalities: respiratory acidosis and alkalosis, and metabolic acidosis and alkalosis. Finally, we briefly look at gas exchange in peripheral tissues and the determinants of the tissue and mixed venous oxygen concentrations. At the end of this chapter, the reader should be able to:

- Describe the main mechanisms for transporting oxygen and carbon dioxide and their relative contributions to the oxygen and carbon dioxide concentrations of the blood
- Identify factors that alter the affinity of oxygen for hemoglobin
- Compare and contrast the dissociation curves for oxygen and carbon dioxide
- Use blood gas data and the Davenport diagram to describe acid-base status
- Predict changes in tissue and mixed venous P_{O_2} based on changes in oxygen delivery and tissue oxygen utilization

In previous chapters, we have considered how air moves to and from the blood-gas barrier, the diffusion of gas across it, the movement of blood to and from the barrier and the important role that matching of ventilation and perfusion plays in efficient gas exchange. In this chapter, we consider how the main respiratory gases, oxygen and carbon dioxide, are transported in the blood, as well as the primary determinants of the acid-base status of the blood and the body as a whole. We begin with the transport of oxygen and carbon dioxide.

OXYGEN

O_2 is carried in the blood in two forms: dissolved and combined with hemoglobin.

Dissolved O_2

This obeys Henry law, that is, the amount dissolved is proportional to the partial pressure (**Figure 6.1**). For each mm Hg of Po_2, there is 0.003 ml O_2 per 100 ml of blood. Thus, normal arterial blood with a Po_2 of 100 mm Hg contains 0.3 ml O_2 per 100 ml.

It is easy to see that this way of transporting O_2 is inadequate. Suppose that the cardiac output during strenuous exercise is 30 liters·min^{-1}. Because arterial blood contains 0.3 ml O_2 per 100 ml blood (i.e., 3 ml O_2·liter^{-1} blood) as dissolved O_2, the total amount delivered to the tissues is only $30 \times 3 = 90$ ml·min^{-1}. Given that the tissue oxygen requirements may be 2,000 ml O_2·min^{-1} or higher, transporting O_2 in solution alone is insufficient and an additional method is required.

Combination with Hemoglobin

Heme is an iron-porphyrin compound that is joined to each of four polypeptide chains that together constitute the protein globin. The chains are of two types, alpha and beta, and differences in their amino acid sequences give rise to various types of human hemoglobin. Normal adult hemoglobin is known as A. Hemoglobin F (fetal) makes up part of the hemoglobin of the newborn infant and is gradually replaced over the first year or so of postnatal life. Fetal hemoglobin has a high oxygen affinity, which is helpful because the environment of the fetus is very hypoxic. Hemoglobin S (sickle) has valine instead of glutamic acid in the beta-chains. This results in a reduced O_2 affinity and a shift in the dissociation curve to the right, but, more important, the deoxygenated form is poorly soluble and crystallizes within the red cell. As a consequence, the cell shape changes from biconcave to crescent or sickle shaped with increased fragility and a tendency to thrombus formation. Many other varieties of hemoglobin have now been described, some with bizarre O_2 affinities, but they are beyond the scope of this text.

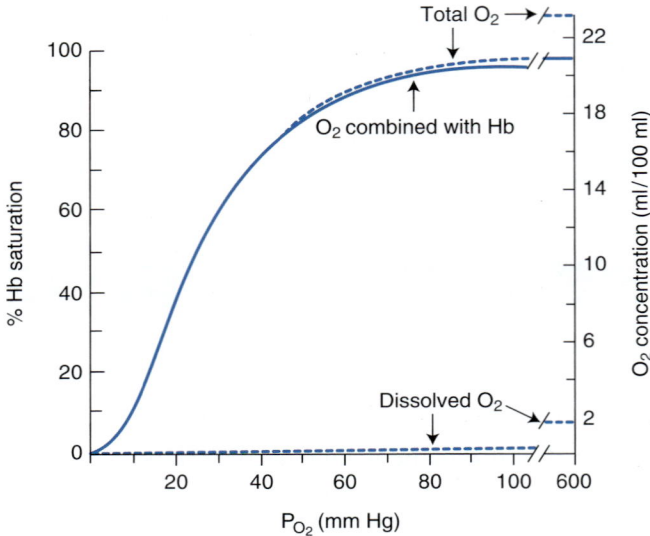

Figure 6.1. O_2 dissociation curve (*solid line*) for pH 7.4, P_{CO_2} 40 mm Hg, and 37°C. The total blood O_2 concentration is also shown for a hemoglobin concentration of 15 g per 100 ml of blood.

Normal hemoglobin A can have its ferrous ion oxidized to the ferric form by various drugs and chemicals, including nitrites, sulfonamides, the antimicrobial agent dapsone, and local anesthetics. This ferric form is known as methemoglobin. There is a congenital cause in which the enzyme methemoglobin reductase is deficient within the red blood cell. Methemoglobin is poor at binding oxygen as well as releasing any bound oxygen to the peripheral tissues. Another abnormal form of hemoglobin is sulfhemoglobin. This is not useful for O_2 carriage.

Hemoglobin

- Has four heme sites that can bind to oxygen.
- Globin has two α and two β chains that can undergo various mutations.
- Adult hemoglobin A has ferrous iron. If this is oxidized to ferric iron, oxygen binding and release of oxygen to the tissues is impaired.
- Fetal hemoglobin F has a high oxygen affinity, which helps the fetus tolerate its hypoxic environment in utero.

O_2 Dissociation Curve

O_2 forms an easily reversible combination with hemoglobin (Hb) to give oxyhemoglobin: $O_2 + Hb \rightleftharpoons HbO_2$. The amount bound at any given time is a function of the P_{O_2}. Suppose we take a number of glass containers (tonometers), each containing a small volume of blood, and add gas with various concentrations of O_2. After allowing time for the gas and blood to reach equilibrium, we measure the P_{O_2} of the gas and the O_2 concentration of the blood. The oxygen concentration is sometimes called the oxygen content. Knowing that 0.003 ml O_2 is dissolved in each 100 ml of blood per mm Hg P_{O_2}, we can calculate the O_2 combined with Hb (Figure 6.1). Note that the amount of O_2 carried by the Hb increases rapidly up to a P_{O_2} of about 60 mm Hg, but above that, the curve becomes much flatter.

The maximum amount of O_2 that can be combined with Hb is called the *O_2 capacity*. This is when all the available binding sites are occupied by O_2. It can be measured by exposing the blood to a very high P_{O_2} (say 600 mm Hg) and subtracting the dissolved O_2. One gram of pure Hb can combine with 1.39 ml O_2,* and because normal blood has about 15 g of Hb per 100 ml, the O_2 capacity is about 20.8 ml O_2 per 100 ml of blood.

The *O_2 saturation* of Hb is the percentage of the available binding sites that have O_2 attached and is given by:

$$\frac{O_2 \text{ combined with Hb}}{O_2 \text{ capacity}} \times 100$$

The O_2 saturation of arterial blood with P_{O_2} of 100 mm Hg is about 97.5%, whereas that of mixed venous blood with a P_{O_2} of 40 mm Hg is about 75%. The change in Hb from the fully oxygenated state to its deoxygenated state is accompanied by a conformational change in the molecule. The oxygenated form is the R (relaxed) state, whereas the deoxy form is the T (tense) state.

In general, the oxygen concentration of blood (in ml O_2 per 100 ml blood) is given by

$$\left(1.39 \times \text{Hb} \times \frac{\text{Sat}}{100}\right) + 0.003 P_{O_2}$$

where Hb is the hemoglobin concentration in gram per 100 ml, Sat is the percentage saturation of the Hb, and P_{O_2} is in mm Hg. In considering this equation, it is important to grasp the relationships among P_{O_2}, O_2 saturation, and O_2 concentration. For example, suppose an individual has a Hb concentration of 15 g per 100 ml of blood and an arterial P_{O_2} of 100 mm Hg. This patient's O_2 capacity will be 20.8 ml per 100 ml, the O_2 saturation will be 97.5% (at normal pH, P_{CO_2}, and temperature), the O_2 combined with Hb will

---

*Some older measurements give 1.34 or 1.36 ml. The reason is that under the normal conditions of the body, some of the hemoglobin is in forms such as methemoglobin that cannot combine with O_2.

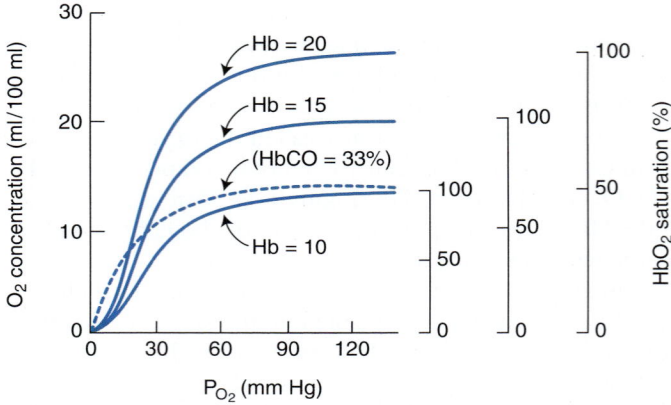

Figure 6.2. Effects of anemia and polycythemia on O_2 concentration and saturation. In addition, the *broken line* shows the O_2 dissociation curve when one-third of the normal hemoglobin is bound to CO. Note that the curve is shifted to the left.

be 20.8 ml per 100 ml and, taking into account the dissolved O_2 of 0.3 mL, the total O_2 concentration will be 20.6 ml per 100 ml of blood. Now suppose this person develops anemia and the Hb concentration falls to 10 g per 100 ml of blood while the Po_2 remains the same. The O_2 saturation will not change, but the O_2 carrying capacity and O_2 concentration will both decrease (**Figure 6.2**).

The curved shape of the O_2 dissociation curve has several physiological advantages. The flat upper portion means that even if the Po_2 in alveolar gas falls somewhat, loading of O_2 will be little affected. In addition, as the red cell takes up O_2 along the pulmonary capillary (Figure 3.3), a large partial pressure difference between alveolar gas and blood continues to exist when most of the O_2 has been transferred. As a result, the diffusion process is hastened. The steep lower part of the dissociation curve means that the peripheral tissues can withdraw large amounts of O_2 for only a small drop in capillary Po_2. This maintenance of blood Po_2 assists the diffusion of O_2 into the tissue cells.

Because reduced Hb is purple, a low arterial O_2 saturation causes *cyanosis*. However, this is not a reliable sign of mild desaturation because its recognition depends on so many variables, such as lighting conditions and skin pigmentation. Because it is the amount of reduced Hb that is important, cyanosis is often marked when polycythemia is present but is difficult to detect in anemic patients.

The O_2 affinity of Hb is not static and, instead, changes due to a variety of factors. The O_2 dissociation curve is shifted to the right, that is, the O_2 affinity of Hb is reduced, by an increase in H^+ concentration, Pco_2, temperature, and the concentration of 2,3-diphosphoglycerate (DPG) in the red cells (**Figure 6.3**). Opposite changes shift it to the left. Most of the effect of Pco_2, which is

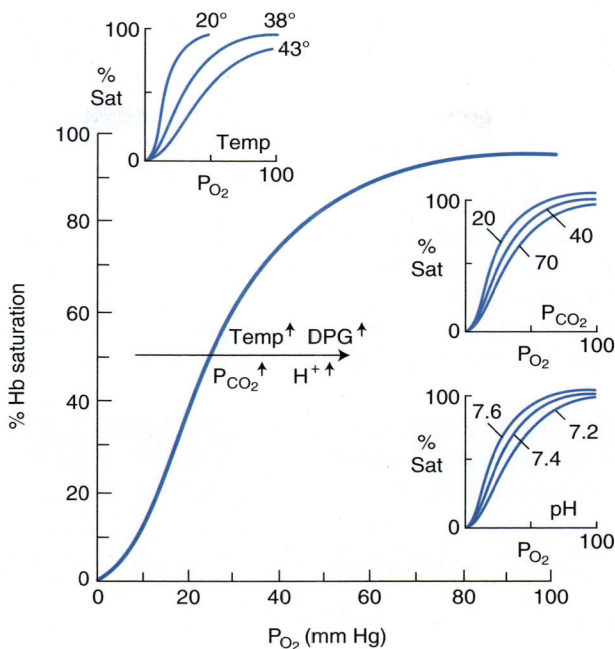

Figure 6.3. Rightward shift of the O_2 dissociation curve by increase of H^+, P_{CO_2}, temperature, and 2,3-diphosphoglycerate (DPG).

known as the *Bohr effect*, can be attributed to its action on H^+ concentration. A rightward shift means more unloading of O_2 at a given P_{O_2} in a tissue capillary. A simple way to remember these shifts is that an exercising muscle is acidic, hypercarbic, and hot, and it benefits from increased unloading of O_2 from the capillary blood.

The environment of the Hb within the red cell also affects the O_2 dissociation curve. An increase in 2,3-DPG, which is an end product of red cell metabolism, shifts the curve to the right. An increase in concentration of this material occurs in chronic hypoxia, for example, at high altitude or in the presence of chronic lung disease. As a result, the unloading of O_2 to peripheral tissues is assisted. By contrast, stored blood in a blood bank may be depleted of 2,3-DPG, which impairs unloading of O_2. A useful measure of the position of the dissociation curve and the affinity of O_2 for Hb is the P_{O_2} for 50% O_2 saturation. This is known as the P_{50}. The normal value for human blood is about 27 mm Hg. Three points on the dissociation curve are useful to remember to convert a given P_{O_2} to its approximate saturation. They are for normal arterial blood: P_{O_2} 100, S_{O_2} 97%; normal mixed venous blood: P_{O_2} 40, S_{O_2} 75%; and P_{50}: 27, S_{O_2} 50%.

Carbon monoxide, which is found in cigarette smoke and automobile exhaust and is elaborated in fires, interferes with the O_2 transport function of blood by combining with Hb to form carboxyhemoglobin (COHb). CO has about 240 times the affinity of O_2 for Hb; this means that CO will combine with the same amount of Hb as O_2 when the CO partial pressure is 240 times lower. In fact, the CO dissociation curve is almost identical in shape to the O_2 dissociation curve of Figure 6.3, except that the Pco axis is greatly compressed. For example, at a Pco of 0.16 mm Hg, about 75% of the Hb is combined with CO as COHb. For this reason, small amounts of CO can tie up a large proportion of the Hb in the blood, thus making it unavailable for O_2 carriage. If this happens, the Hb concentration and Po_2 of blood may be normal, but its O_2 concentration is grossly reduced. The presence of COHb also shifts the O_2 dissociation curve to the left (Figure 6.2), thus interfering with the unloading of O_2. This is an additional feature of the toxicity of CO.

Oxygen Dissociation Curve

- Useful "anchor" points: Po_2 40, So_2 75%; Po_2 100, So_2 97%; P_{50} 27, So_2 50%.
- Curve is right-shifted by increases in temperature, Pco_2, H^+, and 2,3-DPG.
- Small addition of CO to blood causes a left shift and impairs offloading of oxygen.

CARBON DIOXIDE

CO_2 Carriage

CO_2 is carried in the blood in three forms: dissolved, as bicarbonate, and in combination with proteins as carbamino compounds.

1. *Dissolved CO_2*, like O_2, obeys Henry law, but CO_2 is about 24 times more soluble than O_2, its solubility being 0.067 ml·dl⁻¹·mm Hg⁻¹. Although dissolved CO_2 plays a more significant role in its carriage than is the case for oxygen, this is still not sufficient to transport all of the CO_2 produced in the tissues to the lungs.
2. *Bicarbonate* is formed in blood by the following sequence:

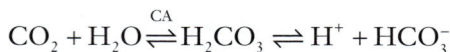

$$CO_2 + H_2O \overset{CA}{\rightleftharpoons} H_2CO_3 \rightleftharpoons H^+ + HCO_3^-$$

The first reaction is very slow in plasma but fast within the red blood cell because of the presence there of the enzyme *carbonic anhydrase* (CA). The second reaction, ionic dissociation of carbonic acid, is fast without an enzyme. When the concentration of these ions rises within the red cell, HCO_3^- moves out, but H^+ cannot easily do this because the cell membrane is relatively impermeable to cations. Thus, to maintain electrical neutrality, Cl^- ions move into the cell from the plasma via a chloride-bicarbonate exchanger, the

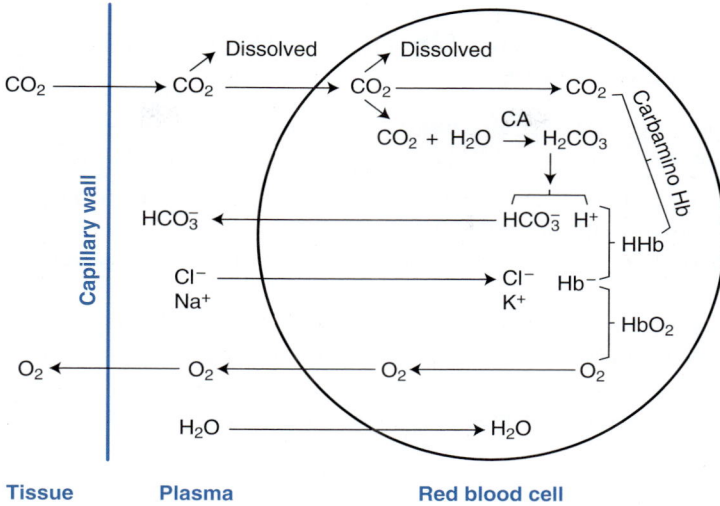

Figure 6.4. Scheme of the uptake of CO_2 and liberation of O_2 in systemic capillaries. Exactly opposite events occur in the pulmonary capillaries.

so-called *chloride shift* (**Figure 6.4**). The movement of chloride is in accordance with the Gibbs-Donnan equilibrium.

Some of the H^+ ions liberated are bound to reduced hemoglobin:

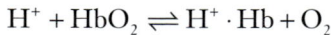

$$H^+ + HbO_2 \rightleftharpoons H^+ \cdot Hb + O_2$$

This occurs because reduced Hb is less acid (i.e., a better proton acceptor) than is the oxygenated form. Thus, the presence of reduced Hb in the peripheral blood helps with the loading of CO_2, whereas the oxygenation that occurs in the pulmonary capillary assists in the unloading. The fact that deoxygenation of the blood increases its ability to carry CO_2 is known as the *Haldane effect*. These events associated with the uptake of CO_2 by blood increase the osmolar content of the red cell, and, consequently, water enters the cell, thus increasing its volume. When the cells pass through the lung and CO_2 is offloaded, they shrink a little.

3. *Carbamino compounds* are formed by the combination of CO_2 with terminal amine groups in blood proteins. The most important protein is the globin of hemoglobin: $Hb \cdot NH_2 + CO_2 \rightleftharpoons Hb \cdot NH \cdot COOH$, giving carbaminohemoglobin. This reaction occurs rapidly without an enzyme, and reduced Hb can bind more CO_2 as carbaminohemoglobin than can HbO_2. Thus, again, unloading of O_2 in peripheral capillaries facilitates the loading of CO_2, whereas oxygenation in the lungs has the opposite effect.

Note that the great bulk of the CO_2 is in the form of bicarbonate. The amount dissolved is small, as is that in the form of carbaminohemoglobin. However, these proportions do not reflect the changes that take place when

CO_2 is loaded or unloaded by the blood. Of the total venous-arterial difference, about 60% is attributable to HCO_3^-, 30% to carbamino compounds, and 10% to dissolved CO_2.

Transport of CO_2 by Blood

- Bicarbonate reactions are the major source of expired CO_2 and depend on carbonic anhydrase in the red cell.
- Transport in solution accounts for about 10% of the CO_2 evolved by the lung.
- Carbamino compounds are formed mainly with hemoglobin and account for about 30% of CO_2 evolved by the lung.
- CO_2 carriage in the form of carbaminohemoglobin is enhanced by deoxygenation of the blood.

CO_2 Dissociation Curve

The relationship between the P_{CO_2} and the total CO_2 concentration of blood is shown in **Figure 6.5**. By analogy with O_2, this is often (though loosely) referred to as the CO_2 dissociation curve, and it is much more linear than is the O_2 dissociation curve (Figure 6.1). Note also that the lower the saturation of Hb with O_2, the larger the CO_2 concentration for a given P_{CO_2}. As we have seen, this *Haldane effect* can be explained by the better ability of reduced Hb to mop up the H^+ ions produced when carbonic acid dissociates, and the greater facility of reduced Hb to form carbaminohemoglobin. **Figure 6.6** shows that

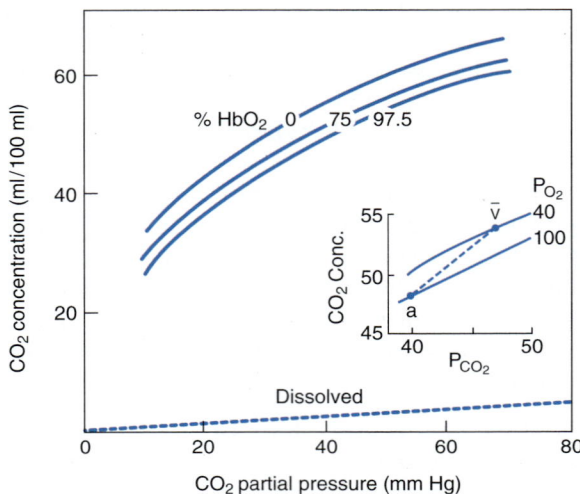

Figure 6.5. CO_2 dissociation curves for blood of different O_2 saturations. Note that oxygenated blood carries less CO_2 for the same P_{CO_2}. The **inset** shows the "physiological" curve between arterial and mixed venous blood.

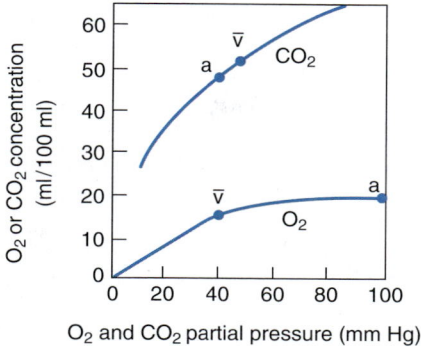

Figure 6.6. Typical O_2 and CO_2 dissociation curves plotted with the same scales. Note that the CO_2 curve is much steeper. "a" and $\bar{V}$ refer to arterial and mixed venous blood, respectively.

the CO_2 dissociation curve is considerably steeper than is that for O_2. For example, in the range of 40 to 50 mm Hg, the CO_2 concentration changes by about 4.7 ml per 100 ml, compared with an O_2 concentration of only about 1.7 ml per 100 ml. This is why the Po_2 difference between arterial and mixed venous blood is large (typically about 60 mm Hg) but the Pco_2 difference is small (about 5 to 7 mm Hg). As noted in Chapter 5, this also explains why a small increase in ventilation returns Pco_2 to normal, but not Po_2, in patients with ventilation-perfusion inequality.

Carbon Dioxide Dissociation Curve

- CO_2 is carried in three forms: dissolved, as bicarbonate, and as carbaminohemoglobin.
- CO_2 curve is steeper and more linear than is the O_2 curve.
- CO_2 curve is right-shifted by increases in So_2 (Haldane effect).

ACID-BASE STATUS

The transport of CO_2 has a profound effect on the acid-base status of the blood and the body as a whole. The lung excretes over 10,000 mEq of carbonic acid per day, compared with less than 100 mEq of fixed acids by the kidney. Therefore, by altering alveolar ventilation and thus the elimination of CO_2, the body has great control over its acid-base balance. This subject will be treated only briefly here because it overlaps the area of renal physiology.

The pH resulting from the solution of CO_2 in blood and the consequent dissociation of carbonic acid is given by the Henderson-Hasselbalch equation. It is derived as follows. In the equation

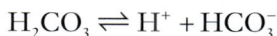

$$H_2CO_3 \rightleftharpoons H^+ + HCO_3^-$$

the law of the mass action gives the dissociation constant of carbonic acid K_a' as

$$\frac{(H^+) \times (HCO_3^-)}{(H_2CO_3)}$$

Because the concentration of carbonic acid is proportional to the concentration of dissolved carbon dioxide, we can change the constant and write

$$K_A = \frac{(H^+) \times (HCO_3^-)}{(CO_2)}$$

Taking logarithms,

$$\log K_A = \log(H^+) + \log\frac{(HCO_3^-)}{(CO_2)}$$

Whence

$$-\log(H^+) = -\log K_A + \log\frac{(HCO_3^-)}{(CO_2)}$$

Because pH is the negative logarithm,

$$pH = pK_A + \log\frac{(HCO_3^-)}{(CO_2)}$$

Because CO_2 obeys Henry law, the CO_2 concentration (in mEq·liter^{-1}) can be replaced by ($Pco_2 \times 0.03$). The equation then becomes:

$$pH = pK_A + \log\frac{(HCO_3^-)}{0.03Pco_2}$$

The value of pK_a is 6.1, and the normal HCO_3^- concentration in arterial blood is 24 mEq·liter^{-1}. Substituting gives

$$pH = 6.1 + \log\frac{24}{0.03 \times 40}$$
$$= 6.1 + \log 20$$
$$= 6.1 + 1.3$$

Therefore,

$$pH = 7.4$$

Note that as long as the ratio of bicarbonate concentration to ($Pco_2 \times 0.03$) remains equal to 20, the pH will remain at 7.4. The bicarbonate concentration is determined chiefly by the kidney, while the Pco_2 is determined primarily by the lung. The normal pH has a range from about 7.38 to 7.42.

The relationships among pH, Pco_2, and HCO_3^- are conveniently shown on a Davenport diagram (**Figure 6.7**). The two axes show HCO_3^- and pH, and lines of equal Pco_2 sweep across the diagram. Normal plasma is represented by point A. The line CAB shows the relationship between HCO_3^- and pH as carbonic acid is added to whole blood, that is, it is part of the titration curve for blood and

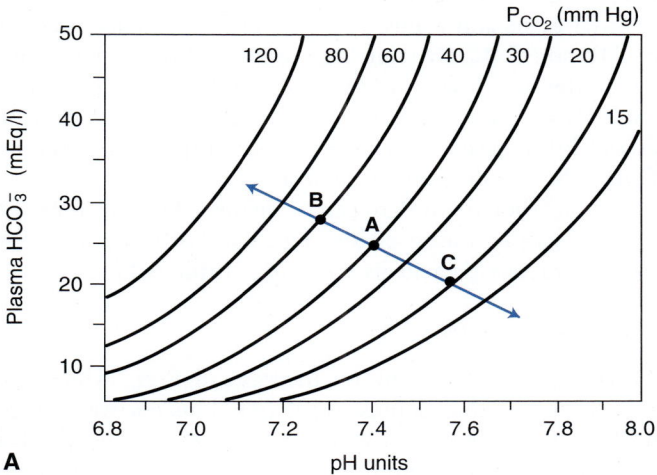

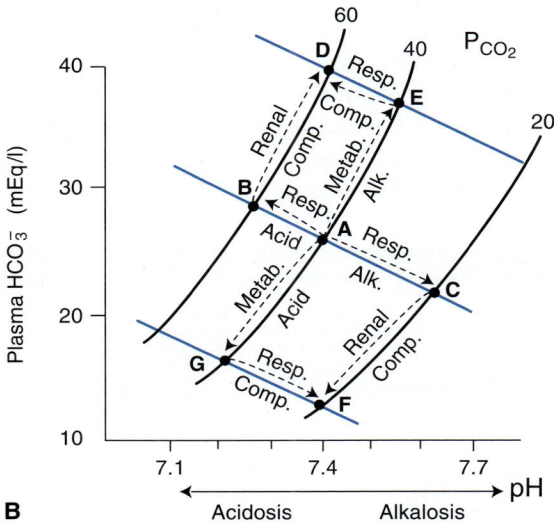

Figure 6.7. Davenport diagram showing the relationships among HCO_3^-, pH, and Pco_2. **A.** Figure shows the normal buffer line BAC. **B.** Figure shows the changes occurring in respiratory and metabolic acidosis and alkalosis (see text). The vertical distance between the buffer lines DE and BAC is the base excess and that between lines GF and BAC is the base deficit (or negative base excess).

is called the *buffer line*. Also, the slope of this line is steeper than is that measured in plasma separated from blood because of the presence of hemoglobin, which has an additional buffering action. The slope of the line measured on whole blood *in vitro* is usually a little different from that found in a patient because of the buffering action of the interstitial fluid and other body tissues.

If the plasma bicarbonate concentration is altered by the kidney, the buffer line is displaced. An increase in bicarbonate concentration displaces the buffer line upward, as shown, for example, by line DE in Figure 6.7. In this case, a *base excess* exists and is given by the vertical distance between the two buffer lines DE and BAC. By contrast, a reduced bicarbonate concentration displaces the buffer line downward (line GF), and there is now a negative base excess, or *base deficit*. A base excess greater than 2 mEq·liter^{-1} indicates a metabolic alkalosis while a base excess less than -2 mEq·liter^{-1} (also referred to as a base deficit) indicates a metabolic acidosis.

The ratio of bicarbonate to P_{CO_2} can be disturbed in four ways: both bicarbonate and P_{CO_2} can be raised or lowered. Each of these four disturbances gives rise to a characteristic acid-base change (**Table 6.1**).

Respiratory Acidosis

Respiratory acidosis is caused by an increase in P_{CO_2}, which reduces the HCO_3^- / P_{CO_2} ratio and thus depresses the pH. This corresponds to a movement from A to B in Figure 6.7. Whenever the P_{CO_2} rises, the bicarbonate must also increase to some extent because of dissociation of the carbonic acid produced. This is reflected by the left upward slope of the blood buffer line in Figure 6.7. However, the ratio HCO_3^-/P_{CO_2} falls. CO_2 retention can be caused by hypoventilation or ventilation-perfusion inequality.

If respiratory acidosis persists, the kidney responds by conserving HCO_3^-. It is prompted to do this by the increased P_{CO_2} in the renal tubular cells, which then excrete a more acid urine by secreting H^+ ions. The H^+ ions are excreted as $H_2PO_4^-$ or NH_4^+; the HCO_3^- ions are reabsorbed. The resulting increase in

Table 6.1	Four Types of Acid-Base Disturbances	
	$$pH = pK + \log \frac{HCO_3^-}{0.03\ P_{CO_2}}$$	
	Primary	**Compensation**
Acidosis		
Respiratory	P_{CO_2} ↑	HCO_3^- ↑
Metabolic	HCO_3^- ↓	P_{CO_2} ↓
Alkalosis		
Respiratory	P_{CO_2} ↓	HCO_3^- ↓
Metabolic	HCO_3^- ↑	Variably present

plasma HCO_3^- then moves the HCO_3^-/P_{CO_2} ratio back up toward its normal level. This corresponds to the movement from B to D along the line $P_{CO_2} = 60$ mm Hg in Figure 6.7 and is known as *compensation for the respiratory acidosis*. Typical events would be

$$pH = 6.1 + \log\frac{24}{0.03 \times 40} = 6.1 + \log 20 = 7.4 \quad (\text{Normal})$$

$$pH = 6.1 + \log\frac{28}{0.03 \times 60} = 6.1 + \log 15.6 = 7.29 \quad (\text{Respiratory acidosis})$$

$$pH = 6.1 + \log\frac{33}{0.03 \times 60} = 6.1 + \log 18.3 = 7.36 \quad (\text{Compensated respiratory acidosis})$$

Renal compensation, which can take several days, is typically not complete, and so the pH does not fully return to its normal level of 7.4. The extent of the renal compensation can be determined from the *base excess*, that is, the vertical distance between the buffer lines BA and DE.

Respiratory Alkalosis

This is caused by a decrease in P_{CO_2}, which increases the HCO_3^-/P_{CO_2} ratio and thus elevates the pH (movement from A to C in Figure 6.7). A decrease in P_{CO_2} is caused by hyperventilation due to, for example, exposure to high altitude (see Chapter 9) or an anxiety attack. Renal compensation occurs by an increased excretion of bicarbonate, thus returning the HCO_3^-/P_{CO_2} ratio back toward normal (C to F along the line $P_{CO_2} = 20$ mm Hg). With prolonged hyperventilation, the renal compensation may be nearly complete. There is a negative base excess, or a *base deficit*.

Metabolic Acidosis

In this context, "metabolic" means a primary change in HCO_3^-, that is, the numerator of the Henderson-Hasselbalch equation. In metabolic acidosis, the ratio of HCO_3^- to P_{CO_2} falls, thus depressing the pH. The HCO_3^- may be lowered by the accumulation of acids in the blood, as in diabetic ketoacidosis, after tissue hypoxia, which releases lactic acid, or with loss of HCO_3^- in severe diarrhea. The corresponding change in Figure 6.7 is a movement from A toward G.

In this instance, respiratory compensation occurs by an increase in ventilation that lowers the P_{CO_2} and raises the depressed HCO_3^-/P_{CO_2} ratio. The stimulus to raise the ventilation is chiefly the action of H^+ ions on the peripheral chemoreceptors (Chapter 8). In Figure 6.7, the point moves in the direction G to F (although not as far as F). There is a base deficit or negative base excess. Respiratory compensation is typically very fast, whereas metabolic compensation for primary respiratory processes is slow.

Table 6.2 Representative Examples of Causes of Primary Acid-Base Abnormalities			
Respiratory Acidosis	**Respiratory Alkalosis**	**Metabolic Acidosis**	**Metabolic Alkalosis**
Opiate overdose	Anxiety attack	Lactic acidosis	Vomiting
Severe chronic obstructive pulmonary disease	High altitude	Diabetic, starvation, or alcoholic ketoacidosis	Loop diuretics
Neuromuscular disease	Hypoxemic lung disease	Uremia	Excess alkali ingestion
Obesity hypoventilation syndrome		Renal tubular acidosis	Hyperaldosteronism
		Severe diarrhea	

Metabolic Alkalosis

Here an increase in HCO_3^- raises the HCO_3^-/P_{CO_2} ratio and, thus, the pH. Excessive ingestion of alkalis and loss of acid gastric secretion by vomiting are causes. In Figure 6.7, the movement is in the direction A to E. Some respiratory compensation sometimes occurs by a reduction in alveolar ventilation that raises the P_{CO_2}. Point E then moves in the direction of D (although not all the way). However, respiratory compensation in metabolic alkalosis is often small and may be absent. Base excess is increased.

Note that mixed respiratory and metabolic disturbances often occur, and it may then be difficult to unravel the sequence of events. Representative examples of processes that cause each of the primary acid-base disturbances are listed in **Table 6.2**.

BLOOD-TISSUE GAS EXCHANGE

Diffusion

O_2 and CO_2 move between the systemic capillary blood and the tissue cells by simple diffusion, just as they move between the capillary blood and alveolar gas in the lung. We saw in Chapter 3 that the rate of transfer of gas through a tissue sheet is proportional to the tissue area and the difference in gas partial pressure between the two sides, and inversely proportional to the thickness. The thickness of the blood-gas barrier is less than 0.5 μm, but the distance between open capillaries in resting muscle is on the order of 50 μm. During exercise, when the O_2 consumption of the muscle increases, additional capillaries open up, thus reducing the diffusion distance and increasing the area for diffusion. Because

CO_2 diffuses about 20 times faster than does O_2 through tissue (Figure 3.1), elimination of CO_2 is much less of a problem than is O_2 delivery.

Tissue Po_2

The way in which the Po_2 falls in tissue between adjacent open capillaries is shown schematically in **Figure 6.8**. As the O_2 diffuses away from the capillary, it is consumed by tissue, and the Po_2 falls. In *A*, the balance between O_2 consumption and delivery (determined by the capillary Po_2 and the intercapillary distance) results in an adequate Po_2 in all the tissue. In *B*, the intercapillary distance or the O_2 consumption has been increased until the Po_2 at one point in the tissue falls to zero. This is referred to as a *critical* situation. In *C*, there is an anoxic region where aerobic (i.e., O_2 utilizing) metabolism is impossible. Under these conditions, the tissue may turn to anaerobic glycolysis with the formation of lactic acid.

There is evidence that much of the fall of Po_2 in peripheral tissues occurs in the immediate vicinity of the capillary wall and that the Po_2 in muscle cells, for example, is very low (1 to 3 mm Hg) and nearly uniform. This pattern can be explained by the presence of myoglobin in the cell that acts as a reservoir for O_2 and enhances its diffusion within the cell.

How low can the tissue Po_2 fall before O_2 utilization ceases? In measurements on suspensions of liver mitochondria *in vitro*, O_2 consumption continues at the same rate until the Po_2 falls to the region of 3 mm Hg. Thus, it appears that the purpose of the much higher Po_2 in capillary blood is to ensure an adequate pressure for diffusion of O_2 to the mitochondria and that at the sites of O_2 utilization, the Po_2 may be very low.

An abnormally low Po_2 in tissues is called tissue hypoxia. This is frequently caused by low O_2 delivery, which can be expressed as the cardiac output multiplied by the arterial O_2 concentration, or $\dot{Q} \times Ca_{O_2}$. The factors that determine were discussed on page 91. Tissue hypoxia can be due to (1) a low Po_2 in arterial blood caused, for example, by pulmonary disease ("hypoxic hypoxia"); (2) a reduced ability of blood to carry O_2, as in anemia or carbon monoxide poisoning ("anemic hypoxia"); or (3) a reduction in tissue blood flow, either generalized, as in shock, or because of local obstruction ("circulatory hypoxia"). A fourth cause is some toxic substance that interferes with the

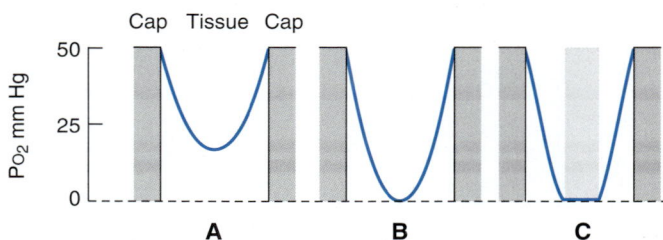

Figure 6.8. Scheme showing the fall of Po_2 between adjacent open capillaries. In *A*, oxygen delivery is adequate; in *B*, critical; and in *C*, inadequate for aerobic metabolism in the central core of tissue.

ability of the tissues to utilize available O_2 ("histotoxic hypoxia"). An example is cyanide, which prevents the use of O_2 by cytochrome oxidase. In this case, the O_2 concentration of venous blood is high and the O_2 consumption of the tissue is extremely low. Cyanide poisoning can be caused by ingestion, for example of rodent pesticides or bitter almonds. It also may occur in fire depending on the material being burned, such as polymer products.

Mixed Venous Po_2

The Po_2 and O_2 concentration of mixed venous blood is determined by the balance between O_2 delivery on the one hand and tissue O_2 utilization on the other. If, for example, O_2 delivery declines, while tissue O_2 utilization remains constant, oxygen extraction from the blood must increase to meet the metabolic needs, thereby decreasing the mixed venous Po_2 and O_2 concentration. In some cases, such as severe sepsis or cyanide intoxication, mitochondrial O_2 utilization is impaired, in which case the mixed venous Po_2 and O_2 concentration increase. **Table 6.3** summarizes some of the features of the different types of hypoxemia and their effects on arterial and mixed venous Po_2 and O_2 concentration.

Table 6.3	Features of Different Types of Hypoxemia or Tissue Hypoxia[a]								
	$P_{A_{O_2}}$	$P_{A_{CO_2}}$	Pa_{O_2}	Pa_{CO_2}	Ca_{O_2}	Sa_{O_2}	$P_{\bar{v}_{O_2}}$	$C_{\bar{v}_{O_2}}$	O_2 Administration Helpful?
Lungs									
Hypoventilation	↓	↑	↓	↑	↓	↓	↓	↓	Yes
Diffusion impairment	O	O	↓	O	↓	↓	↓	↓	Yes
Shunt	O	O	↓	O	↓	↓	↓	↓	Yes[b]
$\dot{V}_A/\dot{Q}$ inequality	Varies	↑ or O	↓	↑ or O	↓	↓	↓	↓	Yes
Blood									
Anemia	O	O	O	O	↓	O	↓	↓	Yes[b]
CO poisoning	O	O	O	O	↓	O[c]	↓	↓	Yes[b]
Methemoglobinemia	O	O	O	O	↓	↓[d]	↓	↓	No
Tissue									
Cyanide poisoning	O	O	O	O	O	O	↑	↑	No

[a]O, normal; ↑ increased; ↓ decreased.
[b]Of some (but limited) value because of increased dissolved oxygen (see Figure 5.4 for shunt.)
[c]If O_2 saturation is calculated for hemoglobin not bound to CO.
[d]When O_2 saturation is measured by pulse oximetry.

KEY CONCEPTS

1. Most of the O_2 transported in the blood is bound to hemoglobin. The maximum amount that can be bound is called the O_2 capacity. The O_2 saturation is the amount combined with hemoglobin divided by the capacity and is equal to the proportion of the binding sites that are occupied by O_2.

2. The O_2 dissociation curve is shifted to the right (i.e., the O_2 affinity of the hemoglobin is reduced) by increases in P_{CO_2}, H^+, temperature, and 2,3-diphosphoglycerate.

3. Most of the CO_2 in the blood is in the form of bicarbonate, with smaller amounts dissolved in blood or in the form of carbamino compounds.

4. The CO_2 dissociation curve is much steeper and more linear than is that for O_2.

5. The acid-base status of the blood is determined by the Henderson-Hasselbalch equation and especially the ratio of bicarbonate concentration to the P_{CO_2}. Acid-base abnormalities include respiratory and metabolic acidosis and alkalosis.

6. The P_{O_2} in some tissues is less than 5 mm Hg, and the purpose of the much higher P_{O_2} in the capillary blood is to provide an adequate gradient for diffusion. Factors determining O_2 delivery to tissues include the blood O_2 concentration and the blood flow.

CLINICAL VIGNETTE

An 85-year-old woman presents to the emergency department with increasing fatigue and shortness of breath on exertion. She is a lifelong nonsmoker and denies cough, chest pain, or sputum production but states that her stools have had a dark, black ("tarry") appearance over the past several weeks. She takes aspirin daily for treatment of stable coronary artery disease. On examination, she had pale palms and conjunctivae. Her lungs were clear to auscultation and, aside from a mild tachycardia (fast heart rate), her cardiac examination was normal. A rectal examination was performed, and the stool tested positive for the presence of red blood cells. A venous blood sample was taken and revealed a hemoglobin concentration of 5 $g \cdot dl^{-1}$ (normal: 14 to 15 $g \cdot dl^{-1}$).

- If you measured her arterial blood gases, what changes would you expect in the P_{O_2} and oxygen saturation?
- What would you expect for her arterial oxygen concentration?
- Why is her heart rate increased?
- What would you expect for the oxygen concentration in her mixed venous blood?

QUESTIONS

For each question, choose the one best answer.

1. A 52-year-old woman presents with a massive upper gastrointestinal hemorrhage and her hemoglobin concentration falls from 13 to 6 g·dl⁻¹. Which of the following pattern of changes in hemoglobin-O_2 saturation, Pa_{CO_2}, arterial oxygen concentration (Ca_{O_2}), and mixed venous oxygen content ($C\bar{v}_{O_2}$) would you expect to see at this time?

Choice	Hb-O_2 Saturation	Pa_{CO_2}	Ca_{O_2}	$C\bar{v}_{O_2}$
A.	Decreased	Increased	Decreased	Decreased
B.	No change	No change	Decreased	Decreased
C.	No change	No change	No change	No change
D.	Decreased	No change	No change	Decreased
E.	No change	Decreased	Decreased	Increased

2. The figure below depicts the relationship between hemoglobin-O_2 saturation and the P_{O_2}.

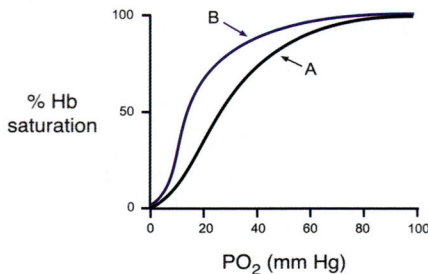

Which of the following factors could account for the shift in the relationship from Curve A to Curve B?
A. Heavy exercise
B. Hypothermia
C. Hypoventilation
D. Increased 2,3-diphosphoglycerate
E. Lactic acidosis

3. A 38-year-old commercial diver presents to the emergency department with decompression sickness. Prior to being placed in a hyperbaric chamber for treatment, he has an arterial Po_2 of 120 mm Hg and an arterial Pco_2 of 41 mm Hg while receiving oxygen by nasal cannula. Once in the chamber, the barometric pressure is raised to 3 atm (2,280 mm Hg), after which his arterial oxygen content rises from 20 ml O_2 per 100 ml blood to 23 ml O_2 per 100 ml blood. Which of the following factors is primarily responsible for the observed improvement in his arterial oxygen content?
   A. Increase in the amount of oxygen dissolved in the plasma
   B. Increase in the hemoglobin-oxygen saturation
   C. Increase in the P50 of hemoglobin
   D. Increase in oxygen binding to terminal hemoglobin amine groups
   E. Leftward shift of the hemoglobin-oxygen dissociation curve

4. A 43-year-old man is brought into the emergency department with altered mental status. He was found in the front seat of his car in his closed garage with the engine still running. While breathing ambient air, his SpO_2 is 99%, his skin color is normal and he has a serum lactate of 8 mmol·liter^{-1} (normal: <2 mmol·liter^{-1}), hemoglobin of 14.5 g·dl^{-1} (normal: 13 to 15 g·dl^{-1}), and arterial Po_2 of 90 mm Hg. A chest radiograph shows no focal opacities. Following admission, a pulmonary artery catheter is placed, after which the mixed venous oxygen saturation is found to be 50%. What is the mechanism for the observed abnormalities in this patient?
   A. Displacement of oxygen from hemoglobin-binding sites
   B. Enhanced activity of mitochondrial cytochrome oxidase
   C. Oxidation of iron in the heme molecule
   D. Rightward shift in the hemoglobin-oxygen dissociation curve
   E. Ventilation-perfusion inequality

5. Which of the following changes is most likely to occur as blood moves across the capillary bed of a muscle from the arterial to the venous side of the circulation?
   A. Decreased bicarbonate concentration
   B. Decreased P_{50} for hemoglobin
   C. Decreased storage of carbon dioxide in physical solution
   D. Increased carbaminohemoglobin
   E. Rightward shift in the relationship between carbon dioxide concentration and Pco_2.

6. The quadriceps muscle Po_2 and oxygen concentration of mixed venous blood ($C_{\bar{v}O_2}$) are measured at two time points as part of an experimental preparation. The values are shown in the table below.

Variable	Time 1	Time 2
Quadriceps P_{O_2} (mm Hg)	5	2
$C\bar{v}_{O_2}$ (ml per 100 ml)	15	12

Which of the following could account for the observed change in these values between Time 1 and Time 2?
A. Cyanide intoxication
B. Decreased hemoglobin concentration
C. Decreased quadriceps temperature
D. Increased cardiac output
E. Increased inspired oxygen fraction

7. A patient with chronic obstructive pulmonary disease presents to the emergency department with increased dyspnea. An arterial blood gas is measured and reveals pH 7.20, Pa_{CO_2} 50 mm Hg, and Pa_{O_2} 50 mm Hg. Which of the following is the most appropriate description of the patient's acid-base status?
A. Fully compensated metabolic acidosis
B. Fully compensated respiratory acidosis
C. Mixed respiratory and metabolic acidosis
D. Uncompensated metabolic acidosis
E. Uncompensated respiratory acidosis

8. The arterial blood gas results for a patient in the intensive care unit are pH 7.25, Pa_{CO_2} 32 mm Hg, and HCO_3^- 25 mEq·liter^{-1}. Which of the following is the most appropriate interpretation of the acid-base status?
A. Acute respiratory acidosis
B. Laboratory error
C. Metabolic acidosis with respiratory compensation
D. Metabolic alkalosis with respiratory compensation
E. Respiratory alkalosis with metabolic compensation

9. A healthy individual ascends by helicopter from sea level to the summit of a mountain that is 4,000 m in elevation. If you were to draw an arterial blood gas while the individual is breathing ambient air immediately following arrival on the summit, which of the following sets of results would you expect to find at this time?

Choice	pH	Pa_{CO_2} (mm Hg)	Pa_{O_2} (mm Hg)	HCO_3^- (mEq·liter^{-1})
A.	7.32	50	55	25
B.	7.39	41	90	24
C.	7.49	32	58	23
D.	7.50	31	92	24
E.	7.43	30	63	20

10. A 46-year-old man is hospitalized after being rescued from a fire in a furniture warehouse. He was short of breath and dizzy on initial evaluation but now has a decreased level of consciousness. His arterial oxygen saturation is 99% while receiving supplemental oxygen. A chest radiograph shows no focal opacities while an electrocardiogram shows only a rapid heart rate. On laboratory studies, his arterial P_{O_2} is 200 mm Hg, hemoglobin is 15 g·dl^{-1}, and he has an elevated lactic acid level. A pulmonary artery catheter is placed, and the mixed venous oxygen saturation is found to be 85%. Which of the following most likely accounts for the patient's clinical condition?
    A. Carboxyhemoglobinemia
    B. Cyanide intoxication
    C. Hypovolemic shock
    D. Methemoglobinemia
    E. Pulmonary edema

11. A 41-year-old woman is receiving mechanical ventilation following a drug overdose. On the 5th day of her admission, she develops fever (39.0°C) and is found to have a blood stream infection. The arterial blood gas that morning had an arterial P_{O_2} of 72 mm Hg that was unchanged compared to blood gas results from the preceding day. Which of the following physiologic changes would you expect?
    A. Decreased carbon dioxide production
    B. Decreased shunt fraction
    C. Increased arterial oxygen concentration
    D. Increased arterial oxygen saturation
    E. Increased P_{50} for hemoglobin

12. An arterial blood gas is performed on a patient in the emergency department and reveals the following: pH 7.48, Pa_{CO_2} 45 mm Hg, and HCO_3^- 32 mEq·liter^{-1}. Which of the following clinical situations could account for these findings?
    A. Anxiety attack
    B. Opiate overdose
    C. Severe chronic obstructive pulmonary disease
    D. Uncontrolled diabetes mellitus
    E. Vomiting

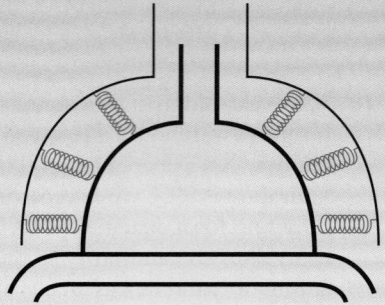

Mechanics of Breathing

How the Lung Is Supported and Moved

7

We now turn to the forces that move the lung and chest wall, and the resistances that they overcome. First, we consider the muscles of respiration, both inspiration and expiration. Then, we look at the factors determining the elastic properties of the lung, including the tissue elements and the air-liquid surface tension. Next, we examine the mechanism of regional differences in ventilation and also the closure of small airways. Just as the lung is elastic, so is the chest wall, and we look at the interaction between the two. The physical principles of airway resistance are then considered, along with its measurement, chief site in the lung, and physiological factors that affect it. Dynamic compression of the airways during a forced expiration is analyzed. Finally, the work required to move the lung and chest wall and the mechanics of positive pressure ventilation are considered. At the end of this chapter, the reader should be able to:

- Compare and contrast the roles of the inspiratory and expiratory muscles of respiration
- Identify factors that increase or decrease pulmonary compliance
- Describe the effect of pulmonary surfactant on surface tension and alveolar stability
- Describe the causes of regional differences in ventilation
- Outline changes in airway and intrapleural pressure during the respiratory cycle
- Identify factors that determine airway resistance
- Describe the mechanism and consequences of dynamic airway compression

MUSCLES OF RESPIRATION

Inspiration

The most important muscle of inspiration is the *diaphragm*. This consists of a thin, dome-shaped sheet of muscle that is inserted into the lower ribs. It is supplied by the phrenic nerves from cervical segments 3, 4, and 5. When it contracts, the abdominal contents are forced downward and forward, and the vertical dimension of the chest cavity is increased. In addition, the rib margins are lifted and moved out, causing an increase in the transverse diameter of the thorax (**Figure 7.1**).

In normal tidal breathing, the level of the diaphragm moves about 1 cm or so, but on forced inspiration and expiration, a total excursion of up to 10 cm may occur. When one side of the diaphragm is paralyzed, it moves *up* rather than *down* with inspiration because the intrathoracic pressure falls. This is known as *paradoxical movement* and can be demonstrated at fluoroscopy when the patient sniffs.

The *external intercostal muscles* connect adjacent ribs and slope downward and forward (**Figure 7.2**). When they contract, the ribs are pulled upward and forward, causing an increase in both the lateral and the anteroposterior diameters of the thorax. The lateral dimension increases because of the "bucket-handle" movement of the ribs. The intercostal muscles are supplied by intercostal nerves that come off the spinal cord at the same level. Paralysis of the intercostal muscles alone does not seriously affect breathing at rest because the diaphragm is so effective.

The *accessory muscles of inspiration* include the scalene muscles, which elevate the first two ribs, and the sternocleidomastoids, which raise the sternum.

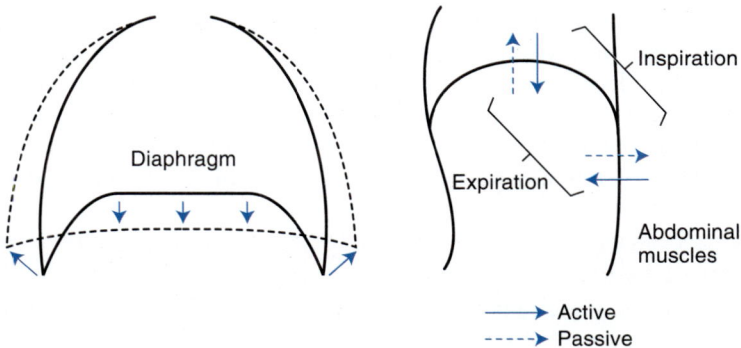

Figure 7.1. On inspiration, the dome-shaped diaphragm contracts, the abdominal contents are forced down and forward, and the rib cage is widened. Both increase the volume of the thorax. On forced expiration, the abdominal muscles contract and push the diaphragm up.

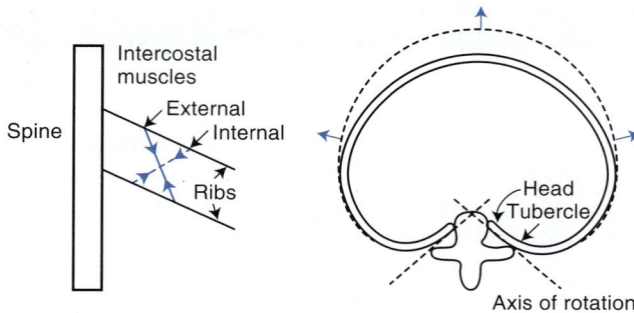

Figure 7.2. When the external intercostal muscles contract, the ribs are pulled upward and forward, and they rotate on an axis joining the tubercle and the head of a rib. As a result, both the lateral and anteroposterior diameters of the thorax increase. The internal intercostals have the opposite action.

There is little, if any, activity in these muscles during quiet breathing, but during exercise, they may contract vigorously. Other muscles that play a minor role include the alae nasi, which cause flaring of the nostrils, and small muscles in the neck and head.

Expiration

This is passive during quiet breathing. The lung and chest wall are elastic and tend to return to their equilibrium positions after being actively expanded during inspiration. During exercise and voluntary hyperventilation, expiration becomes active. The most important muscles of expiration are those of the *abdominal wall*, including the rectus abdominis, internal and external oblique muscles, and transversus abdominis. When these muscles contract, intra-abdominal pressure is raised, and the diaphragm is pushed upward. These muscles also contract forcefully during coughing, vomiting, and defecation.

The *internal intercostal muscles* assist active expiration by pulling the ribs downward and inward (opposite to the action of the external intercostal muscles), thus decreasing the thoracic volume. In addition, they stiffen the intercostal spaces to prevent them from bulging outward during straining. Experimental studies show that the actions of the respiratory muscles, especially the intercostals, are more complicated than this brief account suggests.

Respiratory Muscles

- Inspiration is always active; expiration is passive during rest but active during exercise.
- The diaphragm is the most important muscle of inspiration; it is supplied by phrenic nerves that originate from cervical segments 3, 4, and 5.
- Contraction of the abdominal muscles plays a key role in active expiration.

ELASTIC PROPERTIES OF THE LUNG

Pressure-Volume Curve

Suppose we take an excised animal lung, cannulate the trachea, and place it inside a jar (**Figure 7.3**). When the pressure within the jar is reduced below atmospheric pressure, the lung expands, and its change in volume can be measured with a spirometer. The pressure is held at each level, as indicated by the points, for a few seconds to allow the lung to come to rest. In this way, the pressure-volume curve of the lung can be plotted.

In Figure 7.3, the expanding pressure around the lung is generated by a pump, but in humans, it is developed by an increase in volume of the chest cage. The fact that the intrapleural space between the lung and the chest wall is much smaller than the space between the lung and the bottle in Figure 7.3 makes no essential difference. The intrapleural space contains only a few milliliters of fluid.

Figure 7.3 shows that the curves that the lung follows during inflation and deflation are different. This behavior is known as *hysteresis*. Note that the lung volume at any given pressure during deflation is larger than is that during inflation. Note also that the lung without any expanding pressure has some air inside it. In fact, even if the pressure around the lung is raised above atmospheric pressure, little further air is lost because small airways close, trapping gas in the alveoli (compare Figure 7.9). This *airway closure* occurs at higher lung volumes with increasing age and also in some types of lung disease, including emphysema.

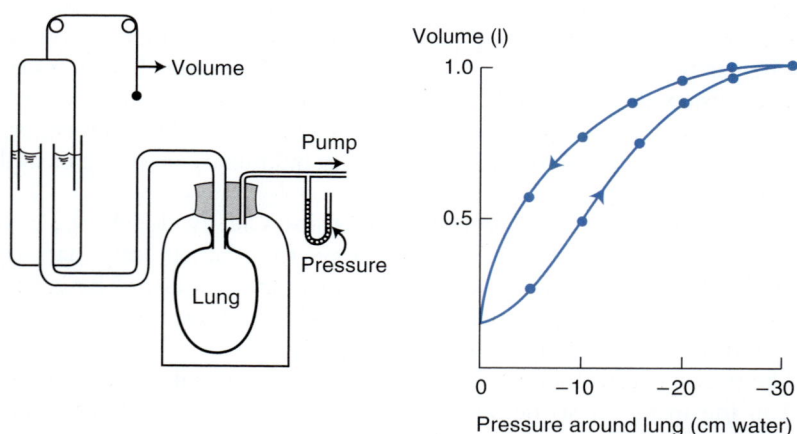

Figure 7.3. Measurement of the pressure-volume curve of excised lung. The lung is held at each pressure for a few seconds while its volume is measured. The curve is nonlinear and becomes flatter at high expanding pressures. Note that the inflation and deflation curves are not the same; this is called hysteresis.

In Figure 7.3, the pressure inside the airways and alveoli of the lung is the same as atmospheric pressure, which is zero on the horizontal axis. Thus, this axis also measures the difference in pressure between the inside and the outside of the lung. This is known as *transpulmonary pressure* and is numerically equal to the pressure around the lung when the alveolar pressure is atmospheric. It is also possible to measure the pressure-volume relationship of the lung shown in Figure 7.3 by inflating it with positive pressure and leaving the pleural surface exposed to the atmosphere. In this case, the horizontal axis could be labeled "airway pressure," and the values would be positive. The curves would be identical to those shown in Figure 7.3.

Compliance

The slope of the pressure-volume curve, or the volume change per unit pressure change, is known as the *compliance*. Therefore, the equation is:

$$\text{Compliance} = \frac{\Delta V}{\Delta P}$$

In the normal range (expanding pressure of about −5 to −10 cm water), the lung is remarkably distensible or very compliant. The compliance of the human lung is about 200 ml·cm H_2O^{-1}. However, at high expanding pressures, the lung is stiffer, and its compliance is smaller, as shown by the flatter slope of the curve.

Compliance is not a fixed property of the lung and, instead, can change as a result of multiple factors. *A reduced* compliance is caused by an increase of fibrous tissue in the lung (pulmonary fibrosis) or by alveolar edema, which prevents the inflation of some alveoli. Compliance also falls if the lung remains unventilated for a long period, especially if its volume is low. This may be partly caused by atelectasis (collapse) of some units, but increases in surface tension also occur (see below). Compliance is also reduced somewhat if the pulmonary venous pressure is increased and the lung becomes engorged with blood. An *increased* compliance occurs in pulmonary emphysema and in the normal aging lung.

The compliance of a lung depends on its size. Clearly, the change in volume per unit change of pressure will be larger for a human lung than, say, a mouse lung. For this reason, the compliance per unit volume of lung, or *specific compliance*, is sometimes measured if we wish to draw conclusions about the intrinsic elastic properties of the lung tissue.

The pressure surrounding the lung is less than atmospheric in Figure 7.3 (and in the living chest) because of the elastic recoil of the lung. What is responsible for the lung's elastic behavior, that is, its tendency to return to its resting volume after distension? One factor is the elastic tissue, which is visible in histological sections. Fibers of elastin and collagen can be seen in the alveolar walls and around vessels and bronchi. Probably the elastic behavior of the lung has less to do with simple elongation of these fibers than it does with their geometrical arrangement. An analogy is a nylon stocking, which is very distensible because of its knitted makeup, although the individual nylon fibers are very difficult to stretch. The changes in elastic recoil that occur in the lung with age and in emphysema are presumably caused by changes in this elastic tissue.

Pressure-Volume Behavior of the Lung

- The pressure-volume curve is nonlinear with the lung becoming stiffer at high volumes.
- The curve shows hysteresis between inflation and deflation.
- Compliance is the slope $\Delta V/\Delta P$.
- Behavior depends on both structural proteins (collagen, elastin) and surface tension.

Surface Tension

Another important factor in the pressure-volume behavior of lung is the surface tension of the liquid film lining the alveoli. Surface tension is the force (e.g., in dynes) acting across an imaginary line 1 cm long in the surface of the liquid (**Figure 7.4A**). It arises because the attractive forces between adjacent molecules of the liquid are much stronger than are those between the liquid and gas, with the result that the liquid surface area becomes as small as possible. This behavior is seen clearly in a soap bubble blown on the end of a tube (**Figure 7.4B**). The two surfaces of the bubble contract as much as they can,

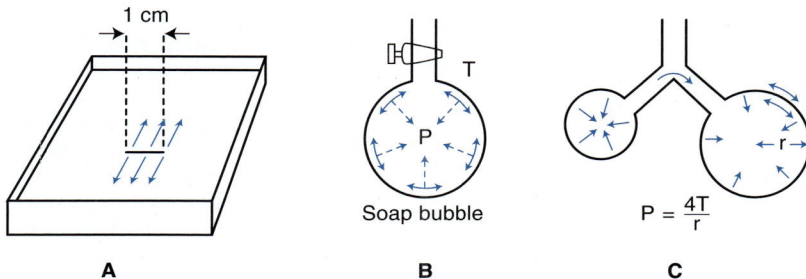

Soap bubble

$$P = \frac{4T}{r}$$

Figure 7.4. **A.** Surface tension is the force (e.g., in dynes) acting across an imaginary line 1 cm long in a liquid surface. **B.** Surface forces in a soap bubble tend to reduce the area of the surface and generate a pressure within the bubble. **C.** Because the smaller bubble generates a larger pressure, it blows up the larger bubble.

forming a sphere (smallest surface area for a given volume) and generating a pressure that can be predicted from Laplace's law:

$$P = \frac{4T}{r}$$

where P is pressure, T is surface tension, and r is radius. When only one surface is involved in a liquid-lined spherical alveolus, the numerator is 2 rather than 4.

The first evidence that surface tension might contribute to the pressure-volume behavior of the lung was obtained when it was found that lungs inflated with saline have a much larger compliance (are easier to distend) than do air-filled lungs (**Figure 7.5**). Because the saline abolished the surface tension forces but presumably did not affect the tissue forces of the lung, this observation meant that surface tension contributed a large part of the static recoil force of the lung. Sometime later, workers studying edema foam coming from the lungs of animals exposed to noxious gases noticed that the tiny air bubbles of the foam were extremely stable. They recognized that this indicated a very low surface tension, an observation that led to the remarkable discovery of pulmonary *surfactant*.

It is now known that some of the cells lining the alveoli secrete a material, surfactant, that profoundly lowers the surface tension of the alveolar lining fluid. Surfactant is a phospholipid whose important constituent is dipalmitoyl phosphatidylcholine (DPPC). Alveolar epithelial cells are of two types. Type I cells have the shape of a fried egg, with long cytoplasmic extensions spreading out thinly over the alveolar walls (Figure 1.1). Type II cells are more compact (**Figure 7.6**), and electron microscopy shows lamellated bodies within them

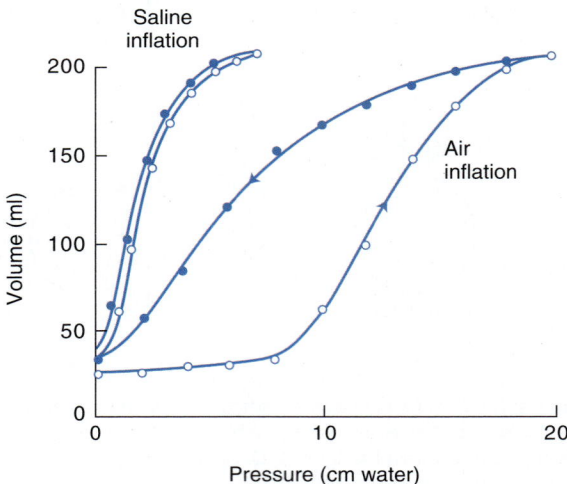

Figure 7.5. Comparison of pressure-volume curves of air-filled and saline-filled lungs (cat). *Open circles,* inflation; *closed circles,* deflation. Note that the saline-filled lung has a higher compliance and also much less hysteresis than the air-filled lung. (From Radford EP. *Tissue Elasticity.* Washington, DC: American Physiological Society; 1957.)

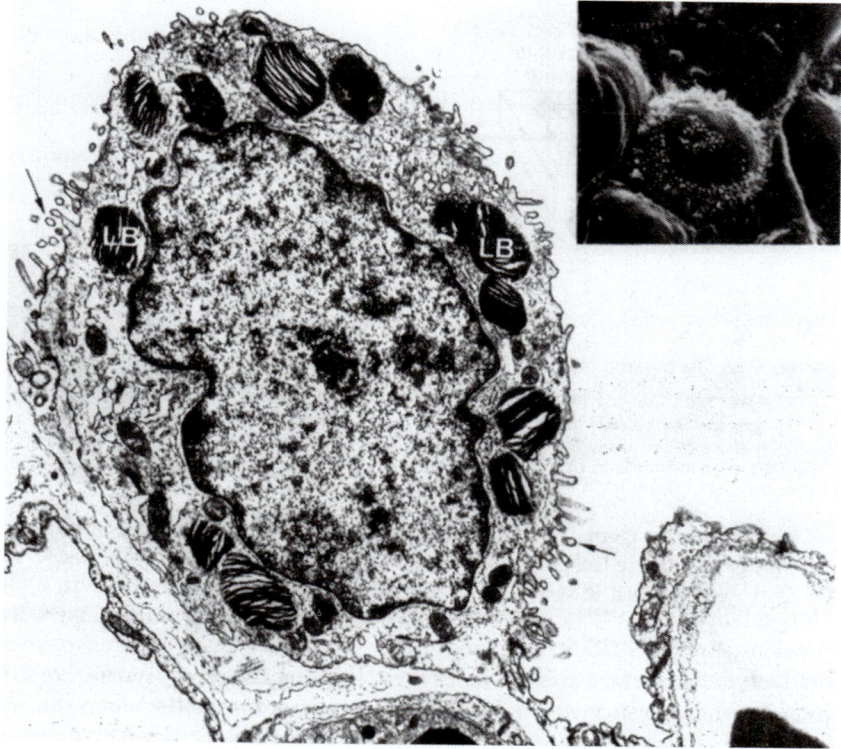

Figure 7.6. Electron micrograph of type II alveolar epithelial cell (×10,000). Note the lamellated bodies (LB), large nucleus, and microvilli (*arrows*). The **inset** *at top right* is a scanning electron micrograph showing the surface view of a type II cell with its characteristic distribution of microvilli (×3,400). (Republished with permission of Springer from Weibel ER, Gil J. In: West JB, ed. *Bioengineering Aspects of the Lung*. New York, NY: Marcel Dekker; 1977; permission conveyed through Copyright Clearance Center, Inc.)

that are extruded into the alveoli and transform into surfactant. Some of the surfactant can be washed out of animal lungs by rinsing them with saline.

The phospholipid DPPC is synthesized in the lung from fatty acids that are either extracted from the blood or are themselves synthesized in the lung. Synthesis is fast, and there is a rapid turnover of surfactant. If the blood flow to a region of lung is abolished as the result of an embolus, for example, the surfactant there may be depleted. Surfactant is formed relatively late in fetal life, and babies born without adequate amounts develop respiratory distress and may die without ventilatory support.

The effects of this material on surface tension can be studied with a surface balance (**Figure 7.7**). This consists of a tray containing saline on which a small amount of test material is placed. The area of the surface is then alternately expanded and compressed by a movable barrier while the surface tension is measured from the force exerted on a platinum strip. Pure saline gives

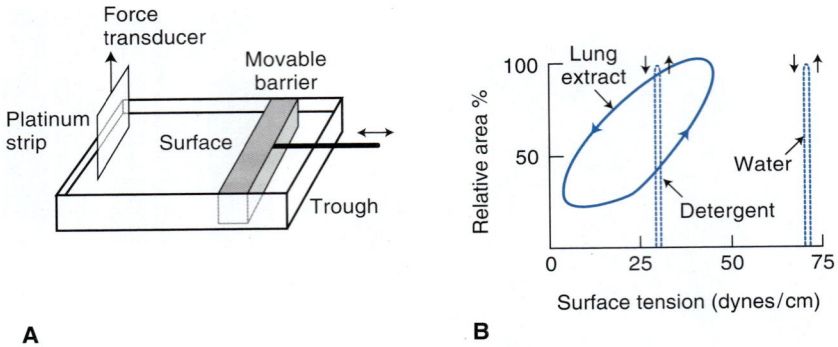

Figure 7.7. **A.** Surface balance. The area of the surface is altered, and the surface tension is measured from the force exerted on a platinum strip dipped into the surface. **B.** Plots of surface tension and area obtained with a surface balance. Note that lung washings show a change in surface tension with area and that the minimal tension is very small. The axes are chosen to allow a comparison with the pressure-volume curve of the lung (Figures 7.3 and 7.5).

a surface tension of about 70 dynes·cm^{-1} (70 mN·m^{-1}), regardless of the area of its surface. Adding detergent reduces the surface tension, but again, this is independent of area. When lung washings are placed on the saline, the curve shown in **Figure 7.7B** is obtained. Note that the surface tension changes greatly with the surface area and that there is hysteresis (compare Figure 7.3). Note also that the surface tension falls to extremely low values when the area is small.

How does surfactant reduce the surface tension so much? The molecules of DPPC are hydrophobic at one end and hydrophilic at the other, and they align themselves in the surface. When this occurs, their intermolecular repulsive forces oppose the normal attracting forces between the liquid surface molecules that are responsible for surface tension. The reduction in surface tension is greater when the film is compressed because the molecules of DPPC are then crowded closer together and repel each other more.

What are the physiological advantages of surfactant? First, a low surface tension in the alveoli increases the compliance of the lung and reduces the work of expanding it with each breath. Next, stability of the alveoli is promoted. The 500 million alveoli appear to be inherently unstable because areas of atelectasis (collapse) often form in the presence of disease. This is a complex subject, but one way of looking at the lung is to regard it as a collection of millions of tiny bubbles (although this is clearly an oversimplification). In such an arrangement, there is a tendency for small bubbles to collapse and blow up large ones. Figure 7.4C shows that the pressure generated by a given surface force in a bubble is inversely proportional to its radius, with the result that if the surface tensions are the same, the pressure inside a small bubble exceeds that in a large bubble. However, Figure 7.7 shows that when lung washings are present, a small surface area is associated with a small surface tension. Thus, the tendency for small alveoli to empty into large alveoli is apparently reduced.

A third role of surfactant is to help to keep the alveoli dry. Just as the surface tension forces tend to collapse alveoli, they also tend to suck fluid out of the capillaries. In effect, the surface tension of the curved alveolar surface reduces the hydrostatic pressure in the tissue outside the capillaries. By reducing these surface forces, surfactant prevents the transudation of fluid.

What are the consequences of loss of surfactant? On the basis of its functions discussed above, we would expect there to be stiff lungs (low compliance), areas of atelectasis, and alveoli filled with transudate. Indeed, these are the pathophysiological features of the neonatal respiratory distress syndrome, which occurs when premature infants are born before adequate quantities of surfactant have been produced. These newborns are treated by instilling synthesized surfactant into the lung.

There is another mechanism that apparently contributes to the stability of the alveoli in the lung. Figures 1.2, 1.7, and 4.3 remind us that all the alveoli (except those immediately adjacent to the pleural surface) are surrounded by other alveoli and are therefore supported by one another. In a structure such as this with many connecting links, any tendency for one group of units to reduce or increase its volume relative to the rest of the structure is opposed. For example, if a group of alveoli has a tendency to collapse, large expanding forces will be developed on them because the surrounding parenchyma is expanded. This support offered to lung units by those surrounding them is termed *interdependence*. The same factors explain the development of low pressures around large blood vessels and airways as the lung expands (Figure 4.2).

Pulmonary Surfactant

- Reduces the surface tension of the alveolar lining layer
- Produced by type II alveolar epithelial cells
- Contains DPPC
- Absence results in reduced lung compliance, alveolar atelectasis, and tendency to pulmonary edema

---

CAUSE OF REGIONAL DIFFERENCES IN VENTILATION

We saw in Figure 2.7 that the lower regions of the lung ventilate more than do the upper zones, and this is a convenient place to discuss the cause of these topographical differences. It has been shown that the intrapleural pressure is less negative at the bottom than the top of the lung (**Figure 7.8**). The reason

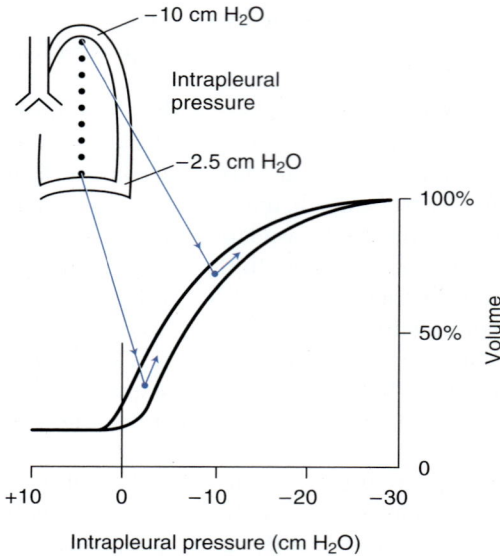

Figure 7.8. Explanation of the regional differences of ventilation down the lung. Because of the weight of the lung, the intrapleural pressure is less negative at the base than at the apex. As a consequence, the basal lung is relatively compressed in its resting state but expands more on inspiration than does the apex. (From West JB. *Ventilation/Blood Flow and Gas Exchange*. 5th ed. Oxford, UK: Blackwell; 1990.)

for this is the weight of the lung. Anything that is supported requires a larger pressure below it than above it to balance the downward-acting weight forces, and the lung, which is partly supported by the rib cage and diaphragm, is no exception. Thus, the pressure near the base is higher (less negative) than at the apex.

Figure 7.8 shows the way in which the volume of a portion of lung (e.g., a lobe) expands as the pressure around it is decreased (compare Figure 7.3). The pressure inside the lung is the same as atmospheric pressure. Note that the lung is easier to inflate at low volumes than at high volumes, where it becomes stiffer. Because the expanding pressure at the base of the lung is small, this region has a small resting volume. However, because it is situated on a steep part of the pressure-volume curve, it expands easily on inspiration. By contrast, the apex of the lung has a big resting volume, is situated on a flatter portion of the pressure-volume curve, has large expanding pressure, and undergoes a small change in volume in inspiration.*

Now when we talk of regional differences in ventilation, we mean the change in volume per unit resting volume. It is clear from Figure 7.8 that the base of the lung has both a larger change in volume and smaller resting volume than does the apex. Thus, its ventilation is greater. Note the paradox that although the base of the lung is relatively poorly expanded compared with the apex, it is better ventilated. The same explanation can

---

*This explanation is an oversimplification because the pressure-volume behavior of a portion of a structure such as the lung may not be identical to that of the whole organ.

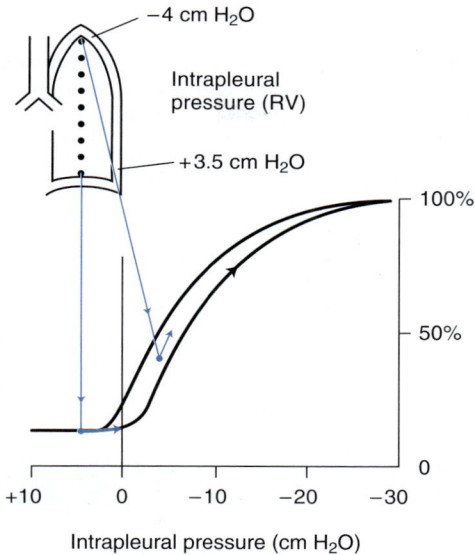

Figure 7.9. Situation at very low lung volumes. Now intrapleural pressures are less negative, and the pressure at the base actually exceeds airway (atmospheric) pressure. As a consequence, airway closure occurs in this region, and no gas enters with small inspirations. (From West JB. *Ventilation/Blood Flow and Gas Exchange.* 5th ed. Oxford, UK: Blackwell; 1990.)

be given for the large ventilation of dependent lung in both the supine and lateral positions.

A remarkable change in the distribution of ventilation occurs at low lung volumes. **Figure 7.9** is similar to Figure 7.8 except that it represents the situation at residual volume (RV) (i.e., after a full expiration; see Figure 2.2). Now the intrapleural pressures are less negative because the lung is not so well expanded and the elastic recoil forces are smaller. However, the differences between apex and base are still present because of the weight of the lung. Note that the intrapleural pressure at the base now actually exceeds airway (atmospheric) pressure. Under these conditions, the lung at the base is not being expanded but compressed, and ventilation is impossible until the local intrapleural pressure falls below atmospheric pressure. By contrast, the apex of the lung is on a favorable part of the pressure-volume curve and ventilates well. Thus, the normal distribution of ventilation is inverted, the upper regions ventilating better than the lower zones.

Regional Differences of Ventilation

- The weight of the upright lung causes a higher (less negative) intrapleural pressure around the base compared with the apex.
- Because of the nonlinear pressure-volume curve, alveoli at the base expand more than do those at the apex.
- If a small inspiration is made from residual volume (RV), the extreme base of the lung is unventilated.

Airway Closure

The compressed region of lung at the base does not have all its gas squeezed out. In practice, small airways, probably in the region of respiratory bronchioles (Figure 1.4), close first, thus trapping gas in the distal alveoli. This *airway closure* occurs only at very low lung volumes in young healthy subjects. However, in elderly, apparently healthy people, airway closure in the lowermost regions of the lung occurs at higher volumes and may be present at functional residual capacity (FRC) (Figure 2.2). The reason is that the aging lung loses some of its elastic recoil, and intrapleural pressures therefore become less negative, thus approaching the situation shown in Figure 7.9. In these circumstances, dependent (i.e., lowermost) regions of the lung may be only intermittently ventilated, and this leads to defective gas exchange (Chapter 5). A similar situation frequently develops in patients with emphysema.

ELASTIC PROPERTIES OF THE CHEST WALL

Just as the lung is elastic, so is the thoracic cage. This can be illustrated by putting air into the intrapleural space (pneumothorax). **Figure 7.10** shows that the normal pressure outside the lung is subatmospheric just as it is in the jar of Figure 7.3. When air is introduced into the intrapleural space, raising the pressure to atmospheric, the lung collapses inward and the chest wall springs outward. This shows that under equilibrium conditions, the chest wall is pulled inward while the lung is pulled outward, the two pulls balancing each other.

These interactions can be seen more clearly if we plot a pressure-volume curve for the lung and chest wall (**Figure 7.11**). For this, the subject inspires or expires from a spirometer and then relaxes the respiratory muscles while the airway pressure is measured ("relaxation pressure"). Incidentally, this is difficult for an untrained subject. Figure 7.11 shows that at FRC, the relaxation pressure of the lung plus chest wall is atmospheric. Indeed, FRC is the equilibrium volume when the elastic recoil of the lung is balanced

Normal   **Pneumothorax**

Figure 7.10. The tendency of the lung to recoil to its deflated volume is balanced by the tendency of the chest cage to bow out. As a result, the intrapleural pressure is subatmospheric. Pneumothorax allows the lung to collapse and the thorax to spring out.

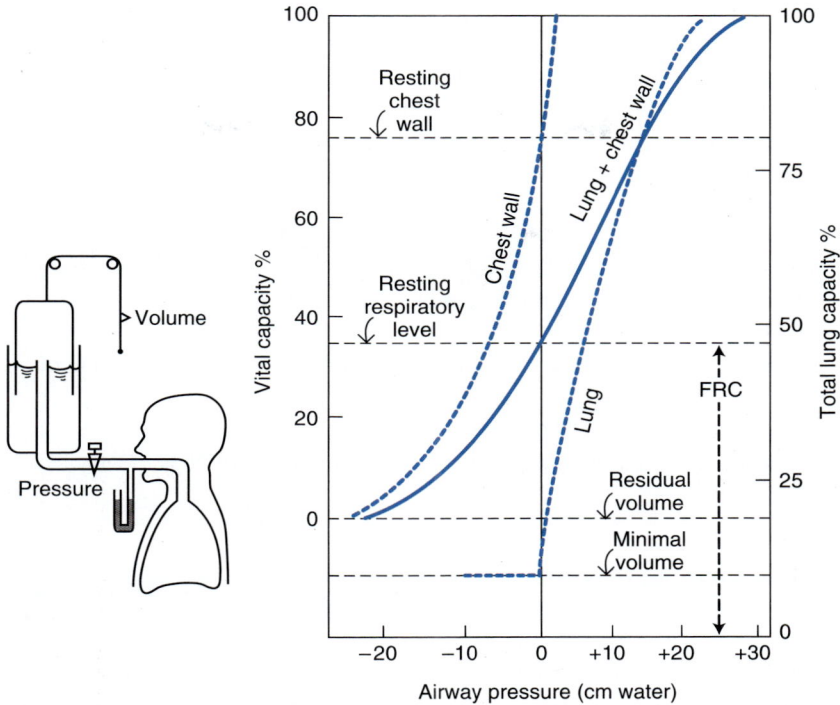

Figure 7.11. Relaxation pressure-volume curve of the lung and chest wall. The subject inspires (or expires) to a certain volume from the spirometer, the tap is closed, and the subject then relaxes the respiratory muscles. The curve for lung + chest wall can be explained by the addition of the individual lung and chest wall curves.

by the normal tendency for the chest wall to spring out. At volumes above this, the pressure is positive, and at smaller volumes, the pressure is subatmospheric.

Figure 7.11 also shows the curve for the lung alone. This is similar to that shown in Figure 7.3, except that for clarity no hysteresis is indicated, and the pressures are positive instead of negative. They are the pressures that would be found from the experiment of Figure 7.3 if, after the lung had reached a certain volume, the line to the spirometer was clamped, the jar opened to the atmosphere (so that the lung relaxed against the closed airway), and the airway pressure measured. Note that at zero pressure, the lung is at its *minimal volume*, which is below RV.

The third curve is for the chest wall only. We can imagine this being measured on a subject with a normal chest wall and no lung. Note that at FRC, the relaxation pressure is negative. In other words, at this volume, the chest cage is tending to spring out. It is not until the volume is increased to about 75% of the vital capacity that the relaxation pressure is atmospheric, that is, that the chest wall has found its equilibrium position. At every volume, the relaxation pressure of the lung plus chest wall is the sum of the pressures for the lung and the chest wall measured separately. Because the pressure (at a given volume) is inversely proportional to compliance, this implies that the total compliance of the lung and chest wall is the sum of the reciprocals of the lung and chest wall compliances measured separately, or $1/C_T = 1/C_L + 1/C_{CW}$.

Relaxation Pressure-Volume Curve

- Elastic properties of both the lung and chest wall determine their combined volume.
- At FRC, the inward pull of the lung is balanced by the outward spring of the chest wall.
- The lung retracts at all volumes above minimal volume.
- The chest wall tends to expand at volumes up to about 75% of vital capacity.

AIRWAY RESISTANCE

Airflow Through Tubes

If air flows through a tube (**Figure 7.12**), a difference in pressure exists between the ends. The pressure difference depends on the rate and pattern of flow. At low flow rates, the stream lines are parallel to the sides of the tube (A). This is known as laminar flow. As the flow rate is increased, unsteadiness develops, especially at branches. Here, separation of the stream lines from the wall may occur, with the formation of local eddies (B). At still higher flow rates, complete disorganization of the stream lines is seen; this is turbulence (C).

The pressure-flow characteristics for *laminar flow* were first described by the French physician Poiseuille. In straight circular tubes, the volume flow rate is given by:

$$\dot{V} = \frac{P\pi r^4}{8nl}$$

where P is the driving pressure (ΔP in Figure 7.12A), r radius, n viscosity, and l length. It can be seen that driving pressure is proportional to flow rate, or $P = K\dot{V}$. Because flow resistance R is driving pressure divided by flow, we have:

$$R = \frac{8nl}{\pi r^4}$$

Note the critical importance of tube radius; if the radius is halved, the resistance increases 16-fold! However, doubling the length only doubles resis-

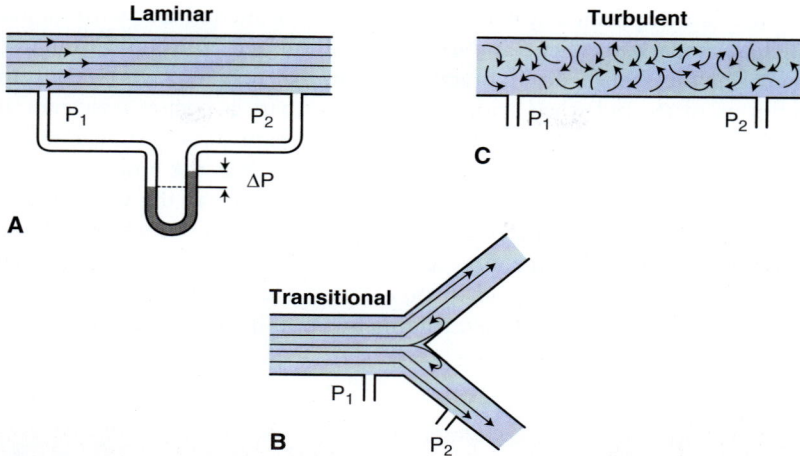

Figure 7.12. Patterns of airflow in tubes. In **(A)**, the flow is laminar; in **(B)**, transitional with eddy formation at branches; and in **(C)**, turbulent. Resistance is $(P_1 - P_2)$/flow.

tance. Note also that the viscosity of the gas, but not its density, affects the pressure-flow relationship under laminar flow conditions.

Another feature of laminar flow when it is fully developed is that the gas in the center of the tube moves twice as fast as the average velocity. Thus, a spike of rapidly moving gas travels down the axis of the tube (Figure 7.12A). This changing velocity across the diameter of the tube is known as the *velocity profile*.

Turbulent flow has different properties. Here pressure is not proportional to flow rate but, approximately, to its square: $P = KV^2$. In addition, the viscosity of the gas becomes relatively unimportant, but an increase in gas density increases the pressure drop for a given flow. Turbulent flow does not have the high axial flow velocity that is characteristic of laminar flow.

Whether flow will be laminar or turbulent depends to a large extent on the Reynolds number, Re. This is given by:

$$Re = \frac{2rvd}{n}$$

where d is density, v average velocity, r radius, and n viscosity. Because density and velocity are in the numerator, and viscosity is in the denominator, the expression gives the ratio of inertial to viscous forces. In straight, smooth tubes, turbulence is probable when the Reynolds number exceeds 2,000. The expression shows that turbulence is most likely to occur when the velocity of flow is high and the tube diameter is large (for a given velocity). Note also that a low-density gas such as helium tends to produce less turbulence.

In such a complicated system of tubes as the bronchial tree with its many branches, changes in caliber, and irregular wall surfaces, the application of the above principles is difficult. In practice, for laminar flow to occur, the entrance conditions of the tube are critical. If eddy formation occurs upstream at a branch point, this disturbance is carried downstream some distance before it disappears. Thus, in a rapidly branching system such as the lung, fully developed laminar flow (Figure 7.12A) probably only occurs in the very small airways where the Reynolds numbers are very low (~1 in terminal bronchioles). In most of the bronchial tree, flow is transitional (*B*), whereas true turbulence may occur in the trachea, especially on exercise when flow velocities are high. In general, driving pressure is determined by both the flow rate and its square: $P = K_1\dot{V} + K_2\dot{V}^2$.

Laminar and Turbulent Flow

- In laminar flow, resistance is inversely proportional to the fourth power of the radius of the tube.
- In laminar flow, the velocity profile shows a central spike of fast gas.
- Turbulent flow is most likely to occur at high Reynolds numbers, that is, when inertial forces dominate over viscous forces.

Measurement of Airway Resistance

Airway resistance is the pressure difference between the alveoli and the mouth divided by a flow rate (Figure 7.12). Mouth pressure is easily measured with a manometer. Alveolar pressure can be deduced from measurements made in a body plethysmograph. More information on this technique is given in Chapter 10.

Pressures During the Breathing Cycle

Suppose we measure the pressures in the intrapleural and alveolar spaces during normal breathing at rest.[†] **Figure 7.13** shows that before inspiration begins, the intrapleural pressure is −5 cm water because of the elastic recoil of the lung (compare Figures 7.3 and 7.10). Alveolar pressure is zero (atmospheric) because with no airflow, there is no pressure drop along the airways. However, for inspiratory flow to occur, the alveolar pressure falls, thus establishing the driving pressure (Figure 7.12). Indeed, the extent of the fall depends on the flow and the resistance of the airways. In normal subjects, the change in alveolar pressure is only 1 cm water or so, but in patients with airway obstruction, it may be many times that.

[†]Intrapleural pressure can be estimated by placing a balloon catheter in the esophagus.

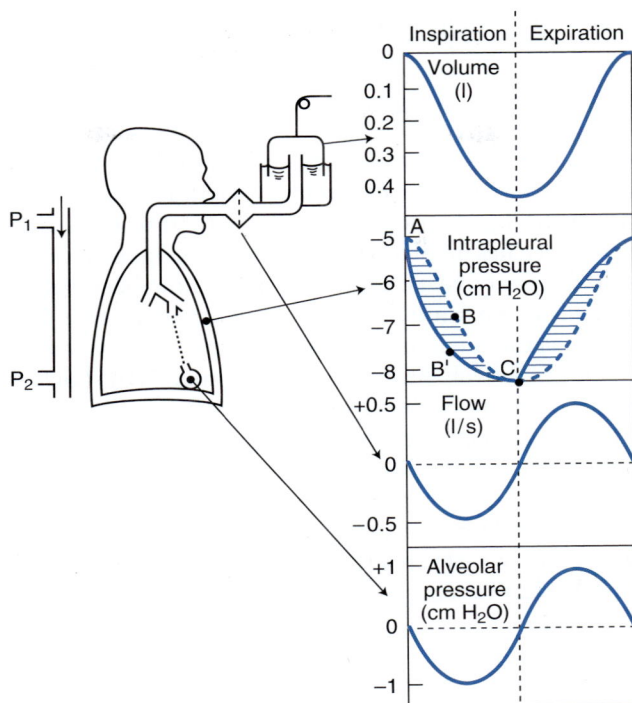

Figure 7.13. Pressures during the breathing cycle. If there was no airway resistance, alveolar pressure would remain at zero and intrapleural pressure would follow the *broken line* ABC, which is determined by the elastic recoil of the lung. The fall in alveolar pressure is responsible for the *hatched* portion of intrapleural pressure (see text).

Intrapleural pressure falls during inspiration for two reasons. First, as the lung expands, its elastic recoil increases (Figure 7.3). This alone would cause the intrapleural pressure to move along the broken line ABC. In addition, however, the reduction in alveolar pressure causes a further fall in intrapleural pressure,[‡] represented by the hatched area, so that the actual path is AB'C. Thus, the vertical distance between lines ABC and AB'C reflects the alveolar pressure at any instant. As an equation of pressures (mouth − intrapleural) = (mouth − alveolar) + (alveolar − intrapleural).

On expiration, similar changes occur. Now intrapleural pressure is *less* negative than it would be in the absence of airway resistance because alveolar pressure is positive. Indeed, with a forced expiration, intrapleural pressure goes above zero.

Note that the shape of the alveolar pressure tracing is similar to that of flow. Indeed, they would be identical if the airway resistance remained constant during the cycle. Also, the intrapleural pressure curve ABC would have

---

[‡]There is also a contribution made by tissue resistance, which is considered later in this chapter.

the same shape as the volume tracing if the lung compliance remained constant.

Chief Site of Airway Resistance

As the airways penetrate toward the periphery of the lung, they become more numerous but much narrower (see Figures 1.3 and 1.5). Based on Poiseuille's equation with its (radius)^4 term, it would be natural to think that the major part of the resistance lies in the very narrow airways. Indeed, this was thought to be the case for many years. However, it has now been shown by direct measurements of the pressure drop along the bronchial tree that the major site of resistance is the medium-sized bronchi and that the very small bronchioles contribute relatively little resistance. **Figure 7.14** shows that most of the pressure drop occurs in the airways up to the seventh generation. Less than 20% can be attributed to airways less than 2 mm in diameter (about generation 8). The reason for this apparent paradox is the prodigious number of small airways.

The fact that the peripheral airways contribute so little resistance is important in the detection of early airway disease. Because they constitute a "silent zone," it is probable that considerable small airway disease can be present

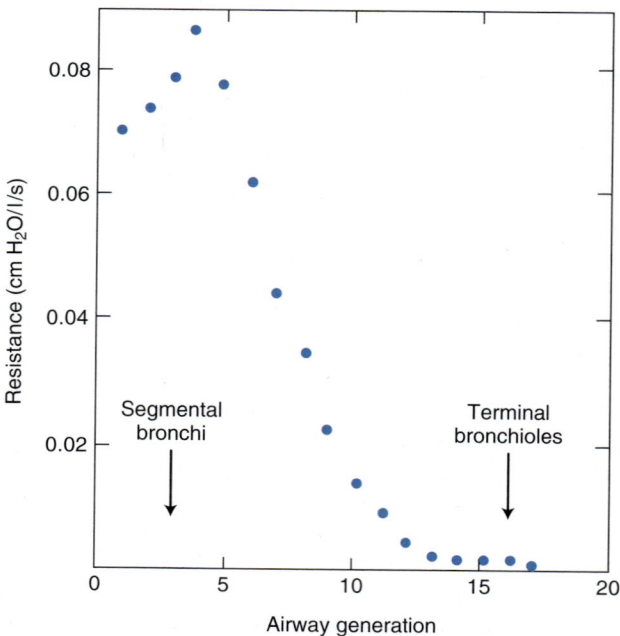

Figure 7.14. Location of the chief site of airway resistance. Note that the intermediate-sized bronchi contribute most of the resistance and that relatively little is located in the very small airways. (Redrawn from Pedley TJ, et al. *Respir Physiol.* 1970;9:387.)

before the commonly used tests of pulmonary function can detect an abnormality. This issue is considered in more detail in Chapter 10.

Factors Determining Airway Resistance

Lung volume has an important effect on airway resistance. Like the extra-alveolar blood vessels (Figure 4.2), the bronchi are supported by the radial traction of the surrounding lung tissue, and their caliber is increased as the lung expands (compare Figure 4.6). **Figure 7.15** shows that as lung volume is reduced, airway resistance rises rapidly. If the reciprocal of resistance (conductance) is plotted against lung volume, an approximately linear relationship is obtained.

At very low lung volumes, the small airways may close completely, especially at the bottom of the lung, where the lung is less well expanded (Figure 7.9). Patients who have increased airway resistance often breathe at high lung volumes; this helps to reduce their airway resistance.

Contraction of *bronchial smooth muscle* narrows the airways and increases airway resistance. This may occur reflexly through the stimulation of receptors in the trachea and large bronchi by irritants such as cigarette smoke. Motor innervation is by the vagus nerve. The tone of the smooth muscle is under the control of the autonomic nervous system. β-adrenergic receptors are of two types: β_1 receptors occur principally in the heart, whereas β_2 receptors relax smooth muscle in the bronchi, blood vessels, and uterus. Stimulation of adrenergic receptors by, for example, epinephrine, causes bronchodilatation. Selective β_2-adrenergic agonists, typically administered via the inhaled route, are extensively used in the treatments of asthma and chronic obstructive pulmonary disease (COPD).

Parasympathetic activity causes bronchoconstriction, as does acetylcholine. Antimuscarinic agents are used in COPD and, occasionally, asthma. A fall of Pco_2 in alveolar gas causes an increase in airway resistance, apparently

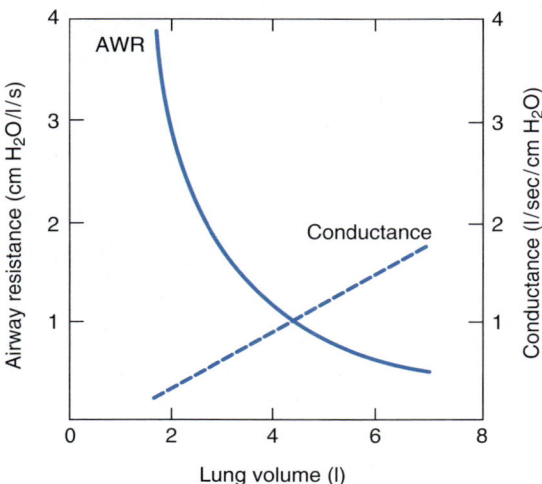

Figure 7.15. Variation of airway resistance (AWR) with lung volume. If the reciprocal of airway resistance (conductance) is plotted, the graph is a straight line. (Redrawn from Briscoe WA, Dubois AB. *J Clin Invest.* 1958;37:1279.)

as a result of a direct action on bronchiolar smooth muscle. The injection of histamine into the pulmonary artery causes constriction of smooth muscle located in the alveolar ducts.

The *density and viscosity* of the inspired gas affect the resistance offered to flow. The resistance is increased during a deep dive because the increased pressure raises gas density. This change in resistance can be mitigated by breathing a helium-O_2 mixture (heliox, Chapter 9). The fact that changes in density rather than viscosity have such an influence on resistance is evidence that flow is not purely laminar in the medium-sized airways, where the main site of resistance lies (Figure 7.14).

Airway Resistance

- Highest in the medium-sized bronchi; low in the very small airways.
- Decreases as lung volume rises because the airways are pulled open.
- Bronchial smooth muscle is controlled by the autonomic nervous system; stimulation of β_2-adrenergic receptors causes bronchodilatation.
- Breathing a dense gas, as when diving, increases resistance.

Dynamic Compression of Airways

Suppose a subject inspires to total lung capacity and then exhales as hard as possible to RV. We can record a *flow-volume curve* like *A* in **Figure 7.16**, which shows that flow rises very rapidly to a high value (peak expiratory flow) but then declines over most of expiration. A remarkable feature of this flow-volume envelope is that it is virtually impossible to penetrate it. In other words, no matter whether we start exhaling slowly and then accelerate, as in B, or make a less forceful expiration, as in C, the descending portion of the flow-volume curve takes virtually the same path. Thus, something powerful is limiting expiratory flow, and over most of the lung volume, flow rate is independent of effort.

We can get more information about this curious state of affairs by plotting the data in another way, as shown in **Figure 7.17**. For this, the subject takes a *series* of maximal inspirations (or expirations) and then exhales (or inhales) fully with varying degrees of effort. If the flow rates and intrapleural pressures are plotted at the *same* lung volume for each expiration and inspiration, so-called *isovolume pressure-flow curves* can be obtained. It can be seen that at high lung volumes, the expiratory flow rate continues to increase with effort, as might be expected. However, at mid or low volumes, the flow rate reaches a plateau and cannot be increased with further increase in intrapleural pressure. Under these conditions, flow is therefore *effort-independent*.

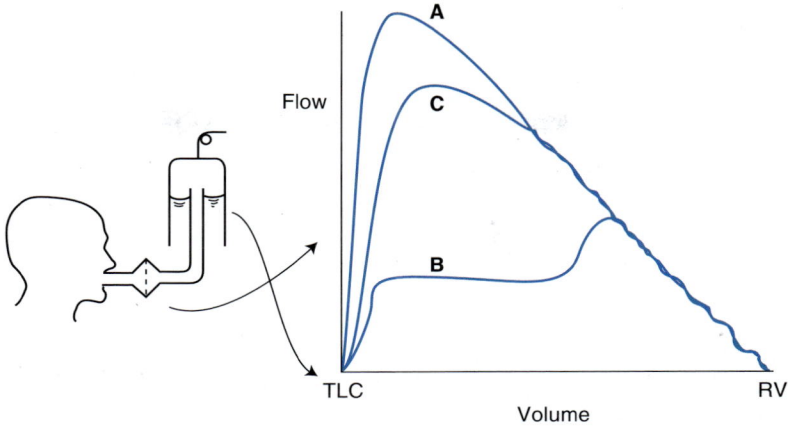

Figure 7.16. Flow-volume curves. In **(A)**, a maximal inspiration was followed by a forced expiration. In **(B)**, expiration was initially slow and then forced. In **(C)**, expiratory effort was submaximal. In all three, the descending portions of the curves are almost superimposed.

The reason for this remarkable behavior is compression of the airways by intrathoracic pressure, referred to as dynamic airway compression. **Figure 7.18** shows schematically the forces acting across an airway within the lung. The pressure outside the airway is shown as intrapleural, although this

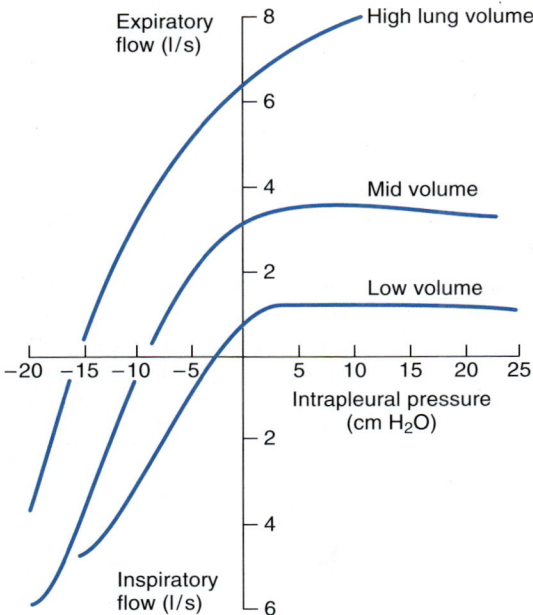

Figure 7.17. Isovolume pressure-flow curves drawn for three lung volumes. Each of these was obtained from a series of forced expirations and inspirations (see text). Note that at the high lung volume, a rise in intrapleural pressure (obtained by increasing expiratory effort) results in a greater expiratory flow. However, at mid and low volumes, flow becomes independent of effort after a certain intrapleural pressure has been exceeded. (Redrawn from Fry DL, Hyatt RE. *Am J Med.* 1960;29:672.)

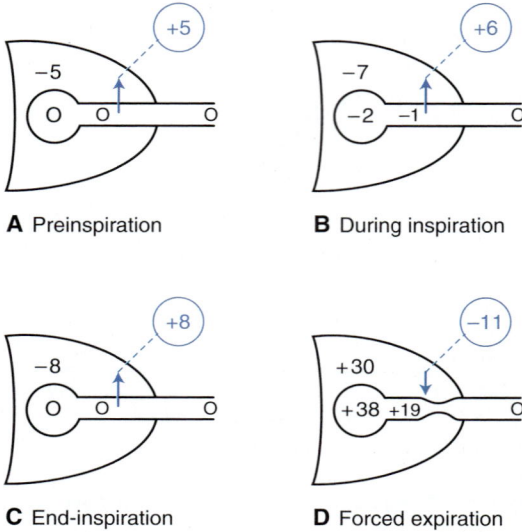

A Preinspiration

B During inspiration

C End-inspiration

D Forced expiration

Figure 7.18 A–D. Scheme showing why airways are compressed during forced expiration. Note that the pressure difference across the airway is holding it open, except during a forced expiration. See text for details.

is an oversimplification. In A, before inspiration has begun, airway pressure is everywhere zero (no flow), and because intrapleural pressure is −5 cm water, there is a pressure of 5 cm water (i.e., a transmural pressure) holding the airway open. As inspiration starts (B), both intrapleural and alveolar pressure fall by 2 cm water (same lung volume as *A*, and tissue resistance is neglected) and flow begins. Because of the pressure drop along the airway, the pressure inside is −1 cm water, and there is a pressure of 6 cm water holding the airway open. At end-inspiration (C), again flow is zero, and there is an airway transmural pressure of 8 cm water.

Finally, at the onset of forced expiration (D), both intrapleural pressure and alveolar pressure increase by 38 cm water (same lung volume as C). Because of the pressure drop along the airway as flow begins, there is now a pressure of −11 cm water, which tends to *close* the airway. Airway compression occurs, and the downstream pressure limiting flow becomes the pressure outside the airway, or intrapleural pressure. Thus, the effective driving pressure becomes alveolar minus intrapleural pressure. This is the same Starling resistor mechanism that limits the blood flow in zone 2 of the lung, where venous pressure becomes unimportant just as mouth pressure does here (Figures 4.8 and 4.9). Note that if intrapleural pressure is raised further by increased muscular effort in an attempt to expel gas, the effective driving pressure is unaltered because the difference between alveolar and intrapleural pressure is determined by lung volume. Thus, flow is independent of effort.

Maximal flow decreases with lung volume (Figure 7.16) because the difference between alveolar and intrapleural pressure decreases and the airways become narrower. Note also that flow is independent of the resistance of the airways downstream of the point of collapse, called the *equal pressure point*. As expiration progresses, the equal pressure point moves distally, deeper into the lung. This occurs because the resistance of the airways rises as lung volume falls, and therefore, the pressure within the airways falls more rapidly with distance from the alveoli.

Dynamic Compression of Airways

- Limits air flow in healthy subjects during a forced expiration.
- May occur in diseased lungs at relatively low expiratory flow rates, thus reducing exercise ability.
- During dynamic compression, flow is determined by alveolar pressure minus intrapleural pressure (not mouth pressure) and is therefore independent of effort.
- Is exaggerated in diseases such as emphysema due to reduced lung elastic recoil and loss of radial traction on airways.

Several factors exaggerate this flow-limiting mechanism. One is any increase in resistance of the peripheral airways because that magnifies the pressure drop along them and thus decreases the intrabronchial pressure during expiration (19 cm water in D). Another is a low lung volume because that reduces the driving pressure (alveolar-intrapleural). This driving pressure is also reduced if recoil pressure is reduced, as in emphysema. Also in this disease, radial traction on the airways is reduced, and they are compressed more readily. Indeed, while this type of flow limitation is seen only during forced expiration in healthy subjects, it may occur during the expirations of normal breathing in patients with severe obstructive lung disease.

Forced Expiration Test

In the pulmonary function laboratory, information about airway resistance in a patient with lung disease can be obtained by measuring the flow rate during a maximal expiration. **Figure 7.19** shows the spirometer record obtained when a subject inspires maximally and then exhales as hard and as completely as he or she can. The volume exhaled in the first second is called the forced expiratory volume, or $FEV_{1.0}$, and the total volume exhaled is the forced vital capacity or FVC (this is often slightly less than the vital capacity measured on a slow exhalation as in Figure 2.2). Normally, the $FEV_{1.0}$ is about 80% of the FVC, although the ratio does decrease with normal aging.

In disease, two general patterns can be distinguished. In *restrictive* diseases such as pulmonary fibrosis, in which the primary problem is expanding the

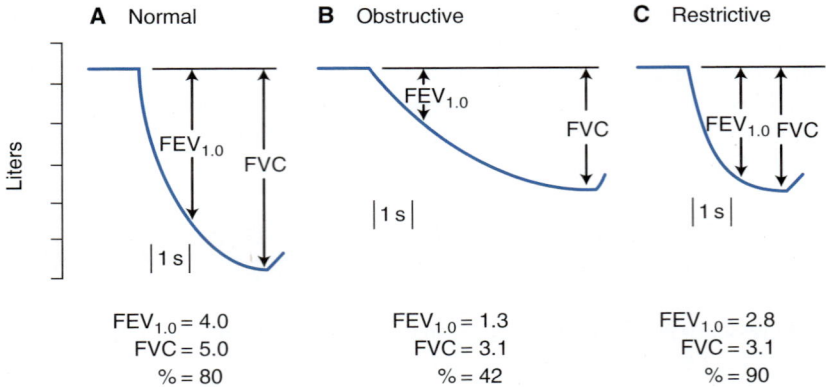

A Normal **B** Obstructive **C** Restrictive

FEV$_{1.0}$ = 4.0
FVC = 5.0
% = 80

FEV$_{1.0}$ = 1.3
FVC = 3.1
% = 42

FEV$_{1.0}$ = 2.8
FVC = 3.1
% = 90

Figure 7.19. Measurement of forced expiratory volume (FEV$_{1.0}$) and forced vital capacity (FVC).

respiratory system on inhalation, both FEV$_{1.0}$ and FVC are reduced, but characteristically the FEV$_{1.0}$/FVC% is normal or increased. In *obstructive* diseases such as COPD or bronchial asthma, where the primary problem is obstruction to airflow on exhalation, the FEV$_{1.0}$ is reduced much more than is the FVC, giving a low FEV$_{1.0}$/FVC%. A mixed restrictive and obstructive pattern can also be seen, although additional measurements of lung volume are necessary to identify such a pattern (Chapter 10).

A related measurement is the *forced expiratory flow rate*, or FEF$_{25\%-75\%}$, which is the average flow rate measured over the middle half of the expiration. Generally, this is closely related to the FEV$_{1.0}$, although occasionally it is reduced when the FEV$_{1.0}$ is normal. Sometimes other indices are also measured from the forced expiration curve. Further details are provided in Chapter 10.

Forced Expiration Test

- Measures the FEV$_{1.0}$ and the FVC
- A simple test used in the evaluation of patients with chronic dyspnea
- Distinguishes between obstructive and restrictive disease

ADDITIONAL CAUSES OF UNEVEN VENTILATION

The cause of the regional differences in ventilation in the lung was discussed earlier. Apart from these topographical differences, there is some additional inequality of ventilation at any given vertical level in the normal lung, which may be exaggerated in many diseases.

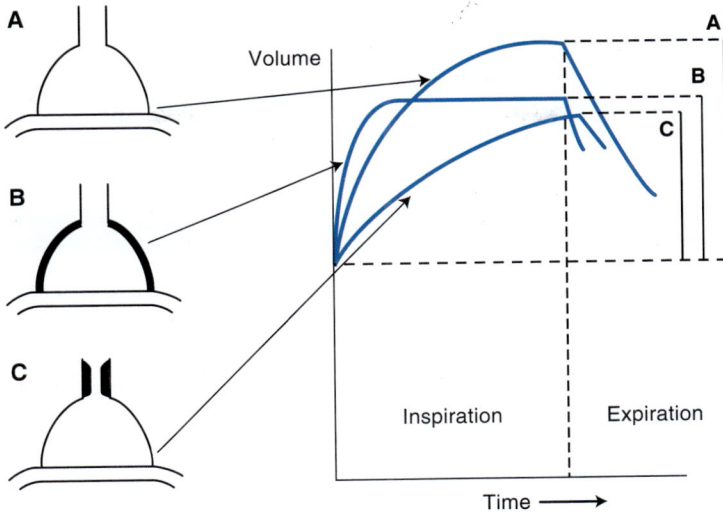

Figure 7.20. Effects of decreased compliance **(B)** and increased airway resistance **(C)** on ventilation of lung units compared with normal **(A)**. In both instances, the inspired volume is abnormally low. (Modified from West JB. *Ventilation/Blood Flow and Gas Exchange.* 5th ed. Oxford, UK: Blackwell; 1990.)

One mechanism of uneven ventilation is shown in **Figure 7.20**. If we regard a lung unit (Figure 2.1) as an elastic chamber connected to the atmosphere by a tube, the amount of ventilation depends on the compliance of the chamber and the resistance of the tube. In Figure 7.20, unit A has a normal distensibility and airway resistance. It can be seen that its volume change on inspiration is large and rapid so that it is complete before expiration for the whole lung begins (*vertical dashed line*). By contrast, unit B has a low compliance, and its change in volume is rapid but small. Finally, unit C has a large airway resistance so that inspiration is slow and not complete before the lung has begun to exhale. Note that the shorter the time available for inspiration (fast breathing rate), the smaller the inspired volume. Such a unit is said to have a long *time constant*, the value of which is given by the product of the compliance and resistance. Thus, inequality of ventilation can result from alterations in either local distensibility or airway resistance, and the pattern of inequality will depend on the frequency of breathing.

Another possible mechanism of uneven ventilation is incomplete diffusion within the airways of the respiratory zone (Figure 1.4). We saw in Chapter 1 that the dominant mechanism of ventilation of the lung beyond the terminal bronchioles is diffusion. Normally, this occurs so rapidly that differences in gas concentration in the acinus are virtually abolished within a fraction of a second. However, if there is dilation of the airways in the region of the respiratory bronchioles, as in some diseases, the distance to be covered by diffusion may be enormously increased. In these circumstances, inspired gas is not distributed uniformly within the respiratory zone because of uneven ventilation *along* the lung units.

TISSUE RESISTANCE

When the lung and chest wall are moved, some pressure is required to overcome the viscous forces within the tissues as they slide over each other. Thus, part of the hatched portion of Figure 7.13 should be attributed to these tissue forces. However, this tissue resistance is only about 20% of the total (tissue + airway) resistance in young normal subjects, although it may increase in some diseases. This total resistance is sometimes called *pulmonary resistance* to distinguish it from airway resistance.

WORK OF BREATHING

Work is required to move the lung and chest wall. In this context, it is most convenient to measure work as pressure × volume.

Work Done on the Lung

This can be illustrated on a pressure-volume curve (**Figure 7.21**). During inspiration, the intrapleural pressure follows the curve ABC, and the work done on the lung is given by the area 0ABCD0. Of this, the trapezoid 0AECD0 represents the work required to overcome the elastic forces, and the hatched area ABCEA represents the work overcoming viscous

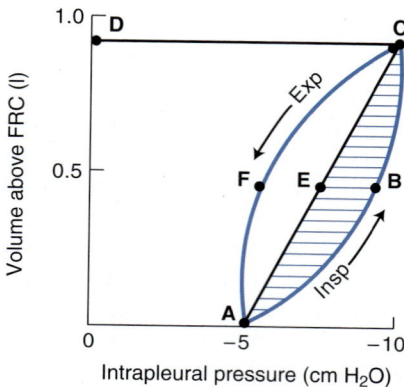

Figure 7.21. Pressure-volume curve of the lung showing the inspiratory work done overcoming elastic forces (*area 0AECD0*) and viscous forces (*hatched area ABCEA*).

(airway and tissue) resistance (compare Figure 7.13). The higher the airway resistance or the inspiratory flow rate, the more negative (rightward) would be the intrapleural pressure excursion between A and C and the larger the area.

On expiration, the area AECFA is work required to overcome airway (+ tissue) resistance. Normally, this falls within the trapezoid 0AECD0, and thus, this work can be accomplished by the energy stored in the expanded elastic structures and released during a passive expiration. The difference between the areas AECFA and 0AECD0 represents the work dissipated as heat.

The higher the breathing rate, the faster the flow rates and the larger the viscous work area ABCEA. On the other hand, the larger the tidal volume, the larger the elastic work area 0AECD0. It is of interest that patients who have a reduced compliance (stiff lungs) tend to take small rapid breaths, whereas patients with severe airway obstruction sometimes breathe slowly. These patterns tend to reduce the work done on the lungs.

Total Work of Breathing

The total work done moving the lung and chest wall is difficult to measure, although estimates have been obtained by artificially ventilating paralyzed patients (or "completely relaxed" volunteers) in an iron-lung type of ventilator. Alternatively, the total work can be calculated by measuring the O_2 cost of breathing and assuming a figure for the efficiency as given by

$$\text{Efficiency } \% = \frac{\text{Work required to ventilate the lung}}{\text{Total energy expended (or } O_2 \text{cost)}} \times 100$$

The efficiency is believed to be about 5% to 10%.

The O_2 cost of quiet breathing is extremely small, being less than 5% of the total resting O_2 consumption. With voluntary hyperventilation, it is possible to increase this to 30%. In patients with obstructive lung disease, the O_2 cost of breathing may limit their exercise ability.

MECHANICS OF POSITIVE PRESSURE VENTILATION

As noted earlier, spontaneously breathing patients generate a driving pressure by increasing the size of the thorax, thereby lowering airway pressure below atmospheric pressure. Patients who develop severe respiratory failure often require mechanical ventilatory support. With modern mechanical ventilators, driving pressure is primarily established by raising the pressure at

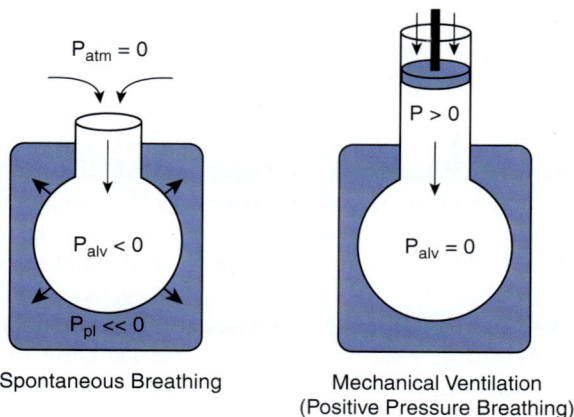

Figure 7.22.
Comparison of spontaneous and positive pressure breathing. At the start of inhalation in spontaneous breathing, alveolar pressure (P_{alv}) falls below atmospheric pressure. At the start of inhalation in mechanical ventilation, pressure at the mouth is raised above alveolar pressure.

Spontaneous Breathing

Mechanical Ventilation
(Positive Pressure Breathing)

the mouth (**Figure 7.22**).[§] This intervention, referred to as positive pressure ventilation, can be done using one of several different methods, or modes, of ventilatory support and markedly reduces the work of breathing performed by the patient. The principles of compliance, airway resistance, and regional differences in ventilation still apply with mechanical ventilation, and patients can even develop dynamic airway compression depending on the ventilator settings and aspects of their pulmonary pathology. The topic of mechanical ventilation is complicated and beyond the scope of this book. Further information can be found in Chapter 10 of *West's Pulmonary Pathophysiology*, 9th edition.

KEY CONCEPTS

1. Inspiration is active, but expiration during rest is passive. The most important muscle of respiration is the diaphragm.

2. The pressure-volume curve of the lung is nonlinear and shows hysteresis. The recoil pressure of the lung is attributable to both its elastic tissue and the surface tension of the alveolar lining layer.

3. Pulmonary surfactant is a phospholipid produced by type II alveolar epithelial cells. Lack of surfactant, as occurs in some premature infants, leads to low compliance and respiratory failure.

[§]In many modes of mechanical ventilation, patients can still initiate breaths by contracting the diaphragm and lowering airway pressure slightly at the start of inhalation. The majority of the driving pressure, however, is generated by raising the pressure at the mouth.

4. The chest wall is elastic like the lung but normally tends to expand. At FRC, the inward recoil of the lung and the outward recoil of the chest wall are balanced.

5. In laminar flow, as exists in small airways, the resistance is inversely proportional to the fourth power of the radius.

6. Lung airway resistance is reduced by increasing lung volume and by stimulation of β_2-adrenergic receptors.

7. Dynamic compression of the airways during a forced expiration results in flow that is effort independent. The driving pressure is then alveolar minus intrapleural pressure. In patients with chronic obstructive lung disease, dynamic compression can occur during mild exercise, thus causing severe disability.

CLINICAL VIGNETTE

A 30-year-old man presents to the emergency department with increasing shortness of breath, chest tightness, and wheezing over the past 2 days. Since the age of 5, he has had asthma, a disease associated with episodic narrowing of the airways. He notes that his symptoms are typically exacerbated by exercise, particularly when done outside in the winter months. On examination, he appears anxious, is using accessory muscles of respiration, and has musical sounds heard throughout both lungs on auscultation. A chest radiograph shows hyperinflated lungs but no focal opacities.

- If one of the small airways in his lung has its diameter reduced by 50%, what is the increase in resistance of this airway?
- What changes would you expect to see in alveolar pressure during inspiration and expiration compared with a normal person?
- How does the observed hyperinflation affect airway resistance during his asthma exacerbation?
- What happens to lung compliance as a result of the overinflation?

QUESTIONS

For each question, choose the one best answer.

1. Maximum inspiratory and expiratory pressures are measured in a patient undergoing evaluation for dyspnea on exertion. The results are displayed in the table below.

Test	Predicted Value	Measured Value	Percent Predicted
Inspiratory pressure (cm H_2O)	120	115	96
Expiratory pressure (cm H_2O)	110	45	41

Weakness of which of the following muscle groups could contribute to the pattern of results observed during this testing?
A. Diaphragm
B. External intercostals
C. Rectus abdominis
D. Scalene
E. Sternocleidomastoid

2. The figure below displays the pressure-volume relationship measured from two different sets of excised lungs, Lung A and Lung B.

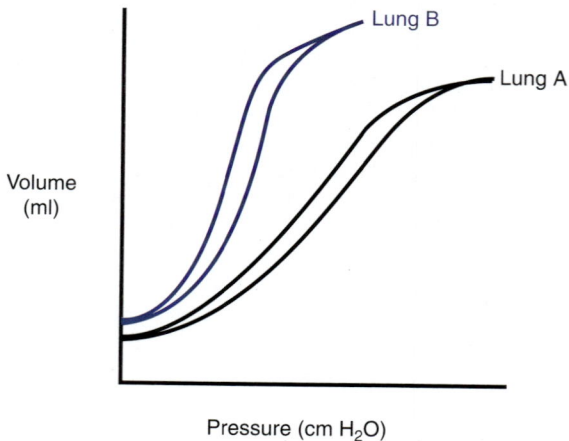

Which of the following factors could account for the position of the pressure-volume relationship for Lung B relative to Lung A
A. Atelectasis of basilar lung segments
B. Decreased airway diameter throughout the lung
C. Decreased number of elastic fibers
D. Decreased surfactant concentration in the alveolar space
E. Increased amount of fibrous tissue

3. Two bubbles have the same surface tension, but bubble X has three times the diameter of bubble Y. The ratio of the pressure in bubble X to that in bubble Y is:
A. 0.3:1
B. 0.9:1
C. 1:1
D. 3:1
E. 9:1

4. Detailed measurements of ventilation, perfusion, and intrapleural pressure are made in the upright position in an astronaut at sea level and again following arrival at the International Space Station. When compared to the sea level values, which of the following would you expect to see following arrival at the space station?
A. Decreased perfusion at the lung apex
B. Increased resting volume at the lung base
C. Increased variability in perfusion between the base and apex
D. Increased variability in ventilation between the base and apex
E. Less negative intrapleural pressure at the lung base

5. A previously healthy 24-year-old man suffered a complete transection of his spinal cord in a motorcycle collision. While recuperating from his injury, he undergoes a variety of assessments of his pulmonary function. On fluoroscopy, the diaphragm descends into the abdomen during inhalation at rest. His maximum expiratory pressure is 25% of that predicted for his age and size, and the strength of his cough is markedly reduced. Based on this pattern of results, which of the following is the highest level at which his spinal cord could be transected?
A. C2
B. C4
C. C6
D. C8
E. T2

6. Which of the following statements best characterizes the state of respiratory system function at the point marked by the arrow in the spirogram below?

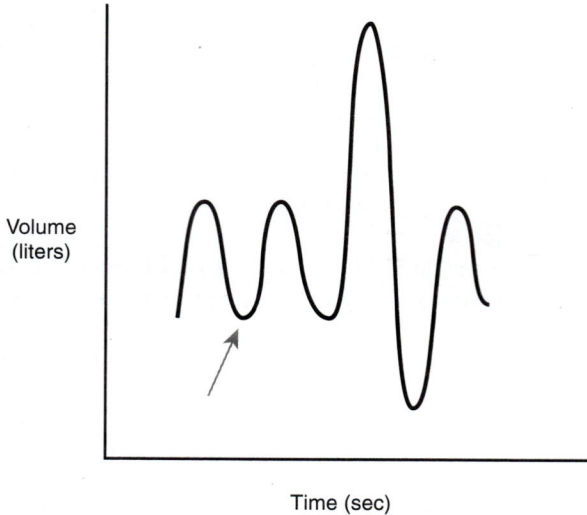

A. Airway resistance is at its minimum value.
B. Elastic recoil of the lung is balanced by the elastic recoil of the chest wall.
C. Intrapleural pressure is greater than atmospheric pressure.
D. Resistance associated with extra-alveolar vessels is at its minimum value.
E. Transmural pressure across the wall of the alveolus is at its maximum value.

7. The figure below depicts inspiratory and expiratory *airflow* during spontaneous breathing at rest in a healthy individual. Points A, B, and C denote different time points during the single respiratory cycle. Which of the following statement is true regarding the time points depicted in this figure?

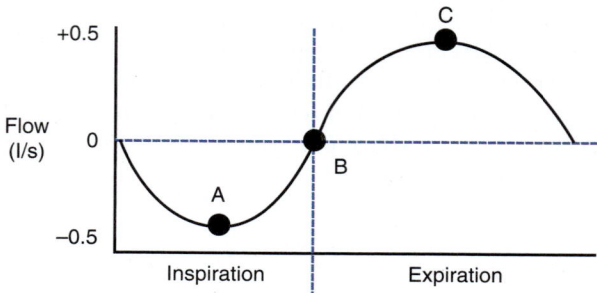

A. Airway resistance is lowest at point B.
B. Alveolar pressure is positive at point A.
C. Driving pressure for airflow is greatest at point B.
D. Driving pressure for airflow is smallest at point C.
E. Intrapleural pressure is at its most negative value at point C.

8. An anesthetized patient with paralyzed respiratory muscles and normal lungs is ventilated by positive pressure. If the anesthesiologist increases the lung volume 2 liters above FRC and holds the lung at that volume for 5 s, the most likely combination of pressures (in cm H_2O) is likely to be:

Choice	Mouth	Alveolar	Intrapleural
A.	0	0	−5
B.	0	+10	−5
C.	+10	+10	−10
D.	+20	+20	+5
E.	+10	0	−10

9. Two lung units, A and B, are inflated from the same starting volume with equal driving pressures. The same change in volume is achieved in each unit and they have the same transpulmonary pressure at the end of inflation. Lung unit B required a longer amount of time to achieve the desired volume change than lung unit A. Which of the following characteristics of lung unit B could account for the differences relative to lung unit A?
    A. Fibrosis
    B. Increased elastic fibers
    C. Increased parasympathetic activity
    D. Pneumonia
    E. Pulmonary edema

10. During an asthma exacerbation, an 18-month-old child develops airway inflammation that results in 1 mm increase in thickness of the airway mucosa around the entire circumference of the lower airways. By how much would airway resistance change in an airway whose lumen was 4 mm in diameter prior to this asthma exacerbation?
    A. 1/2
    B. 2
    C. 4
    D. 16
    E. 64

11. A 30-year-old woman gives birth to a baby girl at only 29 weeks of gestation. Shortly following birth, the baby develops increasing difficulty with breathing and hypoxemia and requires mechanical ventilation. The respiratory therapist notes that her airway resistance

is normal but her compliance is lower than expected. Which of the following factors is likely responsible for respiratory failure in this case?
A. Decreased alveolar macrophage activity
B. Decreased alveolar surfactant concentration
C. Increased airway mucous production
D. Increased airway smooth muscle contraction
E. Increased edema of the airway walls

12. A 20-year-old man is asked to perform spirometry as part of a research project. On the first attempt, he deliberately exhales with only 50% of his maximum effort. On the second attempt, he exhales and gives 100% of his maximum effort. If you analyzed the data from the second attempt, which pattern of changes in peak expiratory flow and flow in the latter part of expiration would you expect to see compared with the first attempt?

Answer Choice	Peak Expiratory Flow	End-Expiratory Flow
A.	No change	No change
B.	Decreased	No change
C.	Increased	Increased
D.	Increased	No change
E.	No change	Increased

13. A 69-year-old man with a long history of smoking complains of worsening dyspnea over a 12-month period. On examination, he is noted to have diffuse expiratory wheezes and a long expiratory phase. A chest radiograph is performed and demonstrates very large lung volumes, flat diaphragms, and increased lucency of the lung, consistent with emphysema. Which of the following patterns would you expect to see on a forced expiration test (spirometry) in this patient?

Answer Choice	$FEV_{1.0}$	FVC	$FEV_{1.0}/FVC$
A.	Normal	Normal	Normal
B.	Decreased	Normal	Normal
C.	Decreased	Decreased	Normal
D.	Decreased	Decreased	Decreased
E.	Normal	Decreased	Normal

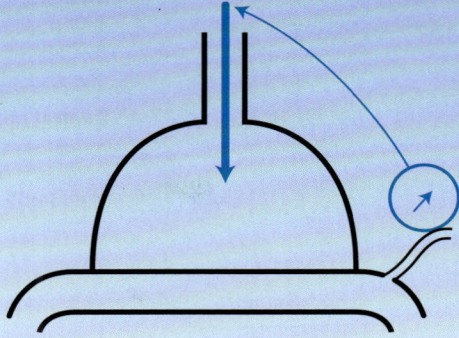

Control of Ventilation

How Gas Exchange Is Regulated

8

- **Central Controller**
  Brainstem
  Cortex
  Other Parts of the Brain

- **Effectors**

- **Sensors**
  Central Chemoreceptors
  Peripheral Chemoreceptors
  Lung Receptors
  Other Receptors

- **Integrated Responses**
  Response to Carbon Dioxide
  Response to Oxygen
  Response to pH
  Response to Exercise

- **Ventilatory Control During Sleep**

- **Abnormal Patterns of Breathing During Sleep**

We have seen that the chief function of the lung is to exchange O_2 and CO_2 between blood and gas and thus maintain normal P_{O_2} and P_{CO_2} in the arterial blood. In this chapter, we shall see that in spite of widely differing demands for O_2 uptake and CO_2 output made by the body, the arterial P_{O_2} and P_{CO_2} are normally kept within close limits. In this chapter, we describe how the careful control of ventilation makes this remarkable regulation of gas exchange possible. First, we look at the central controller and then the various chemoreceptors and other receptors that provide it with information. The integrated responses to carbon dioxide, hypoxia, and pH are then described. At the end of this chapter, the reader should be able to:

- Describe the location and function of the various elements of the central controller
- Describe the primary stimuli and responses of the central and peripheral chemoreceptors
- Outline the mechanisms by which different pulmonary receptors modulate the ventilatory pattern
- Predict changes in ventilation in response to changes in P_{O_2}, P_{CO_2}, pH, and exercise
- Identify an individual with Cheyne-Stokes respiration

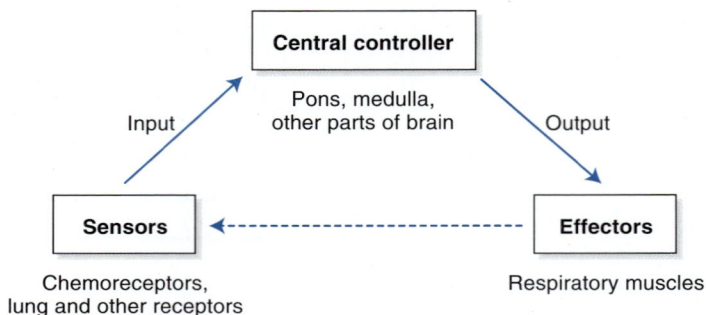

Figure 8.1. Basic elements of the respiratory control system. Information from various sensors is fed to the central controller, the output of which goes to the respiratory muscles. By changing ventilation, the respiratory muscles reduce perturbations of the sensors (negative feedback).

The three basic elements of the respiratory control system (**Figure 8.1**) are as follows:

1. *Sensors* that gather information and feed it to the
2. *Central controller* in the brain, which coordinates the information and, in turn, sends impulses to the
3. *Effectors* (respiratory muscles), which cause ventilation.

We shall see that increased activity of the effectors generally ultimately decreases the sensory input to the brain, for example, by decreasing the arterial P_{CO_2}. This is an example of negative feedback

CENTRAL CONTROLLER

The normal automatic process of breathing originates in impulses that come from the brainstem. The cortex can override these centers if voluntary control is desired. Additional input from other parts of the brain occurs under certain conditions.

Brainstem

The periodic nature of inspiration and expiration is controlled by the central pattern generator that comprises groups of neurons located in the pons and medulla. Three main groups of neurons are recognized.

1. *Medullary respiratory center* in the reticular formation of the medulla beneath the floor of the fourth ventricle. There is a group of cells in the ventrolateral region known as the *Pre-Botzinger complex* that appears to be

essential for the generation of the respiratory rhythm. In addition, a group of cells in the dorsal region of the medulla (*Dorsal Respiratory Group*) is chiefly associated with inspiration, and another group (*Ventral Respiratory Group*) is associated with expiration. These groups of cells have the property of intrinsic periodic firing and are responsible for the basic rhythm of ventilation. When all known afferent stimuli have been abolished, these cells generate repetitive bursts of action potentials that result in nervous impulses going to the diaphragm and other inspiratory muscles. The intrinsic rhythm pattern of the inspiratory area starts with a latent period of several seconds during which there is no activity. Action potentials then begin to appear, increasing in a crescendo over the next few seconds. During this time, inspiratory muscle activity becomes stronger in a "ramp"-type pattern. Finally, the inspiratory action potentials cease, and inspiratory muscle tone falls to its preinspiratory level.

The inspiratory ramp can be "turned off" prematurely by inhibiting impulses from the *pneumotaxic center* (see below). In this way, inspiration is shortened and, as a consequence, the breathing rate increases. The output of the inspiratory cells is further modulated by impulses from the vagus and glossopharyngeal nerves. Indeed, these terminate in the tractus solitarius, which is situated close to the inspiratory area.

The *expiratory area* is quiescent during normal quiet breathing because ventilation is achieved by active contraction of inspiratory muscles (primarily the diaphragm), followed by passive relaxation of the chest wall to its equilibrium position (Chapter 7). However, in more forceful breathing, for example, on exercise, expiration becomes active as a result of the activity of the expiratory cells. Note that there is still not universal agreement on how the intrinsic rhythmicity of respiration is brought about by the medullary centers.

2. *Apneustic center* in the lower pons. This area is so named because if the brain of an experimental animal is sectioned just above this site, prolonged inspiratory gasps (apneuses) interrupted by transient expiratory efforts are seen. Apparently, the impulses from the center have an excitatory effect on the inspiratory area of the medulla, tending to prolong the ramp action potentials. Whether this apneustic center plays a role in normal human respiration is not known, although in some types of severe brain injury, this type of abnormal breathing is seen.

3. *Pneumotaxic center* in the upper pons. As indicated above, this area appears to "switch off" or inhibit inspiration and thus regulates inspiration volume and, secondarily, respiratory rate. This has been demonstrated experimentally in animals by direct electrical stimulation of the pneumotaxic center. Some investigators believe that the role of this center is "fine-tuning" of respiratory rhythm because a normal rhythm can exist in the absence of this center.

> **Respiratory Centers**
>
> - Responsible for generating the rhythmic pattern of inspiration and expiration.
> - Located in the medulla and pons of the brainstem.
> - Receive input from chemoreceptors, lung and other receptors, and the cortex.
> - Major output is to the phrenic nerves, but there are also impulses to other respiratory muscles.

Cortex

Breathing is under voluntary control to a considerable extent, and the cortex can override the function of the brainstem within limits. It is not difficult to halve the arterial P_{CO_2} by hyperventilation, although the consequent alkalosis may cause tetany with contraction of the muscles of the hand and foot (carpopedal spasm). Halving the P_{CO_2} in this way increases the arterial pH by about 0.2 unit (Figure 6.7).

Voluntary hypoventilation is more difficult. The duration of breath-holding is limited by several factors, including the arterial P_{CO_2} and P_{O_2}. A preceding period of hyperventilation increases breath-holding time, especially if oxygen is breathed. However, factors other than chemical are involved. This is shown by the observation that if, at the breaking point of breath-holding, a gas mixture is inhaled that *raises* the arterial P_{CO_2} and *lowers* the P_{O_2}, a further period of breath-holding is possible.

Other Parts of the Brain

Other parts of the brain, such as the limbic system and hypothalamus, can alter the pattern of breathing, for example, in emotional states such as rage and fear.

EFFECTORS

The muscles of respiration include the diaphragm, intercostal muscles, abdominal muscles, and accessory muscles such as the sternocleidomastoids and scalenes. The actions of these were described at the beginning of Chapter 7. Impulses are also sent to the nasopharyngeal muscles to maintain patency of the upper airways. This is particularly important during sleep. In the context of the control of ventilation, it is crucially important that these various muscle groups work in a coordinated manner; this is the responsibility of the central controller. There is evidence that some newborn children, particularly those who are premature, have uncoordinated respiratory muscle activity, especially during sleep. For example, the thoracic muscles may try to inspire while the abdominal muscles expire.

SENSORS

Central Chemoreceptors

A chemoreceptor is a receptor that responds to a change in the chemical composition of the blood or other fluid around it. The most important receptors involved in the minute-by-minute control of ventilation are those situated near the ventral surface of the medulla in the vicinity of the exit of the 9th and 10th nerves. In animals, local application of H^+ or dissolved CO_2 to this area stimulates breathing within a few seconds. At one time, it was thought that the medullary respiratory center itself was the site of action of CO_2, but it is now accepted that the chemoreceptors are anatomically separate. Some evidence suggests that they lie about 200 to 400 μm below the ventral surface of the medulla (**Figure 8.2**).

The central chemoreceptors are surrounded by brain extracellular fluid and respond to changes in its H^+ concentration. An increase in H^+ concentration stimulates ventilation, whereas a decrease inhibits it. The composition of the extracellular fluid around the receptors is governed by the cerebrospinal fluid (CSF), local blood flow, and local metabolism.

Of these, the CSF is apparently the most important. It is separated from the blood by the blood-brain barrier, which is relatively impermeable to H^+ and HCO_3^- ions, although molecular CO_2 diffuses across it easily. When the blood P_{CO_2} rises, CO_2 diffuses into the CSF from the cerebral blood vessels, liberating H^+ ions that stimulate the chemoreceptors. Thus, the CO_2 level in blood regulates ventilation chiefly by its effect on the pH of the CSF,

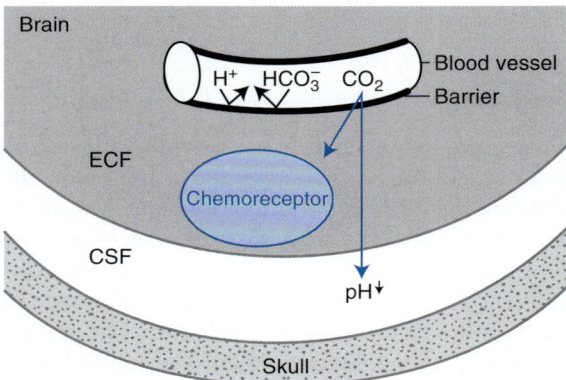

Figure 8.2. Environment of the central chemoreceptors. They are bathed in brain extracellular fluid (ECF), through which CO_2 easily diffuses from blood vessels to cerebrospinal fluid (CSF). The CO_2 reduces the CSF pH, thus stimulating the chemoreceptor. H^+ and HCO_3^- ions cannot easily cross the blood-brain barrier.

although recent evidence suggests CO_2 may also exert a direct effect on the central chemoreceptors independent of changes in H^+. The resulting hyperventilation reduces the P_{CO_2} in the blood and therefore in the CSF. The cerebral vasodilation that accompanies an increased arterial P_{CO_2} enhances diffusion of CO_2 into the CSF and the brain extracellular fluid. The central chemoreceptor does not respond to changes in the P_{O_2}.

The normal pH of the CSF is 7.32, and because the CSF contains much less protein than does blood, it has a much lower buffering capacity. As a result, the change in CSF pH for a given change in P_{CO_2} is greater than in blood. If the CSF pH is displaced over a prolonged period, a compensatory change in HCO_3^- occurs as a result of transport across the blood-brain barrier. However, the CSF pH does not usually return all the way to 7.32. The change in CSF pH occurs more promptly than does the change of the pH of arterial blood by renal compensation (Figure 6.7), a process that takes 2 to 3 days. Because CSF pH returns to near its normal value more rapidly than does blood pH, CSF pH has a more important effect on changes in the level of ventilation and the arterial P_{CO_2}.

One example of these changes is a patient with chronic lung disease and CO_2 retention of long standing who may have a nearly normal CSF pH and, therefore, an abnormally low ventilation for his or her arterial P_{CO_2}. The same pattern may occur in very obese patients who hypoventilate due to a combination of abnormal respiratory mechanics and alterations in ventilatory control. A similar situation is seen in normal subjects who are exposed to an atmosphere containing 3% CO_2 for some days.

Central Chemoreceptors

- Located near the ventral surface of the medulla
- Sensitive to the P_{CO_2} but not P_{O_2} of blood
- Respond to the change in pH of the ECF/CSF when CO_2 diffuses out of cerebral capillaries

---

Peripheral Chemoreceptors

Peripheral chemoreceptors are located in the carotid bodies at the bifurcation of the common carotid arteries and in the aortic bodies above and below the aortic arch. The carotid bodies are the most important in humans. They contain glomus cells of two types. Type I cells show an intense fluorescent staining because of their large content of dopamine. These cells are in close apposition to endings of the afferent carotid sinus nerve (**Figure 8.3**). The carotid body also contains type II cells and a rich supply of capillaries. The precise mechanism of the carotid bodies is still uncertain, but many physiologists

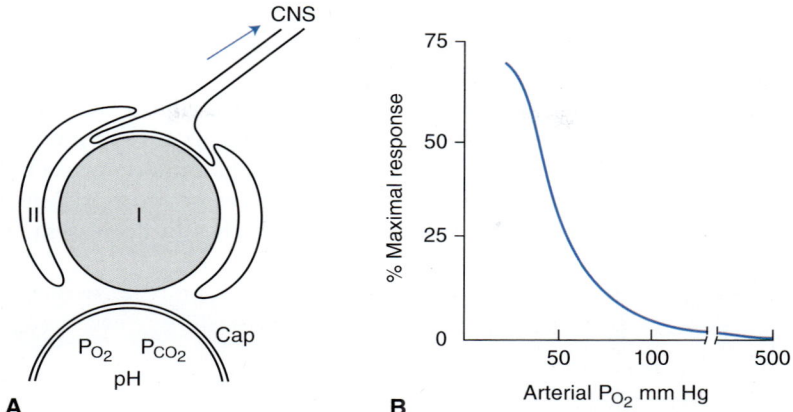

Figure 8.3. **A.** Diagram of a carotid body that contains type I and type II cells with many capillaries (Cap). Impulses travel to the central nervous system (CNS) through the carotid sinus nerve. **B.** The nonlinear response to arterial P_{O_2}. Note that the maximum response occurs below a P_{O_2} of 50 mm Hg.

believe that the glomus cells are the sites of chemoreception and that modulation of neurotransmitter release from the glomus cells by physiological and chemical stimuli affects the discharge rate of the carotid body afferent fibers (Figure 8.3A).

The peripheral chemoreceptors respond to decreases in arterial P_{O_2} and pH and increases in arterial P_{CO_2}. They are unique among tissues of the body in that their sensitivity to changes in arterial P_{O_2} begins around 500 mm Hg. Figure 8.3B shows that the relationship between firing rate and arterial P_{O_2} is very nonlinear; relatively little response occurs until the arterial P_{O_2} is reduced below 100 mm Hg, but then the rate rapidly increases. The carotid bodies have a very high blood flow for their size, and therefore, in spite of their high metabolic rate, the arterial-venous O_2 difference is small. Note that the response is to the P_{O_2}, not the oxygen concentration. The response of these receptors can be very fast; indeed, their discharge rate can alter during the respiratory cycle as a result of the small cyclic changes in blood gases. The peripheral chemoreceptors are responsible for all the increase of ventilation that occurs in humans in response to arterial hypoxemia. Indeed, in the absence of these receptors, severe hypoxemia may depress ventilation, presumably through a direct effect on the respiratory centers. Complete loss of hypoxic ventilatory drive has been shown in patients with bilateral carotid body resection. There is considerable variability between individuals in their hypoxic ventilatory response. Persons who are exposed to chronic hypoxia develop hypertrophy of their carotid bodies.

The response of the peripheral chemoreceptors to arterial P_{CO_2} is less important than is that of the central chemoreceptors. For example, when a normal subject is given a CO_2 mixture to breathe, less than 20% of the ventilatory response can be attributed to the peripheral chemoreceptors. However, their response is more rapid, and they may be useful in matching ventilation to abrupt changes in P_{CO_2}.

In humans, the carotid but not the aortic bodies respond to a fall in arterial pH. This occurs regardless of whether the cause is respiratory or metabolic. As described more below, interaction of the various stimuli occurs, such that increases in chemoreceptor activity in response to decreases in arterial P_{O_2} are potentiated by increases in P_{CO_2} and, in the carotid bodies, by decreases in pH.

Peripheral Chemoreceptors

- Located in the carotid and aortic bodies
- Respond to decreased arterial P_{O_2}, and increased P_{CO_2} and H^+
- Rapidly responding

Lung Receptors

Pulmonary Stretch Receptors

Pulmonary stretch receptors are also known as slowly adapting pulmonary stretch receptors and are believed to lie within airway smooth muscle. They discharge in response to distension of the lung, and their activity is sustained with lung inflation; that is, they show little adaptation. The impulses travel in the vagus nerve via large myelinated fibers.

The main reflex effect of stimulating these receptors is a slowing of respiratory frequency due to an increase in expiratory time. This is known as the Hering-Breuer inflation reflex. It can be well demonstrated in a rabbit preparation in which the diaphragm contains a slip of muscle from which recordings can be made without interfering with the other respiratory muscles. Classic experiments showed that inflation of the lungs tended to inhibit further inspiratory muscle activity. The opposite response is also seen; that is, deflation of the lungs tends to initiate inspiratory activity (deflation reflex). Thus, these reflexes can provide a self-regulatory mechanism or negative feedback.

The Hering-Breuer reflexes were once thought to play a major role in ventilation by determining the rate and depth of breathing. This could be done by using the information from these stretch receptors to modulate the "switching-off" mechanism in the medulla. For example, bilateral vagotomy, which removes the input of these receptors, causes slow, deep breathing in most animals. However, more recent work indicates that the reflexes are largely inactive in adult humans unless the tidal volume exceeds 1 liter, as in exercise. Transient bilateral blockade of the vagus nerves by local anesthesia in awake humans does not change either breathing rate or volume. There is some evidence that these reflexes may be more important in newborn babies.

Irritant Receptors

These are thought to lie between airway epithelial cells, and they are stimulated by noxious gases, cigarette smoke, inhaled dusts, and cold air. The impulses travel up the vagus in myelinated fibers, and the reflex effects include bronchoconstriction and hyperpnea. Some physiologists prefer to call these receptors "rapidly adapting pulmonary stretch receptors" because they show rapid adaptation and are apparently involved in additional mechanoreceptor functions, as well as respond to noxious stimuli on the airway walls. It is possible that irritant receptors play a role in the bronchoconstriction of asthma attacks as a result of their response to released histamine.

J Receptors

These are the endings of nonmyelinated C fibers and sometimes go by this name. The term "juxtacapillary," or J, is used because these receptors are believed to be in the alveolar walls, close to the capillaries. The evidence for this location is that they respond very quickly to chemicals injected into the pulmonary circulation. The impulses pass up the vagus nerve in slowly conducting nonmyelinated fibers and can result in rapid, shallow breathing, although intense stimulation causes apnea. There is evidence that engorgement of pulmonary capillaries and increases in the interstitial fluid volume of the alveolar wall activate these receptors. They may play a role in the rapid, shallow breathing and dyspnea (sensation of difficulty in breathing) associated with left heart failure and interstitial lung disease.

Bronchial C Fibers

These are supplied by the bronchial circulation rather than the pulmonary circulation, as is the case for the J receptors described above. They respond quickly to chemicals injected into the bronchial circulation. The reflex responses to stimulation include rapid shallow breathing, bronchoconstriction, and mucous secretion.

Other Receptors

Nose and Upper Airway Receptors

The nose, nasopharynx, larynx, and trachea contain receptors that respond to mechanical and chemical stimulation. These are an extension of the irritant receptors described above. Various reflex responses have been described, including sneezing, coughing, and bronchoconstriction. Laryngeal spasm may occur if the larynx is irritated mechanically, for example, during insertion of an endotracheal tube with insufficient local anesthesia.

Joint and Muscle Receptors

Impulses from moving limbs are believed to be part of the stimulus to ventilation during exercise, especially in the early stages.

Gamma System

Many muscles, including the intercostal muscles and diaphragm, contain muscle spindles that sense elongation of the muscle. This information is used to reflexly control the strength of contraction. These receptors may be involved in the sensation of dyspnea that occurs when unusually large respiratory efforts are required to move the lung and chest wall, for example, because of airway obstruction.

Arterial Baroreceptors

An increase in arterial blood pressure can cause reflex hypoventilation or apnea through stimulation of the aortic and carotid sinus baroreceptors. Conversely, a decrease in blood pressure may result in hyperventilation.

Pain and Temperature

Stimulation of many afferent nerves can bring about changes in ventilation. Pain often causes a period of apnea followed by hyperventilation. Heating of the skin may result in hyperventilation.

INTEGRATED RESPONSES

Now that we have looked at the various units that make up the respiratory control system (Figure 8.1), it is useful to consider the overall responses of the system to changes in the arterial CO_2, O_2, and pH and to exercise.

Response to Carbon Dioxide

The most important factor in the control of ventilation under normal conditions is the P_{CO_2} of the arterial blood. The sensitivity of this control is remarkable. In the course of daily activity with periods of rest and exercise, the arterial P_{CO_2} is probably held to within 3 mm Hg. During sleep, it may rise a little more.

The ventilatory response to CO_2 is normally measured by having the subject inhale CO_2 mixtures or rebreathe from a bag so that the inspired P_{CO_2} gradually rises. In one technique, the subject rebreathes from a bag that is prefilled with 7% CO_2 and 93% O_2. As the subject rebreathes, metabolic CO_2 is added to the bag, but the O_2 concentration remains relatively high. In such a procedure, the P_{CO_2} of the bag gas increases at the rate of about 4 mm $Hg \cdot min^{-1}$.

Figure 8.4 shows the results of experiments in which the inspired mixture was adjusted to yield a constant alveolar P_{O_2}. (In this type of experiment on normal subjects, alveolar end-tidal P_{O_2} and P_{CO_2} are generally taken to reflect the arterial levels.) It can be seen that with a normal P_{O_2}, the ventilation increases by about 2 to 3 $liters \cdot min^{-1}$ for each 1 mm Hg rise in P_{CO_2}.

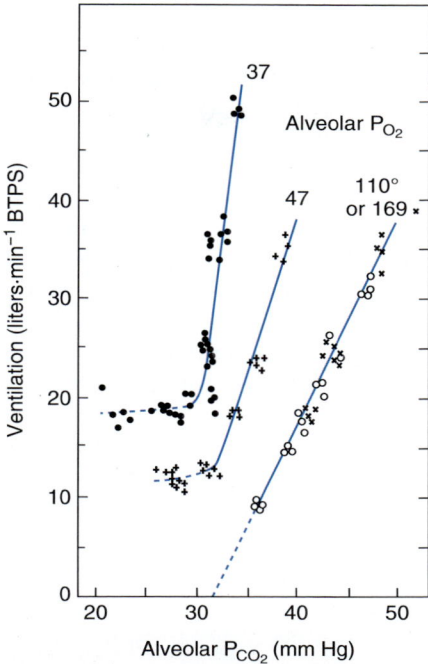

Figure 8.4. Ventilatory response to CO_2. Each curve of total ventilation against alveolar P_{CO_2} is for a different alveolar P_{O_2}. In this study, no difference was found between alveolar P_{O_2} values of 110 and 169 mm Hg, though some investigators have found that the slope of the line is slightly less at the higher P_{O_2}. (From Nielsen M, Smith H. *Acta Physiol Scand*. 1951;24:293.)

Lowering the P_{O_2} produces two effects: ventilation for a given P_{CO_2} is higher and the slope of the line becomes steeper. There is considerable variation between subjects.

Another way of measuring respiratory drive is to record the inspiratory pressure during a brief period of airway occlusion. The subject breathes through a mouthpiece attached to a valve box, and the inspiratory port is provided with a shutter. This is closed during an expiration (the subject being unaware), so that the first part of the next inspiration is against an occluded airway. The shutter is opened after about 0.5 s. The pressure generated during the first 0.1 s of attempted inspiration (known as $P_{0.1}$) is taken as a measure of respiratory center output. This is largely unaffected by the mechanical properties of the respiratory system, although it is influenced by lung volume. This method can be used to study the respiratory sensitivity to CO_2, hypoxemia, and other variables as well.

A reduction in arterial P_{CO_2} is very effective in reducing the stimulus to ventilation. For example, if the reader hyperventilates voluntarily for a few seconds, he or she will find that there is no urge to breathe for a short period. An anesthetized patient will frequently stop breathing for a minute or so if first overventilated by the anesthesiologist. Some swimmers in a sprint race hyperventilate on the starting block to reduce the urge to breathe during the race.

The ventilatory response to CO_2 is reduced by sleep, increasing age, and genetic factors. Trained athletes and divers tend to have a low CO_2 sensitivity. Various drugs depress the respiratory center, including opiates and barbiturates. Patients who have taken an overdose of one of these drugs often have marked hypoventilation. The ventilatory response to CO_2 is also reduced if the work of breathing is increased. This can be demonstrated by having normal subjects breathe through a narrow tube. The neural output of the respiratory center is not reduced, but it is not so effective in producing ventilation. The abnormally small ventilatory response to CO_2 and the CO_2 retention in some patients with chronic lung disease can be partly explained by the same mechanism. In such patients, reducing the airway resistance with bronchodilators often increases their ventilatory response. There is also some evidence that the sensitivity of the respiratory center is reduced in these patients.

As we have seen, the main stimulus to increase ventilation when the arterial P_{CO_2} rises comes from the central chemoreceptors, which respond to the increased H^+ concentration of the brain extracellular fluid near the receptors. An additional stimulus comes from the peripheral chemoreceptors, because of both the rise in arterial P_{CO_2} and the fall in pH.

Ventilatory Response to Carbon Dioxide

- Arterial P_{CO_2} is the most important stimulus to ventilation under most conditions and is normally tightly controlled.
- Most of the stimulus comes from the central chemoreceptors, but the peripheral chemoreceptors also contribute and their response is faster.
- The response is magnified if the arterial P_{O_2} is lowered.
- The response is reduced by sleep and increasing age.

Response to Oxygen

The way in which a reduction of P_{O_2} in arterial blood stimulates ventilation can be studied by having a subject breathe hypoxic gas mixtures. The end-tidal P_{O_2} and P_{CO_2} are used as a surrogate measure of the arterial values. **Figure 8.5** shows that when the alveolar P_{CO_2} is kept at about 36 mm Hg (by altering the inspired mixture), the alveolar P_{O_2} can be reduced to the vicinity of 50 mm Hg before any appreciable increase in ventilation occurs. Raising the P_{CO_2} increases the ventilation at any P_{O_2} (compare Figure 8.4). Note that when the P_{CO_2} is increased, a reduction in P_{O_2} below 100 mm Hg causes some stimulation of ventilation, unlike the situation in which the P_{CO_2} is normal. Thus, the combined effects of both stimuli exceed the sum of each stimulus given separately; this is referred to as interaction between the high CO_2 and

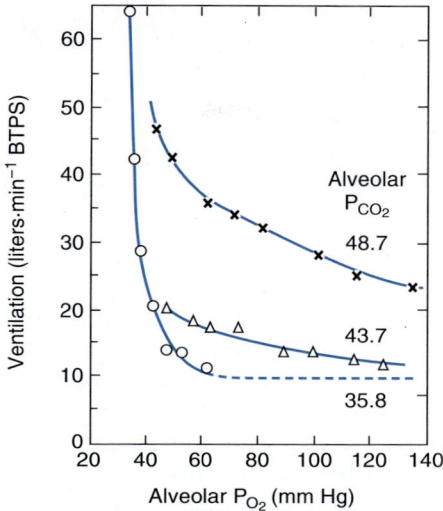

Figure 8.5. Hypoxic response curves. Note that when the P_{CO_2} is 35.8 mm Hg, almost no increase in ventilation occurs until the P_{O_2} is reduced to about 50 mm Hg. (Modified from Loeschke HH, Gertz KH. *Arch Ges Physiol*. 1958;267:460.)

low O_2 stimuli. There are large differences in the magnitude of this response between individuals.

Because the P_{O_2} can normally be reduced so far without evoking a ventilatory response, the role of this hypoxic stimulus in the day-to-day control of ventilation is small. However, in response to hypoxemia due to, for example, pneumonia or ascent to high altitude (Chapter 9), a large increase in ventilation occurs.

In some patients with severe chronic lung disease, the hypoxic drive to ventilation becomes very important. These patients have chronic CO_2 retention, and the pH of their brain extracellular fluid has returned to near normal in spite of a raised P_{CO_2}. Thus, they have lost most of their increase in the stimulus to ventilation from CO_2. In addition, the initial depression of blood pH has been nearly abolished by renal compensation, so there is little pH stimulation of the peripheral chemoreceptors (see below). Under these conditions, arterial hypoxemia is the primary stimulus to additional ventilation beyond the basic level set by the medullary respiratory centers. If such a patient is given a high O_2 mixture to breathe to relieve the hypoxemia, ventilation may decrease significantly. Several other factors are involved including release of hypoxic vasoconstriction and changes in ventilation-perfusion matching. The ventilatory state is best monitored by measuring arterial P_{CO_2}.

As we have seen, hypoxemia reflexly stimulates ventilation by its action on the carotid and aortic body chemoreceptors. It has no action on the central chemoreceptors; indeed, in the absence of peripheral chemoreceptors, hypoxemia depresses respiration. However, prolonged hypoxemia can cause mild cerebral acidosis, which, in turn, can stimulate ventilation.

Ventilatory Response to Hypoxia
• Only the peripheral chemoreceptors are involved.
• There is negligible control during normoxic conditions.
• The control becomes important at high altitude and in long-term hypoxemia caused by chronic lung disease.

Response to pH

A reduction in arterial blood pH stimulates ventilation. In practice, it is often difficult to separate the ventilatory response resulting from a fall in pH from that caused by an accompanying rise in P_{CO_2}. However, in experimental animals in which it is possible to reduce the pH at a constant P_{CO_2}, the stimulus to ventilation can be convincingly demonstrated. Patients with a partly compensated metabolic acidosis (as occurs in diabetic ketoacidosis) who have a low pH and low P_{CO_2} (Figure 6.7) show an increased ventilation. Indeed, this is responsible for the reduced P_{CO_2}.

As we have seen, the chief site of action of a reduced arterial pH is the peripheral chemoreceptors. It is also possible that the central chemoreceptors or the respiratory center itself can be affected by a change in blood pH if it is large enough. In this case, the blood-brain barrier becomes partly permeable to H^+ ions.

Response to Exercise

On exercise, ventilation increases promptly and during strenuous exertion may reach very high levels. Fit young people who attain a maximum O_2 consumption of 4 liters·min^{-1} may have a total ventilation of 150 liters·min^{-1}, that is, more than 15 times their resting level. At low to moderate levels of exercise, the increase in ventilation closely matches the increase in O_2 uptake and CO_2 output. It is remarkable that the cause of the increased ventilation on exercise remains largely unknown.

The arterial P_{CO_2} does not increase during exercise; indeed, during severe exercise, it typically falls as ventilation rises beyond that needed to satisfy metabolic demands in response to the developing lactic acidosis. The arterial P_{O_2} usually increases slightly, although it may fall at very high work levels. The arterial pH remains nearly constant for moderate exercise, although at high levels of exercise it falls because of the lactic acidosis. It is clear, therefore, that none of the mechanisms we have discussed so far can account for the large increase in ventilation observed during light to moderate exercise.

Other stimuli have been suggested. Passive movement of the limbs stimulates ventilation in both anesthetized animals and awake humans. This is a reflex with receptors presumably located in joints or muscles. It may be responsible for the abrupt increase in ventilation that occurs during the first few seconds of exercise. One hypothesis is that oscillations in arterial Po_2 and Pco_2 may stimulate the peripheral chemoreceptors, even though the mean level remains unaltered. These fluctuations are caused by the periodic nature of ventilation and increase when the tidal volume rises, as on exercise. Another theory is that the central chemoreceptors increase ventilation to hold the arterial Pco_2 constant by some kind of servomechanism, just as the thermostat can control a furnace with little change in temperature. The objection that the arterial Pco_2 often falls on exercise is countered by the assertion that the preferred level of Pco_2 is reset in some way. Proponents of this theory believe that the ventilatory response to inhaled CO_2 may not be a reliable guide to what happens on exercise.

Yet another hypothesis is that ventilation is linked in some way to the additional *CO_2 load* presented to the lungs in the mixed venous blood during exercise. In animal experiments, an increase in this load produced either by infusing CO_2 into the venous blood or by increasing venous return has been shown to correlate well with ventilation. However, a problem with this hypothesis is that no suitable receptor has been found.

Additional factors that have been suggested include the *increase in body temperature* during exercise, which stimulates ventilation, and *impulses from the motor cortex*. However, none of the theories proposed so far is completely satisfactory.

VENTILATORY CONTROL DURING SLEEP

There are several important changes in ventilatory control occur during sleep. Voluntary control and other factors that override automatic control of breathing during wakefulness are lost, as is the wakefulness drive to breathe mediated by excitatory inputs to the medullary centers from the reticular formation and hypothalamus. Second, as noted above, ventilatory responses to Pco_2 and Po_2 are decreased. Finally, while not directly related to ventilatory control, the tone of the upper airway dilating muscles (genioglossus and palatal) decrease during sleep, which can predispose to upper airway obstruction and impaired ventilation.

ABNORMAL PATTERNS OF BREATHING DURING SLEEP

Subjects with severe hypoxemia often exhibit a striking pattern of periodic breathing during sleep known as *Cheyne-Stokes respiration*. This is characterized by periods of apnea of 10 to 20 s, separated by approximately equal periods of hyperventilation when the tidal volume gradually waxes and then wanes. This pattern is frequently seen at high altitude, especially at night during sleep (Video 8.1). It is also found in some patients with severe heart failure or neurologic injury. Patients with very severe heart failure may also manifest a waxing and waning pattern of ventilation during exercise.

Cheyne-Stokes respiration is due, in part, to problems with feedback control and, in particular, increased ventilatory responsiveness to changes in P_{CO_2}. The pattern can also be reproduced in experimental animals by lengthening the distance through which blood travels on its way to the brain from the lung. Under these conditions, there is a long delay before the central chemoreceptors sense the alteration in P_{CO_2} caused by a change in ventilation. As a result, the respiratory center hunts for the equilibrium condition, always overshooting it. Other abnormal patterns of breathing can also occur during sleep, such as an ataxic pattern of breathing marked by irregular ventilation and variable periods of apnea seen in patients who use opiate pain medications on a chronic basis.

KEY CONCEPTS

1. The respiratory centers that are responsible for the rhythmic pattern of breathing are located in the pons and medulla of the brainstem. The output of these centers can be overridden by the cortex to some extent.

2. The central chemoreceptors are located near the ventral surface of the medulla and respond to changes in pH of the CSF, which in turn are caused by diffusion of CO_2 from brain capillaries. Alterations in the bicarbonate concentration of the CSF modulate the pH and therefore the chemoreceptor response.

3. The peripheral chemoreceptors, chiefly in the carotid bodies, respond to a reduced P_{O_2} and increases in P_{CO_2} and H^+ concentration. The response to O_2 is small above a P_{O_2} of 50 mm Hg. The response to increased CO_2 is less marked than is that from the central chemoreceptors but occurs more rapidly.

4. Other receptors are located in the walls of the airways and alveoli.

5. The P_{CO_2} of the blood is the most important factor controlling ventilation under normal conditions, and most of the control is via the central chemoreceptors.

6. The P_{O_2} of the blood does not normally affect ventilation, but it becomes important at high altitude and in some patients with lung disease.

7. Exercise causes a large increase in ventilation, but the cause, especially during moderate exercise, is poorly understood.

CLINICAL VIGNETTE

A 23-year-old student ascended over a 1-day period from sea level to a research station located at 3,800 m (12,500 ft, barometric pressure 480 mm Hg). Prior to his departure for the station, an arterial blood sample showed pH of 7.40, P_{CO_2} of 39 mm Hg, P_{O_2} of 93 mm Hg, HCO_3^- 23, and hemoglobin concentration of 15 g·dl^{-1}. After arriving at the research station 8 hours later, another arterial blood sample was taken and showed pH of 7.46, P_{CO_2} of 32 mm Hg, P_{O_2} of 48 mm Hg, and HCO_3^- 22. After a period of 1 week at the research station, a third arterial blood sample revealed pH of 7.41, P_{CO_2} of 27 mm Hg, P_{O_2} of 54 mm Hg, HCO_3^- 17, and hemoglobin concentration 16.5 g·dl^{-1}. For the final component of the research project, he completed an exercise test at the research station in which he pedaled against increasing levels of resistance to his maximum exercise capacity. An arterial blood sample was taken at the end of the test and showed pH of 7.30, P_{CO_2} of 22 mm Hg, and P_{O_2} of 40 mm Hg.

- How do you account for the observed arterial blood gases upon arrival at the research station?
- How do you account for the change in his blood gases over the first week at the research station?
- Why did his hemoglobin concentration increase during his stay at the research station?
- What mechanisms account for the change in his arterial P_{CO_2}, P_{O_2}, and pH during the exercise test?

QUESTIONS

For each question, choose the one best answer.

1. A previously healthy patient is admitted to the intensive care unit following resuscitation from a cardiac arrest due to an arrhythmia. A brain MRI performed after admission shows extensive anoxic injury to the cerebral cortex but no injury to the midbrain, pons, or medulla. Which of the following aspects of ventilatory control will be impaired in this patient?
   A. Central chemoreceptors
   B. Hering-Breuer reflex
   C. Peripheral chemoreceptors
   D. Respiratory rhythm generation
   E. Voluntary control of breathing

2. In an animal model, recordings of diaphragmatic activity are made from a small section of the diaphragm without affecting the function of other respiratory muscles. After lung volume is lowered from 1.0 to 0.5 liter, while systemic blood pressure remains constant at 95/72 mm Hg, the frequency of diaphragmatic contraction is noted to increase. Which of the following receptors is responsible for the observed change in respiratory frequency?
   A. Arterial baroreceptors
   B. Bronchial C fibers
   C. Irritant receptors
   D. Juxtacapillary receptors
   E. Stretch receptors

3. A 41-year-old man is recuperating in the hospital following a surgical procedure. On the fifth hospital day, he develops a gastrointestinal hemorrhage due to a gastric ulcer. His hemoglobin concentration decreases from 13 to 9 $g \cdot dl^{-1}$. His oxygen saturation remains 98% during this time, while an arterial blood gas drawn at the time of this event while breathing ambient air shows a pH of 7.39, Pco_2 of 41 mm Hg, Po_2 of 85 mm Hg, and bicarbonate of 25 $mEq \cdot liter^{-1}$. The arterial Po_2 is unchanged from the arterial blood gas taken the previous day. Which of the following would you expect to see as a result of his gastrointestinal hemorrhage?
   A. Decreased central chemoreceptor output
   B. Increased central chemoreceptor output
   C. Increased juxtacapillary receptor output
   D. Increased peripheral chemoreceptor output
   E. No change in peripheral chemoreceptor output

4. As part of an evaluation for abnormal breathing patterns during sleep, a 25-year-old woman undergoes a test in which she inhales a gas mixture with an inspired CO_2 fraction of 3.5% for several minutes. The figure below shows the changes in her minute ventilation as the end-tidal partial pressure of CO_2—a surrogate value for the arterial Pco_2—increases. For the purposes of comparison, data from a healthy control are displayed on the left. Based on these data, which of the following components of this patient's respiratory control system is most likely abnormal?

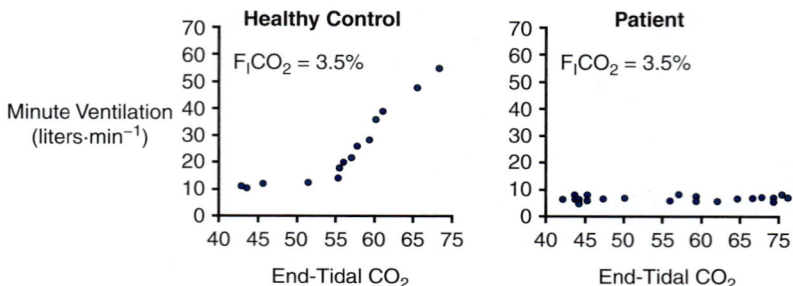

A. Central chemoreceptors
B. Juxtacapillary receptors
C. Peripheral chemoreceptors
D. Pneumotaxic center
E. Pulmonary stretch receptors

5. During an evaluation in pulmonary clinic, a 67-year-old woman with chronic obstructive pulmonary disease was found to have an FEV_1 of 0.9 liter (45% predicted) and an arterial blood gas showing a pH of 7.35, Pco_2 of 55 mm Hg, and HCO_3^- of 30 mEq·liter^{-1}. Two weeks later, she presents to the emergency department with chest pain and is found to have an oxygen saturation of 85% breathing ambient air. She is placed on supplemental oxygen and her oxygen saturation rises to 100%. Which of the following would you expect to occur as a result of this intervention?
   A. Decreased juxtacapillary receptor output
   B. Decreased P_{50} for hemoglobin
   C. Increased arterial Pco_2
   D. Increased pulmonary vascular resistance
   E. Increased ventral respiratory group output

6. After ascending to a mountain hut at 4,559 m, an otherwise healthy man is noted by his friends to have an abnormal breathing pattern while sleeping. His chest wall movement increases over successive breaths before decreasing over another few breaths and eventually ceasing altogether. After a period of about 20 s without respiratory effort, he starts breathing again and repeats the pattern described above. This continues for several hours. Which of the following mechanisms contributes to this breathing pattern during sleep?
   A. Blunted peripheral chemoreceptor responses to changes in arterial Po_2
   B. Hering-Breuer reflex
   C. Hypoxic injury to the medullary respiratory center
   D. Increased ventilatory responsiveness to changes in arterial Pco_2
   E. Stimulation of juxtacapillary receptors

7. A 27-year-old woman presents to the emergency department with nausea, vomiting, and polyuria over a several day period. On examination, she is noted to be taking deep breaths at an increased respiratory rate. Her laboratory studies reveal a bicarbonate of 12 mEq·liter^{-1}, glucose of 457 mg·dl^{-1}, white blood cell count of 9×10^3 cells·µl^{-1}, and hematocrit of 47%. Her chest radiograph shows no lung opacities. Given this presentation, which of the following physiologic responses would you expect to observe in this patient?
   A. Decreased Juxtacapillary ("J") receptor output
   B. Decreased P_{50} for hemoglobin

C. Decreased Pre-Botzinger complex output
D. Increased CSF P_{CO_2}
E. Increased peripheral chemoreceptor output

8. A 59-year-old man with poorly controlled hypertension is admitted to the ICU with a cerebrovascular accident due to occlusion of the vertebral and basilar arteries. He is intubated for airway protection given his severely altered mental status. The following morning, he remains intubated and is not initiating any breathing movements on his own despite not receiving any sedative or neuromuscular blockade medications. On an arterial blood gas, his P_{CO_2} is 40 mm Hg. Ischemic injury to which of the following areas of the brain is most likely responsible for his respiratory status?
   A. Cerebellar hemisphere
   B. Globus pallidus
   C. Medulla
   D. Midbrain
   E. Thalamus

9. A 59-year-old man with severe chronic obstructive pulmonary disease has an arterial blood sample taken while breathing ambient air to determine if he qualifies for home oxygen therapy. The blood sample reveals a pH of 7.35 and a P_{CO_2} of 53 mm Hg. Which of the following changes would you expect to see in his cerebrospinal fluid compared to normal values?
   A. Decreased hydrogen ion concentration
   B. Decreased P_{CO_2}
   C. Increased bicarbonate concentration
   D. Increased lactate concentration
   E. Increased pH

10. A 64-year-old man underwent bilateral carotid artery surgery for treatment of carotid atherosclerotic disease during which both of his carotid bodies were removed. He is planning trek to high altitude with some friends during which they will travel above 3,000 m in elevation. If you drew an arterial blood gas on him at this elevation, what difference would you expect to see compared to his healthy travel partners?
    A. Higher arterial P_{CO_2}
    B. Higher arterial pH
    C. Higher alveolar P_{O_2}
    D. Higher arterial P_{O_2}
    E. Lower bicarbonate

11. A 23-year-old woman participates in a research project in which measurements are made at sea level while she is inhaling gas mixtures with varying concentrations of carbon dioxide. If you repeat the experiment immediately upon her arrival at an elevation of 4,000 m while she is breathing ambient air and compared the results with her sea level responses, which of the following would you expect to see at any given alveolar CO_2?
    A. Decreased arterial pH
    B. Decreased peripheral chemoreceptor output
    C. Decreased pulmonary artery pressure
    D. Increased serum bicarbonate
    E. Increased total ventilation

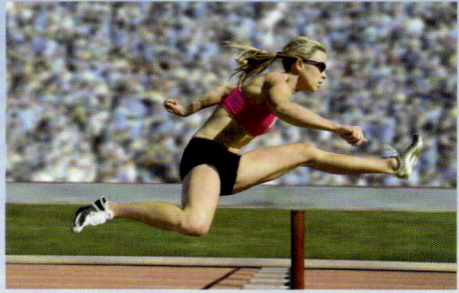

Respiratory System Under Stress

9

How Gas Exchange Is Accomplished During Exercise, at Low and High Pressures, and at Birth

The normal lung has enormous reserves at rest, and these enable it to meet the greatly increased demands for gas exchange during exercise. In addition, the lung serves as our principal physiological link with the environment in which we live; its surface area is some 30 times greater than that of the skin. The human urge to climb higher and dive deeper puts the respiratory system under great stress, although these situations are minor insults compared with the process of being born! At the end of this chapter, the reader should be able to:

- Describe the changes in respiratory and hemodynamic variables during exercise
- Outline the expected physiologic responses to high altitude
- Explain the mechanism for absorption atelectasis
- Identify complications of SCUBA diving
- Describe the mechanisms by which inhaled particulate matter is trapped in the airways
- Outline the key features of the fetal circulation and describe changes that occur after birth

EXERCISE

The gas exchange demands of the lung are enormously increased by exercise. Typically, the resting oxygen consumptions of 300 ml·min^{-1} can rise to about 3,000 ml·min^{-1} in a moderately fit subject (and as high as 6,000 ml·min^{-1} in an elite athlete). Similarly, the resting CO_2 output of, say, 250 ml·min^{-1} increases to about 3,000 ml·min^{-1}. Typically, the respiratory exchange ratio (R) rises from about 0.8 at rest to 1.0 during exercise. This increase reflects a greater reliance on carbohydrate rather than fat to produce the required energy. Indeed, R often reaches even higher levels during the unsteady state of severe exercise when lactic acid is produced by anaerobic glycolysis, and additional CO_2 is therefore eliminated from bicarbonate. In addition, there is increased CO_2 elimination because the increased H^+ concentration stimulates the peripheral chemoreceptors, thus increasing ventilation.

Exercise is conveniently studied on a treadmill or stationary bicycle. As work rate (or power) is increased, oxygen uptake increases linearly (**Figure 9.1A**). However, above a certain work rate, $\dot{V}O_2$ becomes constant; this is known as the $\dot{V}O_{2max}$. An increase in work rate above this level can occur only through anaerobic glycolysis. Individuals cannot sustain this level of work for very long.

Ventilation also increases linearly initially when plotted against work rate or $\dot{V}O_2$, but at high $\dot{V}O_2$ values, it increases more rapidly because lactic acid is liberated, thereby increasing the ventilatory stimulus (**Figure 9.1B**). Sometimes,

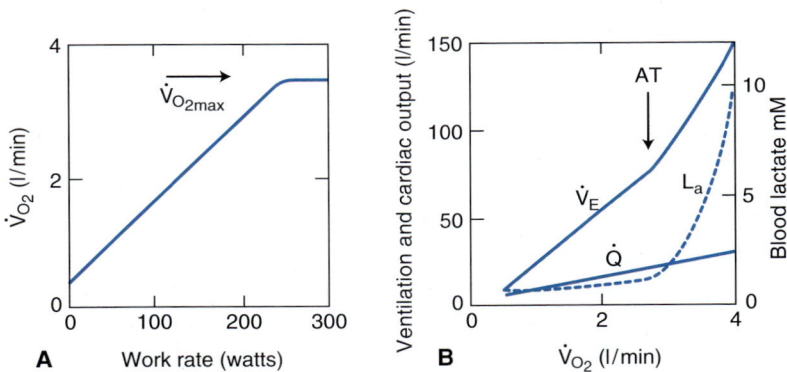

Figure 9.1. **A.** O_2 consumption ($\dot{V}O_2$) increases nearly linearly with work rate until the $\dot{V}O_{2max}$ is reached. **B.** Ventilation initially increases linearly with O_2 consumption but rises more rapidly when substantial amounts of blood lactate are formed. If there is a clear break, this is sometimes called the anaerobic or ventilatory threshold (AT). Cardiac output increases more slowly than does ventilation.

there is a clear change in the slope; this has been called the *anaerobic threshold* or *ventilation threshold* although the term is somewhat controversial. The anaerobic threshold occurs at relatively low work levels in unfit individuals, whereas well-trained individuals reach this threshold at a higher percentage of their maximum exercise capacity. While lactic acidosis contributes to the increase in ventilation, as we saw in Chapter 8, the very large increase in ventilation that occurs during exercise is largely unexplained. However, the net result of the change in ventilation is that the P_{CO_2} and pH are little affected by moderate exercise, whereas very high work levels, P_{CO_2} often falls, alveolar P_{O_2} rises and pH falls because of lactic acidosis.

Many functions of the respiratory system change in response to exercise. The diffusing capacity of the lung increases because of increases in both the diffusing capacity of the membrane, D_M, and the volume of blood in the pulmonary capillaries, V_c. These changes are brought about by recruitment and distension of pulmonary capillaries, particularly in the upper parts of the lung. Typically, the diffusing capacity increases at least threefold. In healthy individuals, the amount of ventilation-perfusion inequality decreases during moderate exercise because of the more uniform topographical distribution of blood flow. However, because the degree of ventilation-perfusion inequality in healthy individuals is trivial, this is of little consequence. In the majority of individuals, the arterial P_{O_2} remains constant through exercise. However, some elite athletes at extremely high work levels show a fall in arterial P_{O_2} probably caused by diffusion limitation because of the reduced time available for the loading of oxygen in the pulmonary capillary (Figure 3.3). Ventilation-perfusion inequality, possibly because of mild degrees of interstitial pulmonary edema, may also play a role. Certainly, fluid must move out of pulmonary capillaries because of the increased pressure within them.

Cardiac output increases approximately linearly with work level as a result of increases in both heart rate and stroke volume, with the latter increasing due to increases in venous return and cardiac inotropy. The change in cardiac output is only about a quarter of the increase in ventilation (in liter·min^{-1}). This makes sense because it is much easier to move air than to move blood. If we look at the Fick equation, $\dot{V}_{O_2} = \dot{Q}(Ca_{O_2} - C_{\bar{v}_{O_2}})$, the increase in $\dot{V}_{O_2}$ is brought about by both an increase in cardiac output and a rise in the arterial-venous O_2 difference because of the fall in the oxygen concentration of mixed venous blood. By contrast, if we look at the analogous equation for ventilation, $\dot{V}_{O_2} = \dot{V}_E(F_{I_{O_2}} - F_{E_{O_2}})$, the difference between inspired and expired O_2 concentrations does not change. This is consistent with the much larger increase in ventilation than blood flow. The increase in cardiac output is associated with elevations of both the pulmonary arterial and pulmonary venous pressures, although pulmonary artery pressure does not rise nearly as high as systemic systolic pressure because pulmonary vascular resistance falls due to recruitment and distension of pulmonary capillaries.

The oxygen dissociation curve moves to the right in exercising muscles because of the increase in P_{CO_2}, H^+ concentration, and temperature. This assists the unloading of oxygen to the muscles. When the blood returns to the lung, the temperature of the blood falls a little and the curve shifts leftward somewhat.

In peripheral tissues, additional capillaries open up, thus reducing the diffusion path length to the mitochondria. Peripheral vascular resistance falls because the large increase in cardiac output is not associated with much of an increase in mean arterial pressure during dynamic exercise such as running, although systolic pressure often rises considerably. During static exercise such as weight lifting, large increases in systemic arterial pressure often occur. Exercise training increases the number of capillaries and mitochondria in skeletal muscle.

Exercise

- O_2 uptake increases linearly with work rate.
- Ventilation increases linearly with O_2 uptake until the ventilatory (or anaerobic) threshold is reached after which ventilation increases more rapidly.
- Cardiac output increases but much less than ventilation.
- Elite athletes may show diffusion limitation of O_2 transfer at maximal exercise, and some develop ventilation-perfusion inequality possibly caused by interstitial edema.

HIGH ALTITUDE

The barometric pressure decreases with distance above the earth's surface in an approximately exponential manner (**Figure 9.2**). The pressure at 5,800 m (19,000 ft) is only one-half the normal 760 mm Hg, so the P_{O_2} of moist inspired gas is $(380 - 47) \times 0.2093 = 70$ mm Hg (47 mm Hg is the partial pressure of water vapor at body temperature). At the summit of Mount Everest (altitude 8,848 m, or 29,028 ft), the inspired P_{O_2} is only 43 mm Hg. At 19,200 m (63,000 ft), the barometric pressure is 47 mm Hg, so the inspired P_{O_2} is zero.

In spite of the hypoxia associated with high altitude, some 200 million people live at elevations over 2,500 m (8,000 ft), and permanent residents live higher than 5,000 m (16,400 ft) in the Andes. A remarkable degree of acclimatization occurs when humans ascend to these altitudes; indeed, climbers have lived for several days at altitudes that would cause unconsciousness within a few seconds in the absence of acclimatization.

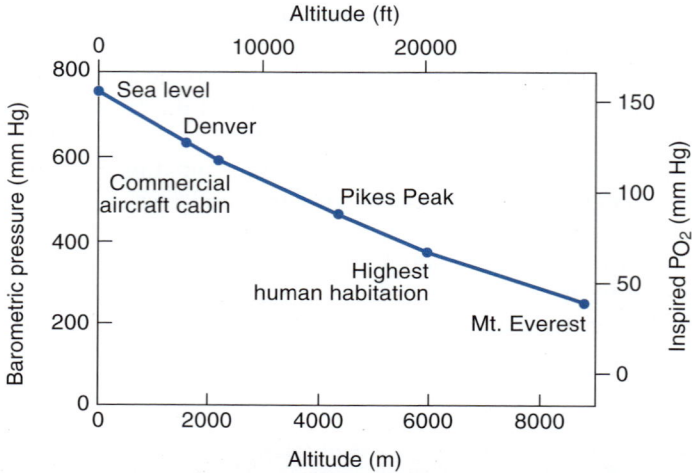

Figure 9.2. Relationship between altitude and barometric pressure. Note that the P_{O_2} of moist inspired gas is about 130 mm Hg at 1,520 m (5,000 ft) (Denver, CO) but is only 43 mm Hg on the summit of Mount Everest.

Hyperventilation

The most important feature of acclimatization to high altitude is hyperventilation. Its physiological value can be seen by considering the alveolar gas equation for a climber on the summit of Mount Everest. If the climber's alveolar P_{CO_2} was 40 and respiratory exchange ratio 1, the climber's alveolar P_{O_2} would be $43 - (40/1)^* = 3$ mm Hg! However, by increasing the climber's ventilation fivefold, and thus reducing the P_{CO_2} to 8 mm Hg (see p. 21), the alveolar P_{O_2} is increased to $43 - 8 = 35$ mm Hg.

The mechanism of the hyperventilation is stimulation of the peripheral chemoreceptors by hypoxemia. The resulting low arterial P_{CO_2} and alkalosis tend to inhibit this increase in ventilation, but after a day or so, the cerebrospinal fluid (CSF) pH is brought partly back toward normal by movement of bicarbonate out of the CSF, and after 2 or 3 days, the pH of the arterial blood is returned nearer to normal by renal excretion of bicarbonate. These brakes on ventilation are then reduced, and it increases further. In addition, there is now evidence that the sensitivity of the carotid bodies to hypoxia increases during acclimatization. Interestingly, people who are born at high altitude have a diminished ventilatory response to hypoxia that is only slowly corrected by subsequent residence at sea level.

---

*When R = 1, the correction factor (F) shown on p. 87 vanishes.

Polycythemia

Another apparently valuable feature of acclimatization to high altitude is an increase in the red blood cell concentration of the blood. The resulting rise in hemoglobin concentration, and therefore O_2-carrying capacity, means that although the arterial P_{O_2} and O_2 saturation are diminished, the O_2 concentration of the arterial blood may be normal or even above normal. For example, in some permanent residents at 4,600 m (15,000 ft) in the Peruvian Andes, the arterial P_{O_2} is only 45 mm Hg, and the corresponding arterial O_2 saturation is only 81%. Ordinarily, this would considerably decrease the arterial O_2 concentration, but because of the polycythemia, the hemoglobin concentration is increased from 15 to 19.8 g·100 ml⁻¹, giving an arterial O_2 concentration of 22.4 g·100 ml⁻¹, which is actually higher than the normal sea level value. The polycythemia also tends to maintain the P_{O_2} of mixed venous blood, and typically in Andean natives living at 4,600 m (15,000 ft), this P_{O_2} is only 7 mm Hg below normal (**Figure 9.3**).

The initial increase in hemoglobin concentration is caused by hemoconcentration due to a reduction in plasma volume. Subsequent increases

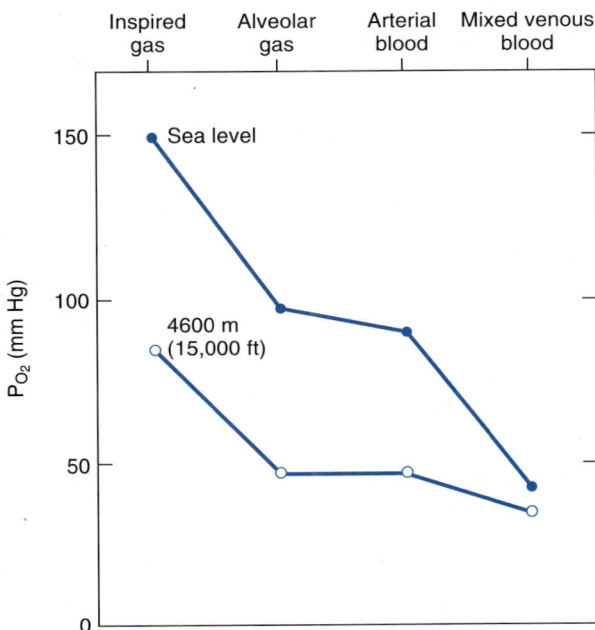

Figure 9.3. P_{O_2} values from inspired air to mixed venous blood at sea level and in residents at an altitude of 4,600 m (15,000 ft). Note that in spite of the much lower inspired P_{O_2} at altitude, the P_{O_2} of the mixed venous blood is only 7 mm Hg lower. (From Hurtado A. In: Dill DB, ed. *Handbook of Physiology, Adaptation to the Environment*. Washington, DC: American Physiological Society; 1964.)

occur because hypoxemia triggers increased release of erythropoietin from the kidney within 2 to 3 days of exposure to high altitude, which stimulates bone marrow activity and increased red blood cell production. The latter mechanism is one reason polycythemia can be seen in many patients with chronic hypoxemia caused by lung disease or cyanotic congenital heart disease.

Although the polycythemia of high altitude increases the O_2-carrying capacity of the blood, it also raises the blood viscosity. This can be deleterious, and some physiologists believe that the marked polycythemia that is sometimes seen is an inappropriate response.

Other Physiological Changes at High Altitude

There is a rightward shift of the O_2 dissociation curve at moderate altitudes that results in a better unloading of O_2 in venous blood at a given Po_2. The cause of the shift is an increase in concentration of 2,3-diphosphoglycerate, which develops primarily because of the respiratory alkalosis. At higher altitudes, there is a *leftward shift* in the dissociation curve caused by the respiratory alkalosis, and this assists in the loading of O_2 in the pulmonary capillaries. The *number of capillaries per unit volume* in peripheral tissues increases and changes occur in the *oxidative enzymes* inside the cells. The *maximum breathing capacity* increases because the air is less dense, and this assists the very high ventilations (up to 200 liters·min^{-1}) that occur on exercise. However, the maximum O_2 uptake declines rapidly above 4,600 m (15,000 ft).

Pulmonary vasoconstriction occurs in response to alveolar hypoxia (Figure 4.10). This increases the pulmonary arterial pressure and the work done by the right heart. The hypertension is exaggerated by the polycythemia, which raises the viscosity of the blood. With prolonged exposure, hypertrophy of the right heart can be seen, with characteristic changes in the electrocardiogram. There is no physiological advantage in this response, except that the topographical distribution of blood flow becomes more uniform. The pulmonary hypertension is sometimes associated with pulmonary edema, although the pulmonary venous pressure is normal. The probable mechanism is that the arteriolar vasoconstriction is uneven, and leakage occurs in unprotected, damaged capillaries. The edema fluid has a high protein concentration, indicating that the permeability of the capillaries is increased.

Newcomers to high altitude frequently complain of headache, fatigue, dizziness, palpitations, insomnia, loss of appetite, and nausea. This is known as *acute mountain sickness* and is attributable to the hypoxemia and alkalosis. In rare cases, cerebral edema can occur, leading to severe neurologic dysfunction.

Acclimatization to High Altitude

- Most important feature is hyperventilation.
- Polycythemia is slow to develop, but over time, it can raise the arterial oxygen concentration substantially.
- Other features include increases in cellular oxidative enzymes and the concentration of capillaries in some tissues.
- Hypoxic pulmonary vasoconstriction is not beneficial at high altitude.

Permanent Residents of High Altitude

In some parts of the world, notably Tibet and the South American Andes, large numbers of people have lived at high altitude for many generations. It is now known that Tibetans exhibit features of natural selection to the hypoxia of high altitude. For example, there are differences in birth weight, hemoglobin concentrations, and arterial oxygen saturation in infants and exercising adults compared with lowlanders who go to high altitude. Recent studies show that Tibetans have developed differences in their genetic makeup. For example, the gene that encodes the hypoxia-inducible factor 2α (HIF-2α) is more frequent in Tibetans than Han Chinese. HIF-2α is a transcription factor that regulates many physiological responses to hypoxia. Long-term residents sometimes develop an ill-defined syndrome, known as *chronic mountain sickness*, which is characterized by marked polycythemia, fatigue, reduced exercise tolerance, and severe hypoxemia.

O_2 TOXICITY

The usual problem is getting enough O_2 into the body, but it is possible to have too much. When high concentrations of O_2 are breathed for many hours, damage to the lung may occur. If guinea pigs are placed in 100% O_2 at atmospheric pressure for 48 h, they develop pulmonary edema. The first pathological changes are seen in the endothelial cells of the pulmonary capillaries (see Figure 1.1). Evidence of impaired gas exchange has been demonstrated in humans after 30 h of inhalation of 100% O_2 while healthy volunteers who breathe 100% O_2 at atmospheric pressure for 24 h complain of substernal distress that is aggravated by deep breathing. They also develop a diminution of vital capacity of 500 to 800 ml, which is probably caused by absorption atelectasis (see below). Increasing clinical evidence has also suggested that overly high arterial Po_2 in patients receiving invasive mechanical ventilation may worsen patient outcomes.

Another hazard of breathing 100% O_2 is seen in premature infants who develop blindness because of retinopathy of prematurity, that is, fibrous tissue formation behind the lens. Here, the mechanism is local vasoconstriction caused by the high P_{O_2} in the incubator. It can be avoided if the arterial P_{O_2} is kept below 140 mm Hg.

Absorption Atelectasis

This is another danger of breathing 100% O_2. Suppose that an airway is obstructed by mucus (**Figure 9.4**). The total pressure in the trapped gas is close to 760 mm Hg (it may be a few mm Hg less as it is absorbed because of elastic forces in the lung). But the sum of the partial pressures in the venous blood is far less than 760 mm Hg. This is because the P_{O_2} of the venous blood remains relatively low, even when O_2 is breathed. In fact, the rise in O_2 *concentration* of arterial and venous blood when O_2 is breathed will be the same if cardiac output remains unchanged, but because of the shape of the O_2 dissociation curve (see Figure 6.1), the increase in venous P_{O_2} is only about 10 to 15 mm Hg. Thus, because the sum of the partial pressures in the alveolar gas greatly exceeds that in the venous blood, gas diffuses into the blood, and rapid collapse of the alveoli occurs. Reopening such an atelectatic area may be difficult because of surface tension effects in such small units.

Absorption atelectasis also occurs in a blocked region even when air is breathed, although here the process is slower. Figure 9.4B shows that again

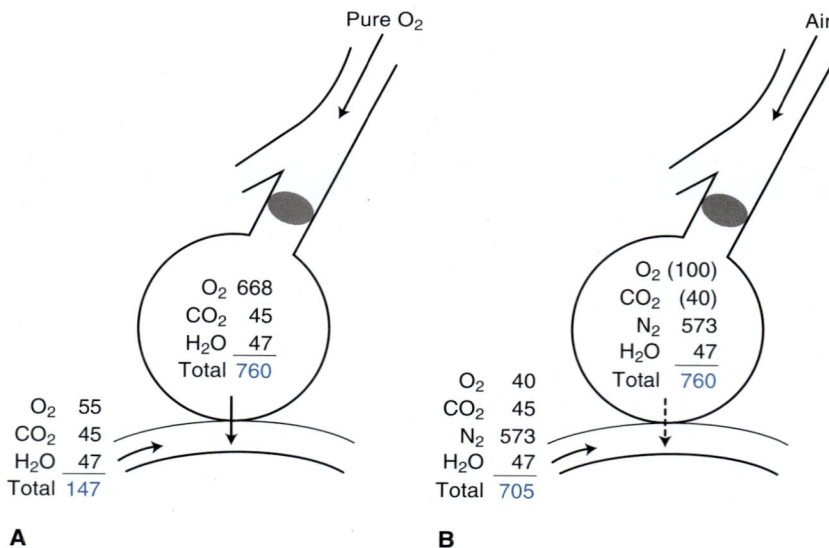

Figure 9.4. Reasons for atelectasis of alveoli beyond blocked airways when O_2 **(A)** and when air **(B)** is breathed. Note that in both cases, the sum of the gas partial pressures in the mixed venous blood is less than in the alveoli. In **(B)**, the P_{O_2} and P_{CO_2} are shown in *parentheses* because these values change with time. However, the total alveolar pressure remains within a few mm Hg of 760.

the sum of the partial pressures in venous blood is less than 760 mm Hg because the fall in P_{O_2} from arterial to venous blood is much greater than the rise in P_{CO_2} (this is a reflection of the steeper slope of the CO_2 compared with the O_2 dissociation curve—see Figure 6.6). Because the total gas pressure in the alveoli is near 760 mm Hg, absorption is inevitable. Actually, the changes in the alveolar partial pressures during absorption are somewhat complicated, but it can be shown that the rate of collapse is limited by the rate of absorption of N_2. Because this gas has a low solubility, its presence acts as a "splint" that, as it were, supports the alveoli and delays collapse. Even relatively small concentrations of N_2 in alveolar gas have a useful splinting effect. Nevertheless, postoperative atelectasis is a common problem in patients who are treated with high O_2 mixtures. Collapse is particularly likely to occur at the bottom of the lung, where the parenchyma is least well expanded (see Figure 7.8) or the small airways are actually closed (see Figure 7.9). This same basic mechanism of absorption is responsible for the gradual disappearance of a pneumothorax, or a gas pocket introduced under the skin.

SPACE FLIGHT

The absence of gravity causes a number of physiological changes, and some of these affect the lung. The distribution of ventilation and blood flow become more uniform, with a small corresponding improvement in gas exchange (see Figures 5.8 and 5.10), though some inequality remains because of non-gravitational factors. The deposition of inhaled aerosol is altered because of the absence of sedimentation. In addition, thoracic blood volume initially increases because blood does not pool in the legs. This raises pulmonary capillary blood volume and diffusing capacity. Postural hypotension occurs on return to earth; this is known as *cardiovascular deconditioning*. Decalcification of bone and muscle atrophy may occur, presumably through disuse. There is also a small reduction in red cell mass. Space sickness during the first few days of flight can be a serious operational problem.

INCREASED PRESSURE

During diving, the pressure increases by 1 atm for every 10 m (33 ft) of descent. It is extremely difficult and dangerous for an individual to attempt to breathe underwater with a long tube running to the surface because the high pressure limits expansion of the chest and compresses the lung. Also the pressure in the pulmonary capillaries increases leading to pulmonary edema. SCUBA equipment provides a solution to these challenges and allows people to remain at great depths for long periods of time, but poses important risks.

Barotrauma

By breathing air at increased pressure from an air tank, SCUBA divers prevent compression of the lung while at depth. With travel back to the surface, barometric pressure decreases and the gas in the alveolar space will expand according to the principles of Boyle's Law. For this reason, SCUBA divers must exhale as they ascend to prevent overinflation and possible rupture of the lungs. This is known as barotrauma and can take the form of either pneumomediastinum or pneumothorax. Other gas cavities such as the middle ear or intracranial sinus may also be subject to compression or overexpansion if they fail to communicate with the outside.

Decompression Sickness

During diving, the high partial pressure of N_2 forces this poorly soluble gas into solution in body tissues. This particularly occurs in fat, which has a relatively high N_2 solubility. However, the blood supply of adipose tissue is meager, and the blood can carry little N_2. In addition, the gas diffuses slowly because of its low solubility. As a result, equilibration of N_2 between the tissues and the environment takes hours.

During ascent, N_2 is slowly removed from the tissues. If decompression is unduly rapid, bubbles of gaseous N_2 form, just as CO_2 is released when a bottle of champagne is opened. Some bubbles can occur without physiological disturbances, but large numbers of bubbles and the fact that they increase in size during ascent can cause pain, especially in the region of joints ("bends"). In severe cases, there may be respiratory problems such as chest pain and dyspnea, as well as neurological disturbances including deafness, impaired vision, and even paralysis caused by bubbles in the central nervous system (CNS) that obstruct blood flow.

The treatment of decompression sickness is recompression. This reduces the volume of the bubbles and forces them back into solution, and often results in a dramatic reduction of symptoms. Prevention is by careful decompression in a series of regulated steps. Schedules, based partly on theory and partly on experience, exist that show how rapidly a diver can come up and minimize the risk of developing bends. Even those who adhere tightly to these schedules can still develop the bends, however. A short but very deep dive may require hours of gradual decompression. It is now known that bubble formation during ascent is very common. Therefore, the aim of the decompression schedules is to prevent the bubbles from growing too large.

The risk of decompression sickness following very deep dives can be reduced if a helium-O_2 mixture is breathed during the dive. Helium is about one-half as soluble as is N_2, so less is dissolved in tissues. In addition, it has one-seventh of the molecular weight of N_2 and therefore diffuses out more rapidly through tissue (Figure 3.1). Both these factors reduce the risk of bends. Another advantage of a helium-O_2 mixture for divers is its low density, which reduces the work of breathing. Pure O_2 or enriched O_2 mixtures cannot be used at depth because of the dangers of O_2 toxicity (see below).

Decompression Sickness

- Caused by the formation of N_2 bubbles during ascent from a deep dive.
- May result in pain ("bends") and neurological disturbances.
- Can be prevented by a slow, staged ascent.
- Treated by recompression in a chamber.
- Incidence is reduced by breathing a helium-oxygen mixture.

Commercial divers who are working at great depths, for example, on pipelines, sometimes use *saturation diving*. When they are not in the water, they live in a high-pressure chamber on the supply ship for several days, which means that they do not return to normal atmospheric pressure during this time. In this way, they avoid decompression sickness. However, at the end of the period at high pressure, they may take many days to decompress safely.

Inert Gas Narcosis

Although we usually think of N_2 as a physiological inert gas, at high partial pressures, it affects the CNS. At a depth of about 50 m (160 ft), there is a feeling of euphoria (not unlike that following a glass or two of alcohol), and scuba divers have been known to offer their mouthpieces to fish! At higher partial pressures, loss of coordination and eventually coma may develop. The mechanism of action is not fully understood but may be related to the high fat-to-water solubility of N_2, which is a general property of anesthetic agents. Other gases, such as helium and hydrogen, can be used at much greater depths without narcotic effects.

O_2 Toxicity

We saw earlier that inhalation of 100% O_2 at 1 atm can damage the lung. Another form of O_2 toxicity is stimulation of the CNS, leading to convulsions, when the Po_2 considerably exceeds 760 mm Hg. The convulsions may be preceded by premonitory symptoms such as nausea, ringing in the ears, and twitching of the face.

The likelihood of convulsions depends on the inspired Po_2 and the duration of exposure, and it is increased if the subject is exercising. At a Po_2 of 4 atm, convulsions frequently occur within 30 min. For increasingly deep dives, the O_2 concentration is progressively reduced to avoid toxic effects and may eventually be less than 1% for a normal inspired Po_2! The amateur scuba diver should *never* fill his or her tanks with O_2 alone because of the danger of a convulsion underwater. However, pure O_2 is sometimes used by the military for shallow dives because a closed breathing circuit with a CO_2 absorber leaves no telltale bubbles. The biochemical basis for the deleterious effects of a high Po_2 on the CNS is not fully understood but is probably the inactivation of certain enzymes, especially dehydrogenases containing sulfhydryl groups.

Hyperbaric O_2 Therapy

Increasing the arterial Po_2 to a very high level by raising barometric pressure is useful in some clinical situations. In addition to its role in treating decompression sickness, it can be used for severe CO poisoning in which most of the hemoglobin is bound to CO and is therefore unavailable to carry O_2. By raising the inspired Po_2 to 3 atm in special chambers, the amount of dissolved O_2 in arterial blood can be increased to about 6 ml per 100 ml (see Figure 6.1), and thus, the needs of the tissues can be met without functioning hemoglobin. Severe anemia is sometimes managed in this way in patients who refuse blood transfusions.

Fire and explosions are serious hazards of a 100% O_2 atmosphere, especially at increased pressure. For this reason, O_2 in a pressure chamber is given by mask, and the chamber itself is filled with air.

POLLUTED ATMOSPHERES[†]

Atmospheric pollution is an increasing problem in many countries as the number of motor vehicles and industries increases. The chief pollutants are various oxides of nitrogen and sulfur, ozone, carbon monoxide, various hydrocarbons, and particulate matter. Of these, nitrogen oxides, hydrocarbons, and CO are produced in large quantities by the internal combustion engine, the sulfur oxides mainly come from fossil fuel power stations, and ozone is chiefly formed in the atmosphere by the action of sunlight on nitrogen oxides and hydrocarbons. The concentration of atmospheric pollutants is greatly increased by a temperature inversion that prevents the normal escape of the warm surface air to the upper atmosphere.

Nitrogen oxides cause inflammation of the upper respiratory tract and eye irritation, and they are responsible for the yellow haze of smog. Sulfur oxides and ozone also cause bronchial inflammation, and ozone in high concentrations can produce pulmonary edema. The danger of CO is its propensity to tie up hemoglobin, and cyclic hydrocarbons are potentially carcinogenic. Both these pollutants exist in tobacco smoke, which is inhaled in far higher concentrations than any other atmospheric pollutant. There is evidence that some pollutants act synergistically, that is, their combined actions exceed the sum of their individual actions.

[†]For a more detailed account, see West JB, Luks AM. *West's Pulmonary Pathophysiology: The Essentials*. 9th ed. Wolters Kluwer; 2018.

Many pollutants exist as *aerosols*, that is, very small particles that remain suspended in the air. When an aerosol is inhaled, its fate depends on the size of the particles. Large particles are removed by *impaction* in the nose and pharynx. This means that the particles are unable to turn the corners rapidly because of their inertia, and they impinge on the wet mucosa and are trapped. Medium-sized particles deposit in small airways and elsewhere because of their weight. This is called *sedimentation* and occurs especially where the flow velocity is suddenly reduced because of the enormous increase in combined airway cross section (Figure 1.5). For this reason, deposition is heavy in the terminal and respiratory bronchioles, and this region of a coal miner's lung shows a large dust concentration. The smallest particles (<0.1 μm in diameter) may reach the alveoli, where some deposition occurs through *diffusion* to the walls. Many small particles are not deposited at all but are exhaled with the next breath.

Once deposited, most of the particles are removed by various clearance mechanisms. Particles that deposit on bronchial walls are swept up the moving staircase of mucus that is propelled by cilia, and they are either swallowed or expectorated. This is sometimes called the mucociliary ladder. However, the ciliary action can be paralyzed by inhaled irritants, such as cigarette smoke. Particles deposited in the alveoli are chiefly engulfed by macrophages that leave via the blood or lymphatics.

PERINATAL RESPIRATION

Placental Gas Exchange

During fetal life, gas exchange takes place through the placenta. Its circulation is in parallel with that of the peripheral tissues of the fetus (**Figure 9.5**), unlike the situation in the adult, in which the pulmonary circulation is in series with the systemic circulation. Maternal blood enters the placenta from the uterine arteries and surges into small spaces called intervillous sinusoids that function like the alveoli in the adult. Fetal blood from the aorta (Ao) is supplied to capillary loops that protrude into the intervillous spaces. Gas exchange occurs across the blood-blood barrier, which is approximately 3.5 μm thick.

This arrangement is much less efficient for gas exchange than in the adult lung. Maternal blood apparently swirls around the sinusoids somewhat haphazardly, and there are probably large differences of Po_2 within these blood spaces. Contrast this situation with the air-filled alveoli, in which rapid gaseous diffusion stirs up the alveolar contents. The result is that the Po_2 of the fetal blood leaving the placenta is only about 30 mm Hg (Figure 9.5).

This blood mixes with venous blood draining from the fetal tissues and reaches the right atrium (RA) via the inferior vena cava. Because of streaming within the right atrium, most of this blood then flows directly into the

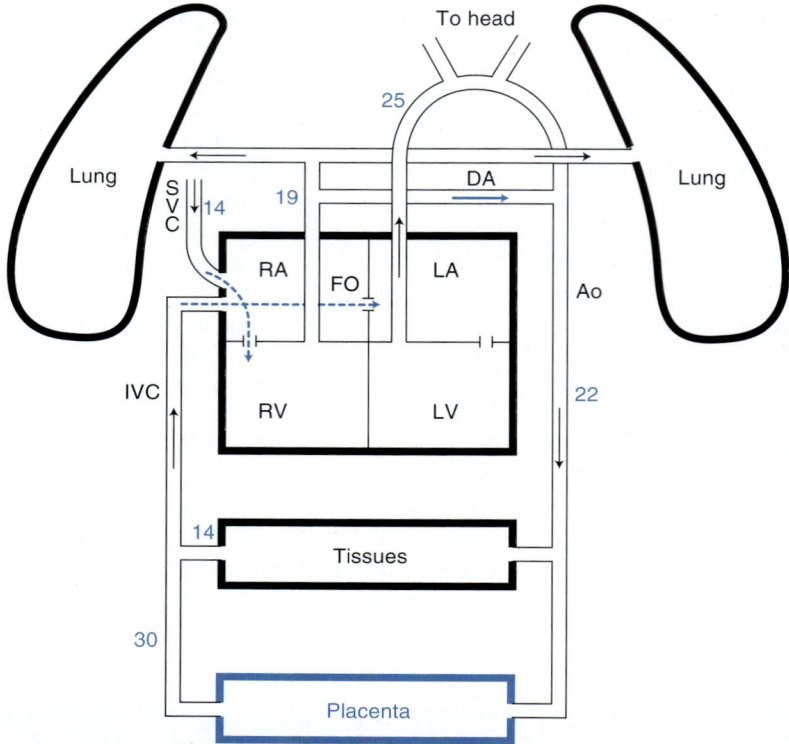

Figure 9.5. Blood circulation in the human fetus. The *numbers* show the approximate Po₂ of the blood in mm Hg. See text for details. Ao, aorta; DA, ductus arteriosus; FO, foramen ovale; IVC, inferior vena cava; LA, left atrium; LV, left ventricle; RA, right atrium. RV, right ventricle; SVC, superior vena cava.

left atrium (LA) through the open foramen ovale (FO) and thus is distributed via the ascending aorta to the brain and heart. Less well-oxygenated blood returning to the right atrium via the superior vena cava finds its way to the right ventricle, but only a small portion reaches the lungs. Most is shunted to the aorta through the ductus arteriosus (DA). The net result of this complex arrangement is that the best-oxygenated blood reaches the brain and heart, and the non–gas-exchanging lungs receive only about 15% of the cardiac output. Note that the arterial Po₂ in the descending aorta is only about 22 mm Hg. The fetus can still carry sufficient oxygen in the blood to support its development despite this very low Po₂ because it has a special form of hemoglobin, hemoglobin F, with a very high affinity for oxygen.

To summarize the three most important differences between the fetal and adult circulations:

1. The placenta is in parallel with the circulation to the tissues, whereas the lung is in series in the adult.

2. The ductus arteriosus shunts most of the blood from the pulmonary artery to the descending aorta.
3. Streaming within the right atrium means that the oxygenated blood from the placenta is preferentially delivered to the left atrium through the foramen ovale and therefore via the ascending aorta to the brain.

The First Breath

The emergence of a baby into the outside world is perhaps the most cataclysmic event of his or her life. The baby is suddenly bombarded with a variety of external stimuli. In addition, the process of birth interferes with placental gas exchange, with resulting hypoxemia and hypercapnia. Finally, the sensitivity of the chemoreceptors apparently increases dramatically at birth, although the mechanism is unknown. As a consequence of all these changes, the baby makes the first gasp.

The fetal lung is not collapsed but is inflated with liquid to about 40% of total lung capacity. This fluid is continuously secreted by alveolar cells during fetal life and has a low pH. Some of it is squeezed out as the infant moves through the birth canal, but the remainder helps in the subsequent inflation of the lung. As air enters the lung, large surface tension forces have to be overcome. By increasing the radius of curvature of the alveolar spaces, the residual fluid lowers the pressures necessary to inflate the lung (see Figure 7.4). Nevertheless, the intrapleural pressure during the first breath may fall to −40 cm water before any air enters the lung, and peak inspiratory pressures as low as −100 cm water during the first few breaths have been recorded. These very large transient pressures are partly caused by the high viscosity of the lung liquid compared with air. The fetus makes very small, rapid breathing movements in the uterus over a considerable period before birth.

Expansion of the lung is very uneven at first. However, pulmonary surfactant, which is formed relatively late in fetal life, is available to stabilize open alveoli, and the lung liquid is removed by the lymphatics and capillaries. Within a short time, the functional residual capacity has almost reached its normal value, and an adequate gas-exchanging surface has been established. However, it is several days before uniform ventilation is achieved.

Circulatory Changes

A dramatic fall in pulmonary vascular resistance follows the first few breaths. In the fetus, the pulmonary arteries are exposed to the full systemic blood pressure via the ductus arteriosus, and their walls are very muscular. As a result, the resistance of the pulmonary circulation is exquisitely sensitive to such vasoconstrictor agents as hypoxemia, acidosis, and serotonin and to vasodilators such as acetylcholine. Several factors account for the fall in pulmonary vascular resistance at birth, including the abrupt rise in alveolar Po_2 that abolishes hypoxic vasoconstriction and the increased volume of the lung that widens the caliber of the extra-alveolar vessels (see Figure 4.2).

With the resulting increase in pulmonary blood flow, left atrial pressure rises and the flaplike foramen ovale quickly closes. A rise in aortic pressure resulting from the loss of the parallel umbilical circulation also increases left atrial pressure. In addition, right atrial pressure falls as the umbilical flow ceases. The ductus arteriosus begins to constrict a few minutes later in response to the direct action of the increased Po_2 on its smooth muscle. This constriction is aided by reductions in the levels of local and circulating prostaglandins. Flow through the ductus arteriosus soon reverses as the resistance of the pulmonary circulation falls. Nonsteroidal anti-inflammatory drugs can be given to inhibit prostaglandin synthesis and promote closure when the ductus remains patent after birth. In rare circumstances, prostaglandins are actually administered to infants with certain congenital heart defects to keep the ductus open.

Changes at or Shortly After Birth

- Baby makes strong inspiratory efforts and takes its first breath.
- Large fall in pulmonary vascular resistance.
- Ductus arteriosus closes, as does the foramen ovale.
- Lung liquid is removed by lymphatics and capillaries.

RESPIRATION IN INFANCY

Even after the critical changes noted above are completed, the infant's respiratory system differs in important ways from that of adults. This poses ongoing challenges, particularly during times of stress.

Mechanics and Airflow

Because of the high compliance of their chest walls, FRC is lower in infants than in adults. The ribs are also more horizontal than in adults, limiting the increase in thoracic volume on inhalation. Thoracic volume change is also limited by the fact that the infant diaphragm is higher in the chest and has more horizontal insertion points, and therefore, a smaller zone of apposition. The relatively small respiratory muscle mass and low number of fatigue-resistant fibers limit their ability to sustain high workloads during periods of stress. Airway diameter is quite small; thus, problems such as mucous or mucosal edema that narrow airway caliber have a marked effect on airway resistance.

Gas Exchange

The full complement of alveoli is not present until many years after birth. Infants are prone to rapid development of hypoxemia in the setting of respiratory compromise. This is due to their low FRC, as well as their high metabolic rate, which predisposes them to large decreases in alveolar P_{O_2} whenever ventilation is reduced.

Control of Breathing

Development of the ventilatory control system starts early in gestation but is not complete by birth. Newborn infants have reduced ventilatory responses to changes in P_{CO_2} and a biphasic ventilatory response to hypoxemia; whereas older infants and adults experience sustained increases in ventilation, newborns experience a transient rise in ventilation followed by a return to baseline and, in some cases, depressed ventilation. Premature infants may become apneic. The adult pattern of responses to hypoxemia is present about two weeks after birth.

KEY CONCEPTS

1. Exercise greatly increases O_2 uptake and CO_2 output. O_2 consumption increases linearly with work rate up to the $\dot{V}_{O_2}$ max. There is a large rise in ventilation, but cardiac output increases less.

2. The most important feature of acclimatization to high altitude is hyperventilation, which results in very low arterial P_{CO_2} values at extreme altitude. Polycythemia increases the O_2 concentration of the blood but is slow to develop. Other features of acclimatization include changes in oxidative enzymes and an increased capillary concentration in some tissues.

3. Patients who breathe a high concentration of O_2 are liable to develop atelectasis if an airway is obstructed, for example, by mucus. Atelectasis can also occur with air breathing, but this is much slower.

4. Following SCUBA diving to great depths, decompression sickness may occur as a result of the formation of N_2 bubbles in the blood. These can cause pain in joints ("bends") and also respiratory and CNS effects. Prevention is by gradual ascent, and treatment is by recompression.

5. Atmospheric pollutants frequently exist as aerosols that are deposited in the lung by impaction, sedimentation, or diffusion depending on the size of the particles. They are subsequently removed from the airways by the mucociliary escalator and from the alveoli by macrophages.

6. The environment of the fetus is very hypoxic, with the P_{O_2} in the descending aorta being less than 25 mm Hg. The transition from

placental to pulmonary gas exchange results in dramatic changes in the circulation, including a striking fall in pulmonary vascular resistance and eventual closure of the ductus arteriosus and foramen ovale. Important differences with the adult respiratory system are found after birth and pose challenges in periods of stress.

CLINICAL VIGNETTE

A 25-year-old competitive cyclist completes an exercise test as part of his training. He pedals on a cycle ergometer as the work rate is steadily increased until he is exhausted. Total ventilation, oxygen consumption, carbon dioxide elimination, arterial oxygen saturation (by pulse oximetry), and pulmonary artery systolic pressure (by echocardiography) are measured, and the results are shown.

Variable	Rest	Midexercise	Maximum Exercise
O_2 Consumption (ml·min^{-1})	250	2,000	4,000
CO_2 Output (ml·min^{-1})	200	1,950	4,500
Ventilation (liters·min^{-1})	6	60	150
Systemic blood pressure (mm Hg)	110/70	180/75	230/80
Pulmonary artery systolic pressure (mm Hg)	25	28	35
Arterial P_{O_2} (mm Hg)	90	90	89
Arterial P_{CO_2} (mm Hg)	40	39	31
pH	7.4	7.39	7.10

A graph of the changes in oxygen uptake and total ventilation over the course of the test is shown below:

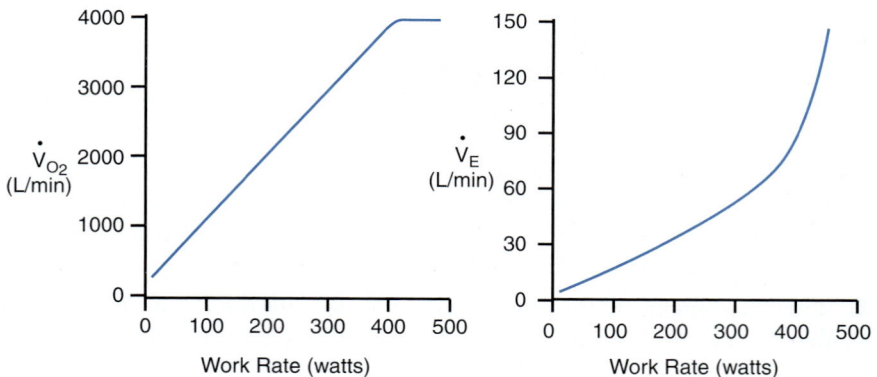

- Why does maximum oxygen consumption reach a plateau in late exercise?
- What explains the pattern of total ventilation over the course of the test?
- What happens to alveolar-arterial P_{O_2} difference in late exercise?
- What is the explanation of the observed changes in acid-base status over the course of the exercise test?

QUESTIONS

For each question, choose the one best answer.

1. A previously healthy, sedentary woman undergoes a cardiopulmonary exercise test at sea level to evaluate increasing dyspnea on exertion. The table below displays data obtained at rest prior to the test and at maximum exercise. Which of the variables demonstrates an abnormal pattern of response to progressive exercise?

Variable	Rest	Maximum Exercise
Blood pressure (mm Hg)	110/78	170/105
Heart rate (beats·min^{-1})	90	180
Arterial P_{CO_2} (mm Hg)	40	33
Arterial P_{O_2} (mm Hg)	90	60
Ventilation (liters·min^{-1})	8	140

- A. Arterial P_{CO_2}
- B. Arterial P_{O_2}
- C. Blood pressure
- D. Heart rate
- E. Ventilation

2. A newborn infant is noted to have increased work of breathing several days following birth. After a heart murmur is found on examination, an echocardiogram reveals that the blood flow is present in the ductus arteriosus. If there are no other congenital heart defects, which of the following would you expect to find in this infant?
- A. Decreased blood flow in the pulmonary circulation
- B. Increased arterial P_{CO_2}
- C. Increased pulmonary vascular resistance
- D. Left atrial dilation
- E. Patent foramen ovale

3. A 40-year-old is receiving invasive mechanical ventilation with an inspired oxygen fraction of 1.0 after presenting with septic shock. Which of the following would you expect to occur if a mucous plug completely blocks the opening to the right middle lobe?
   A. Atelectasis of the right middle lobe
   B. Increased arterial P_{CO_2}
   C. Increased blood flow to the right middle lobe
   D. Increased ventilation-perfusion ratio in the right middle lobe
   E. Right pneumothorax

4. Which of the following correctly describes a normal path for blood flow in the fetal circulation?
   A. Aorta → ductus arteriosus → pulmonary artery
   B. Aorta → tissue capillaries → placenta
   C. Left ventricle → foramen ovale → right ventricle
   D. Placenta → tissue capillaries → inferior vena cava
   E. Right atrium → foramen ovale → left atrium

5. An astronaut is in the seated position as her rocket launches as part of a mission to the International Space Station. Which of the following would you expect to occur as the ship leaves the earth's atmosphere and she transitions from 1G to 0G?
   A. Decreased blood flow to the apex of the lung
   B. Decreased deposition of medium-sized particles in the terminal bronchioles
   C. Decreased thoracic blood volume
   D. Decreased ventilation to the apex of the lung
   E. Increased ventilation-perfusion ratio in the apex of the lung

6. A 45-year-old man is placed in a hyperbaric chamber set to 3 atm for treatment of injuries suffered as a result of a house fire. He was intubated due to altered mental status and inhalation injury and remains on mechanical ventilation with an F_IO_2 of 0.5 while in the chamber. Sixty minutes after being placed in the chamber, he has twitching of his lips followed by a 1 min generalized seizure. Which of the following is most likely responsible for this adverse event?
   A. Cerebral arterial gas embolism
   B. Increased partial pressure of carbon monoxide
   C. Increased partial pressure of nitrogen
   D. Increased partial pressure of oxygen
   E. Nitrogen bubble formation

7. The figure below demonstrates the change in minute ventilation during a cardiopulmonary exercise test in a healthy individual. Which of the following accounts for the rate of rise in minute ventilation in Phase B compared to that seen in Phase A.

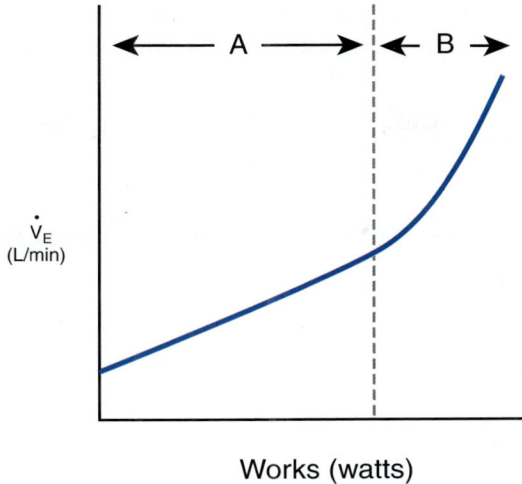

Works (watts)

A. Bronchodilation
B. Decreased arterial P_{CO_2}
C. Increased arterial P_{O_2}
D. Increased serum lactate concentration
E. Rightward shift of the hemoglobin-oxygen dissociation curve

8. A 45-year-old man goes SCUBA diving while on vacation in Hawaii. Concerned that he was running out of gas in his SCUBA tank, he ascends quickly to the surface of the water where, over a period of several hours after emerging, he develops severe pain in his knees and elbows, pruritus (itchiness), followed by difficulty breathing and problems with his hearing and vision. Which of the following mechanisms most likely explains these problems?
   A. Bubbles of gaseous nitrogen
   B. Excessive partial pressure of carbon dioxide while at depth
   C. Excessive partial pressure of oxygen while at depth
   D. Failure to exhale on ascent
   E. Middle ear and sinus compression

9. A 23-year-old woman ascends from sea level to a mountain hut at 4,559 m as part of a research project. An arterial blood sample is taken shortly following arrival on the summit and again on the morning of the 5th day at the hut. If she remains healthy during the course of her stay, which of the following changes in blood gas values would you expect to see on the 5th day compared to the sample drawn immediately following arrival?
   A. Decreased arterial P_{CO_2}
   B. Decreased arterial P_{O_2}
   C. Increased base excess
   D. Increased pH
   E. Increased serum bicarbonate

10. A 48-year-old woman cycles to her maximum exercise capacity during a cardiopulmonary exercise test at sea level and again following ascent to an altitude of 5,400 m. Arterial blood gases were measured at rest and maximum exercise and the arterial Po_2 values in mm Hg are shown below. Which of the following mechanisms most likely accounts for the observed changes in her arterial Po_2?

Test Location	Rest	Maximum Exercise
Sea level	90	90
5,400 m	50	38

A. Decreased dead space fraction
B. Decreased hemoglobin concentration
C. Hypoventilation
D. Increased shunt fraction
E. Shortened red blood cell capillary transit time

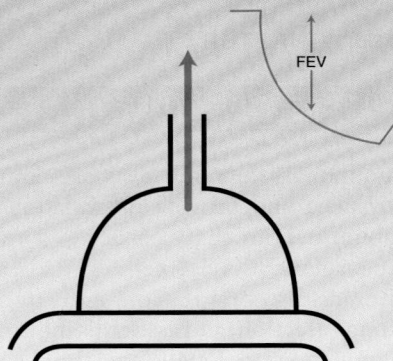

FEV

Tests of Pulmonary Function

10

How Respiratory Physiology Is Applied to Measure Lung Function*

This final chapter deals with pulmonary function testing, which is an important practical application of respiratory physiology in the clinic. First, we look at the forced expiration, a very simple but nevertheless very useful test. Then, there are sections on ventilation-perfusion relationships, blood gases, lung mechanics, control of ventilation, and exercise testing. By understanding the principles of respiratory physiology contained in Chapters 1 to 9, the reader can comprehend the details and utility of the testing discussed in the chapter. At the end of this chapter, the reader should be able to:

- Describe the uses pulmonary function testing
- Use the $FEV_{1.0}$, FVC, and flow volume loops to differentiate between obstructive and restrictive diseases
- Describe the different methods for assessing ventilation-perfusion inequality
- Use the alveolar-arterial P_{O_2} difference to determine the cause of hypoxemia
- Outline methods for estimating lung compliance, airway resistance, and closing volume
- Describe the role of cardiopulmonary exercise testing in the evaluation of patients with chronic dyspnea

*This chapter is only a brief introduction to pulmonary function tests. A more detailed description can be found in West JB, Luks AM, *West's Pulmonary Pathophysiology: The Essentials*. 9th ed. Wolters Kluwer; 2018.

USES OF PULMONARY FUNCTION TESTING

Pulmonary function tests are commonly used in the evaluation of chronic dyspnea and provide information on the nature of a patient's physiologic abnormalities that can be used to guide further diagnostic evaluation and management. They can also be used to assess response to treatment, monitor disease progression, evaluate fitness for surgical procedures, such as a lung resection, and assess disability for the purposes of insurance and workers' compensation. Finally, they can be used as part of research or epidemiological surveys to assess industrial hazards or to document the prevalence of disease in the community.

When used for diagnostic purposes, the primary role of these tests is in the evaluation of *chronic* respiratory problems rather than *acute* respiratory compromise. Arterial blood gases are one important exception as, along with chest imaging, echocardiography, and electrocardiography, they play a key role in the evaluation of acute dyspnea or hypoxemia.

While pulmonary function tests are useful diagnostic tools, it is important to keep their role in the proper perspective. These tests provide information about the primary physiologic issues in a given patient and point the way for further evaluation but rarely provide a definitive diagnosis. Testing may indicate, for example, that a patient has obstruction to air flow or decreased compliance, but other clinical and radiographic data are necessary to determine the cause of these physiologic derangements. These issues are considered further in *West's Pulmonary Pathophysiology*, 9th edition.

Some of the tests described below can only be performed in a sophisticated pulmonary function laboratory while others, such as spirometry, are easily performed in an outpatient clinic.

VENTILATION

Forced Expiration

As discussed in Chapter 7 (Figure 7.19), the forced expiratory maneuver, or spirometry, provides measurements of the forced expiratory volume (FEV) and forced vital capacity (FVC). These parameters are useful for identifying a patient's primary physiologic abnormality. The FVC may be reduced at its top or bottom end (see **Figure 10.1**). In *restrictive* diseases, inspiration is limited by the reduced compliance of the lung or chest wall, or weakness of the inspiratory muscles. In *obstructive* disease, the total lung capacity is typically abnormally large, but expiration ends prematurely. The reason for this is early airway closure brought about by increased smooth muscle tone of the bronchi, as in asthma, or loss of radial traction from surrounding parenchyma, as

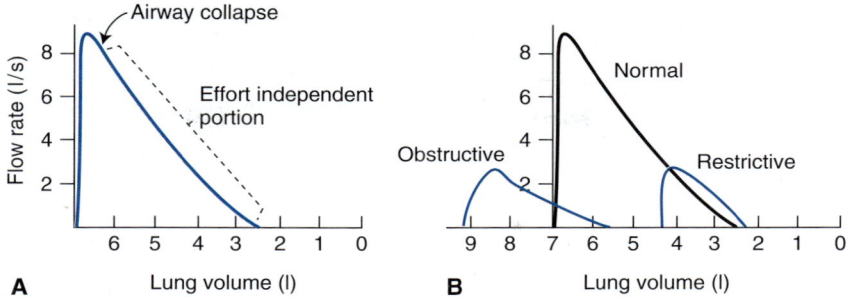

Figure 10.1. Flow-volume curves obtained by recording flow rate against volume during a forced expiration from maximum inspiration. The figures show absolute lung volumes, although these cannot be measured from single expirations. See text for details.

in emphysema. Other causes include edema of the bronchial walls or secretions within the airways.

The $FEV_{1.0}$ (or $FEF_{25\%-75\%}$) is reduced by an increase in airway resistance or a reduction in elastic recoil of the lung. It is remarkably independent of expiratory effort. The reason for this is the dynamic compression of airways, which was discussed earlier (see Figure 7.18). This mechanism explains why the flow rate is independent of the resistance of the airways downstream of the collapse point but is determined by the elastic recoil pressure of the lung and the resistance of the airways upstream of the collapse point. The location of the collapse point is in the large airways, at least initially. Thus, both the increase in airway resistance and the reduction of lung elastic recoil pressure can be important factors in the reduction of the $FEV_{1.0}$, as, for example, in pulmonary emphysema or asthma.

The ratio of these two variables ($FEV_{1.0}/FVC$) is also calculated and used to inform diagnosis. Reductions in the ratio are seen in patients with airflow obstruction but not restriction, with the lower limit of normal varying somewhat depending on the guidelines used for test interpretation.

In addition to these variables, spirometry provides another useful piece of information, the *flow-volume curve* (see Figure 7.16). Figure 10.1 reminds us that after a relatively small amount of gas has been exhaled, flow is limited by airway compression and is determined by the elastic recoil force of the lung and the resistance of the airways upstream of the collapse point. In *restrictive* diseases, the maximum flow rate is reduced, as is the total volume exhaled. However, if flow is related to the absolute lung volume (i.e., including the residual volume, which cannot be measured from a single expiration), the flow rate is often abnormally high during the latter part of expiration (Figure 10.1B). This can be explained by the increased lung recoil and the increased radial traction holding the airways open. By contrast, in *obstructive* diseases, the flow rate is very low in relation to lung volume, and a scooped-out appearance is often seen following the point of maximum flow.

Spirometry is sometimes performed both before and after administration of an inhaled short-acting bronchodilator. Changes in $FEV_{1.0}$ and FVC following administration of the medication provide further insight into the individual's airway function.

Lung Volumes

The determination of lung volumes by spirometry and the measurement of functional residual capacity (FRC) by helium dilution and body plethysmography were discussed earlier (see Figures 2.2 through 2.4).

The FRC can also be found by having the subject breathe 100% O_2 for several minutes and washing all the N_2 out of the subject's lung. Suppose that the lung volume is V_1 and that the total volume of gas exhaled over 7 min is V_2 and that its concentration of N_2 is C_2. We know that the concentration of N_2 in the lung before washout was 80%, and we can measure the concentration left in the lung by sampling end-expired gas with an N_2 meter at the lips. Call this concentration C_3. Then, assuming no net change in the amount of N_2, we can write $V_1 \times 380 = (V_1 \times C_3) + (V_2 \times C_2)$. Thus, V_1 can be derived. A disadvantage of this method is that the concentration of nitrogen in the gas collected over 7 min is very low, and a small error in its measurement leads to a larger error in calculated lung volume. In addition, some of the N_2 that is washed out comes from body tissues, and this should be allowed for. This method, like the helium dilution technique, measures only ventilated lung volume, whereas, as we saw in the discussion of Figure 2.4, the body plethysmograph method includes gas trapped behind closed airways.

The measurement of anatomic dead space by Fowler's method was described earlier (see Figure 2.6).

DIFFUSION

The principles of the measurement of the diffusing capacity for carbon monoxide by the single-breath method were discussed on p. 39. The diffusing capacity for O_2 is very difficult to measure, and it is only done as a research procedure.

BLOOD FLOW

The measurement of total pulmonary blood flow by the Fick's principle and by the indicator dilution method was discussed on pp. 52–53.

VENTILATION-PERFUSION RELATIONSHIPS

Topographical Distribution of Ventilation and Perfusion

Regional differences of ventilation and blood flow can be measured using radioactive xenon, as briefly described earlier (see Figures 2.7 and 4.7).

Inequality of Ventilation

This can be measured by single-breath and multiple-breath methods. The *single-breath method* is very similar to that described by Fowler's for measuring anatomic dead space (Figure 2.6). There we saw that if the N_2 concentration at the lips is measured following a single breath of O_2, the N_2 concentration of the expired alveolar gas is almost uniform, giving a nearly flat "alveolar plateau." This reflects the approximately uniform dilution of the alveolar gas by the inspired O_2. By contrast, in patients with lung disease, the alveolar N_2 concentration continues to rise during expiration. This is caused by the uneven dilution of the alveolar N_2 by inspired O_2.

The reason the concentration rises is that the poorly ventilated alveoli (those in which the N_2 has been diluted least) always empty last, presumably because they have long time constants (see Figures 7.20 and 10.4). In practice, the change in N_2 percentage concentration between 750 and 1,250 ml of expired volume is often used as an index of uneven ventilation. This is a simple, quick, and useful test.

The *multiple-breath method* is based on the rate of washout of N_2, as shown in **Figure 10.2**. The subject is connected to a source of 100% O_2, and a fast-responding N_2 meter samples gas at the lips. If the ventilation of the lung were uniform, the N_2 concentration would be reduced by the same *fraction* with each breath. For example, if the tidal volume (excluding dead space) were equal to the FRC, the N_2 concentration would halve with each breath. In general, the N_2 concentration is $FRC/[FRC + (V_T - V_D)]$ times that of the previous breath, where V_T and V_D are the tidal volume and anatomic dead space, respectively. Because the N_2 is reduced by the same fraction with each breath, the plot of log N_2 concentration against breath number would be a straight line (see Figure 10.2) if the lung behaved as a single, uniformly ventilated compartment. This is very nearly the case in healthy individuals.

In patients with lung disease, however, the nonuniform ventilation results in a curved plot because different lung units have their N_2 diluted at different rates. Thus, fast-ventilated alveoli cause a rapid initial fall in N_2, whereas slow-ventilated spaces are responsible for the long tail of the washout (see Figure 10.2).

Inequality of Ventilation-Perfusion Ratios

One way of assessing the mismatch of ventilation and blood flow within the diseased lung is that introduced by Riley. This is based on measurements of Po_2 and Pco_2 in arterial blood and expired gas (the principles were briefly

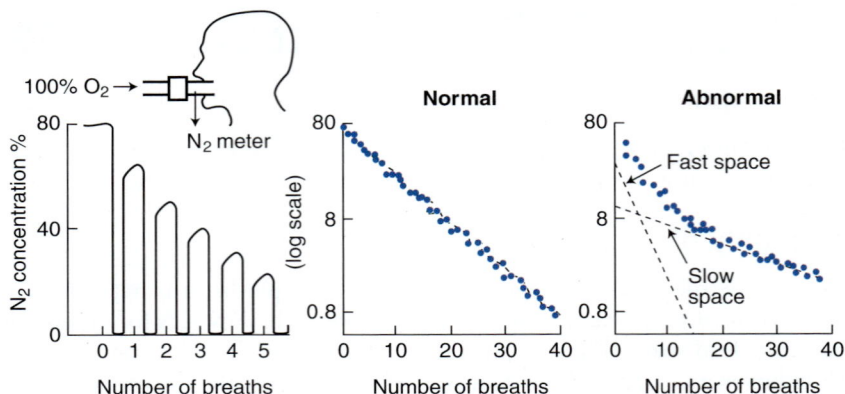

Figure 10.2. N_2 washout obtained when an individual breathes 100% O_2. Normal lungs give an almost linear plot of N_2 concentration against number of breaths on semilogarithmic paper, but this plot is nonlinear when uneven ventilation is present.

described in Chapter 5). In practice, expired gas and arterial blood are collected simultaneously from the patient, and various indices of ventilation-perfusion inequality are computed.

One useful measurement is the *alveolar-arterial* P_{O_2} difference. We saw in Figure 5.11 how this develops because of regional differences of gas exchange in the normal lung. **Figure 10.3** is an O_2-CO_2 diagram that allows us to examine this development more closely. First, suppose that there is no ventilation-perfusion inequality and that all the lung units are represented by a single point (i) on the ventilation-perfusion line. This is known as the "ideal" point. Now as ventilation-perfusion inequality develops, the lung units begin to spread away from i toward both $\bar{v}$ (low ventilation-perfusion ratios) and I (high ventilation-perfusion ratios) (compare Figure 5.7). The bar over v refers to mixed venous blood. When this happens, the mixed capillary blood (a) and mixed alveolar gas (A) also diverge from i. They do so along lines i to $\bar{v}$ and i to I, which represent a constant respiratory exchange ratio (CO_2 output/O_2 uptake), because this is determined by the metabolism of the body tissues.[†]

The horizontal distance between A and a represents the (*mixed*) *alveolar-arterial* P_{O_2} difference. In practice, this can only be measured easily if ventilation is essentially uniform but blood flow is uneven, because only then can a representative sample of mixed alveolar gas be obtained. This is sometimes the case in pulmonary embolism. More frequently, the P_{O_2} difference between ideal alveolar gas and arterial blood is calculated—the (*ideal*) *alveolar-arterial* P_{O_2} difference. The ideal alveolar P_{O_2} can be calculated from the alveolar gas equation that relates the P_{O_2} of any lung unit to the composition of the inspired gas, the respiratory exchange ratio, and the P_{CO_2} of the unit. In the case of ideal alveoli, the P_{CO_2} is taken to be the same as arterial blood

---

[†]In this necessarily simplified description, some details are omitted. For example, the mixed venous point alters when ventilation-perfusion inequality develops.

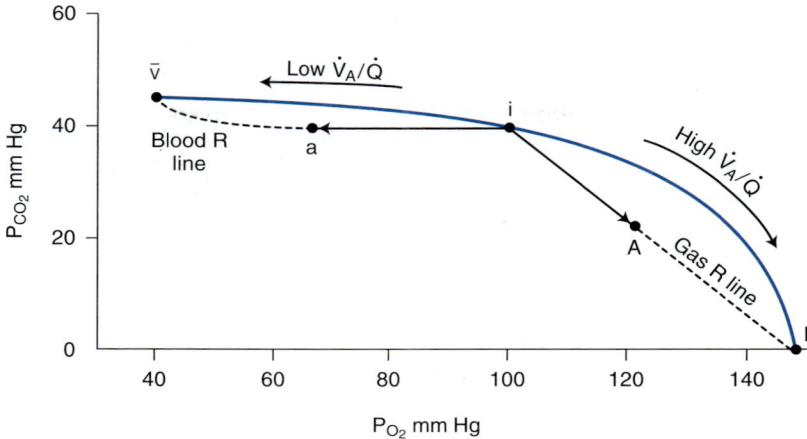

Figure 10.3. O_2-CO_2 diagram showing the ideal point (i), that is, the hypothetical composition of alveolar gas and end-capillary blood when no ventilation-perfusion inequality is present. As inequality develops, the arterial (a) and alveolar (A) points diverge along their respective R (respiratory exchange ratio) lines. The mixed alveolar-arterial P_{O_2} difference is the horizontal distance between the points.

because the line along which point i moves is so nearly horizontal. Note that this alveolar-arterial P_{O_2} difference is caused by units between i and $\bar{v}$, that is, those with low ventilation-perfusion ratios. In calculating the ideal alveolar P_{O_2}, it is necessary to know the inspired P_{O_2}, which can be difficult, for example, if the patient is receiving oxygen by nasal cannula or some other oxygen delivery devices. This information is more easily obtained if the individual is breathing ambient air or receiving oxygen via mechanical ventilation.

Two more indices of ventilation-perfusion inequality are frequently derived. One is *physiologic shunt* (also called *venous admixture*). For this, we pretend that all of the leftward movement of the arterial point (a) away from the ideal point (i) (i.e., the hypoxemia) is caused by the addition of mixed venous blood ($\bar{v}$) to ideal blood (i). This is not so fanciful as it first seems, because units with very low ventilation-perfusion ratios put out blood that has essentially the same composition as mixed venous blood (see Figures 5.6 and 5.7). In practice, the shunt equation (see Figure 5.3) is used in the following form:

$$\frac{\dot{Q}_{PS}}{\dot{Q}_T} = \frac{Ci_{O_2} - Ca_{O_2}}{Ci_{O_2} - C\bar{v}_{O_2}}$$

where $\dot{Q}_{PS}/\dot{Q}_T$ refers to the ratio of the physiologic shunt to total flow. The O_2 concentration of ideal blood is calculated from the ideal P_{O_2} and O_2 dissociation curve.

The other index is *alveolar dead space*. Here, we pretend that all of the movement of the alveolar point (A) away from the ideal point (i) is caused by the addition of inspired gas (I) to ideal gas. Again, this is not such an outrageous notion as it may first appear because units with very high ventilation-perfusion ratios behave very much like point I. After all, a unit with an infinitely high ventilation-perfusion ratio contains gas that has the same composition as does inspired air (see Figures 5.6 and 5.7). The Bohr equation for dead space (see p. 23) is used in the following form:

$$\frac{VD_{alv}}{V_T} = \frac{Pi_{CO_2} - PA_{CO_2}}{Pi_{CO_2}}$$

where A refers to expired alveolar gas. The result is called *alveolar dead space* to distinguish it from the *anatomic dead space*, that is, the volume of the conducting airways. Because expired alveolar gas is often difficult to collect without contamination by the anatomic dead space, the mixed expired CO_2 is often measured. The result is called the *physiologic dead space*, which includes components from the alveolar dead space and anatomic dead space. Because the Pco_2 of ideal gas is very close to that of arterial blood (see Figure 10.3), the equation for physiologic dead space is

$$\frac{V_{D_{phys}}}{V_T} = \frac{Pa_{CO_2} - P_{E_{CO_2}}}{Pa_{CO_2}}$$

The normal value for physiologic dead space is about 30% of the tidal volume at rest and consists almost completely of anatomic dead space. In healthy individuals, it decreases with exercise, whereas in acute and chronic lung diseases, it may increase to 50% or more due to the presence of ventilation-perfusion inequality.

BLOOD GASES AND pH

Po_2, Pco_2, and pH are easily measured in blood samples with blood-gas electrodes. A glass electrode is used to measure the pH of whole blood. The Pco_2 electrode is, in effect, a tiny pH meter in which a bicarbonate buffer solution is separated from the blood sample by a thin membrane. When carbon dioxide diffuses across the membrane from the blood, the pH of the buffer changes in accordance with the Henderson-Hasselbalch relationship. The pH meter then reads out the Pco_2. The O_2 electrode is a polarograph, that is, a device which, when supplied with a suitable voltage, gives a minute current that is proportional to the amount of dissolved O_2. In practice, all three electrodes are arranged to give their outputs on the same meter by appropriate switching, and a complete analysis on a blood sample can be done in a few minutes. Sometimes the arterial and mixed venous O_2 saturation are also measured with an instrument called a co-oximeter. Co-oximetry can also be used to measure the amount of carboxy- and methemoglobin.

We saw in Chapter 5 that there are four causes of low arterial Po_2 or hypoxemia: (1) hypoventilation, (2) diffusion impairment, (3) shunt, and (4) ventilation-perfusion inequality. The arterial Po_2 can also be reduced if the inspired value is low, as is the case, for example, at high altitude.

In distinguishing between these causes, keep in mind that hypoventilation is *always* associated with a raised arterial Pco_2 and that only when a shunt is present does the arterial Po_2 fail to rise to the expected level when 100% O_2 is administered. In diseased lungs, impaired diffusion is always accompanied by ventilation-perfusion inequality, and, indeed, it is usually impossible to determine how much of the hypoxemia is attributable to defective diffusion.

There are two causes of an increased arterial Pco_2: (1) hypoventilation and (2) ventilation-perfusion inequality. The latter does not *always* cause CO_2 retention, because any tendency for the arterial Pco_2 to rise signals the respiratory center via the chemoreceptors to increase ventilation and thus hold the Pco_2 down. The fact that the CO_2 dissociation curve is steep and nearly straight in the physiologic range helps lower the Pco_2 when ventilation increases. However, in the absence of this increased ventilation, the Pco_2 must rise. Changes in the blood gases in different types of hypoxemia are summarized in Table 6.3.

The assessment of the acid-base status of the blood was discussed in Chapter 6.

MECHANICS OF BREATHING

Lung Compliance

Compliance is defined as the volume change per unit of pressure change across the lung. To obtain this, we need to know intrapleural pressure. In practice, esophageal pressure is measured by having the subject swallow a small balloon on the end of a catheter. Esophageal pressure is not identical to intrapleural pressure but reflects its pressure changes fairly well. The measurement is not reliable in supine subjects because of interference by the weight of the mediastinal structures.

A simple way of measuring compliance is to have the subject breathe out from total lung capacity into a spirometer in steps of, say, 500 ml and measure the esophageal pressure simultaneously. The glottis should be open, and the lung should be allowed to stabilize for a few seconds after each step. In this way, a pressure-volume curve similar to the upper line in Figure 7.3 is obtained. The whole curve is the most informative way of reporting the elastic behavior of the lung. Indices of the shape of the curve can be derived. Notice that the compliance, which is the slope of the curve, will vary depending on what lung volume is used. It is conventional to report the slope over the liter above FRC measured during deflation. Even so, the measurement is not very repeatable.

Lung compliance can also be measured during resting breathing, as shown in Figure 7.13. Here, we make use of the fact that at no-flow points (end of inspiration or expiration), the intrapleural pressure reflects only the elastic recoil forces and not those associated with airflow. Thus, the volume difference divided by the pressure difference at these points is the compliance.

This method is not valid in patients with airway disease because the variation in time constants throughout the lung means that flow still exists within the lung when it has ceased at the mouth. **Figure 10.4** shows that if we consider a lung region that has a partially obstructed airway, it will always lag behind the rest of the lung (compare Figure 7.20). In fact, it may continue to fill when the rest of the lung has begun to empty, with the result that gas moves into it from adjoining lung units—so-called *pendelluft* (swinging air). As the breathing frequency is increased, the proportion of the tidal volume that

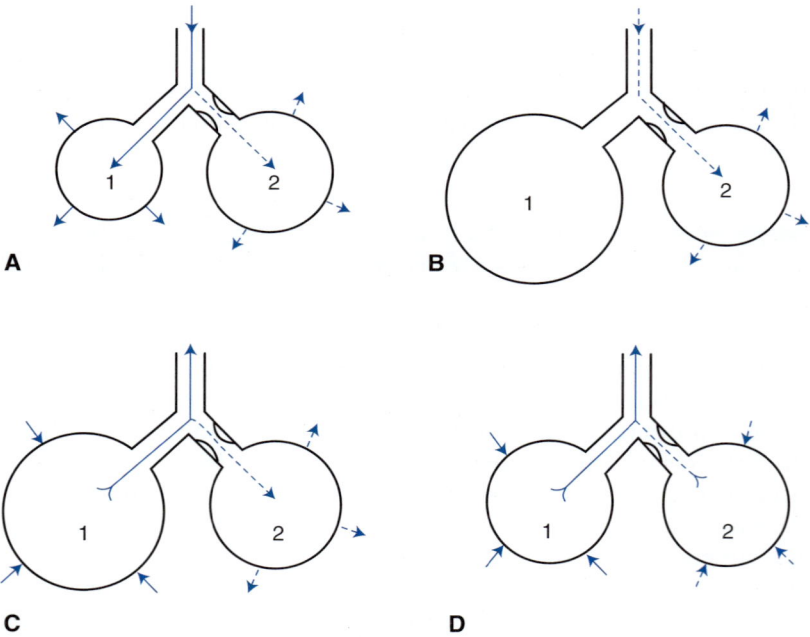

Figure 10.4. Effects of uneven time constants on ventilation. Compartment 2 has a partially obstructed airway and, therefore, a long time constant (compare Figure 7.20). During inspiration **(A)**, gas is slow to enter it, and it therefore continues to fill after the rest of the lung (*1*) has stopped moving **(B)**. Indeed, at the beginning of the expiration **(C)**, the abnormal region (*2*) may still be inhaling while the rest of the lung has begun to exhale. In **(D)**, both regions are exhaling, but compartment 2 lags behind compartment 1. At higher frequencies, the tidal volume to the abnormal region becomes progressively smaller.

goes to this partially obstructed region becomes smaller and smaller. Thus, less and less of the lung is participating in the tidal volume changes, and therefore, the lung appears to become less compliant.

Maximum inspiratory and expiratory pressures can also be measured to determine whether a patient with a restrictive pattern on spirometry has a neuromuscular disorder. Patients with isolated diaphragmatic weakness have reduced inspiratory pressure only, whereas those with diffuse neuromuscular disease have reduced inspiratory and expiratory pressures.

Airway Resistance

Airway resistance is the pressure difference between the alveoli and the mouth per unit of airflow. It can be measured in a body plethysmograph (**Figure 10.5**).

Before inspiration, the box pressure is atmospheric. At the onset of inspiration, the pressure in the alveoli falls as the alveolar gas expands by a volume ΔV. This compresses the gas in the box, and from its change in pressure, ΔV can be calculated (compare Figure 2.4). If lung volume is known, ΔV can be converted into alveolar pressure using Boyle's law. Flow is measured simultaneously, and thus, airway resistance is obtained. The measurement is made during expiration in the same way. Lung volume is determined as described in Figure 2.4.

Airway resistance can also be measured during normal breathing from an intrapleural pressure record as obtained with an esophageal balloon (see Figure 7.13). However, in this case, tissue viscous resistance is included as well (see p. 142). Intrapleural pressure reflects two sets of forces, those opposing the elastic recoil of the lung and those overcoming resistance to air and tissue flow. It is possible

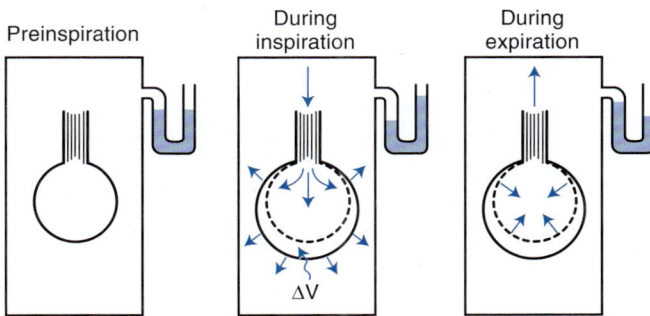

Figure 10.5. Measurement of airway resistance with the body plethysmograph. During inspiration, the alveolar gas is expanded, and box pressure therefore rises. From this, alveolar pressure can be calculated. The difference between alveolar and mouth pressure, divided by flow, gives airway resistance (see text). (Modified from Comroe JH. *The Lung: Clinical Physiology and Pulmonary Function Tests.* 2nd ed. Chicago, IL: Year Book; 1965. Copyright © 1965 Elsevier. With permission.)

to subtract the pressure caused by the recoil forces during quiet breathing because this is proportional to lung volume (if compliance is constant). The subtraction is done with an electrical circuit. We are then left with a plot of pressure against flow that gives (airway + tissue) resistance. This method is not satisfactory in lungs with severe airway disease because the uneven time constants prevent all regions from moving together (see Figure 10.4).

Closing Volume

Early disease in small airways can be sought by using the single-breath N_2 washout (see Figure 2.6) and thus exploiting the topographical differences of ventilation (see Figures 7.8 and 7.9). Suppose a subject takes a vital capacity (VC) breath of 100% O_2, and during the subsequent exhalation, the N_2 concentration at the lips is measured (**Figure 10.6**). Four phases can be recognized.

First, pure dead space is exhaled (1), followed by a mixture of dead space and alveolar gas (2), and then pure alveolar gas (3). Toward the end of expiration, an abrupt increase in N_2 concentration is seen (4). This signals closure of airways at the base of the lung (see Figure 7.9) and is caused by preferential emptying of the apex, which has a relatively high concentration of N_2. The reason for the higher N_2 at the apex is that during a VC breath of O_2, this region expands less (see Figure 7.9), and, therefore, the N_2 there is less diluted

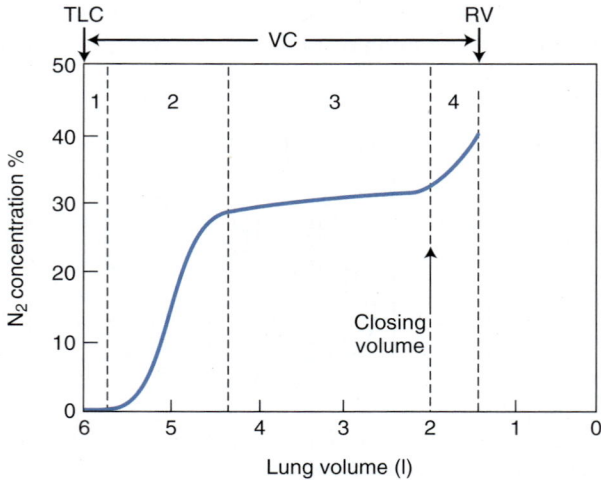

Figure 10.6. Measurement of the closing volume. If a vital capacity inspiration of 100% O_2 is followed by a full expiration, four phases in the N_2 concentration measured at the lips can be recognized (see text). The last is caused by preferential emptying of the upper part of the lung after the lower-zone airways have closed.

with O_2. Thus, the volume of the lung at which dependent airways begin to close can be read off the tracing.

In young normal subjects, the closing volume is about 10% of the VC. It increases steadily with age and is equal to about 40% of the VC, that is, the FRC, at about the age of 65 years. Relatively small amounts of disease in the small airways apparently increase the closing volume. Sometimes the *closing capacity* is reported. This is the closing volume plus the residual volume.

CONTROL OF VENTILATION

The responsiveness of the chemoreceptors and respiratory center to CO_2 can be measured by having the subject rebreathe into a rubber bag, as discussed on p. 160. We saw that the alveolar Po_2 also affects ventilation, so that if the response to CO_2 alone is required, the inspired Po_2 should be kept above 200 mm Hg to avoid any hypoxic drive. The ventilatory response to hypoxia can be measured in a similar way if the subject rebreathes from a bag with a low Po_2 but constant Pco_2.

EXERCISE

Additional information about cardiac and pulmonary function can often be obtained with cardiopulmonary exercise testing. As discussed at the beginning of Chapter 9, the resting lung has enormous reserves; its ventilation, blood flow, O_2 and CO_2 transfer, and diffusing capacity can be increased severalfold on exercise. Exercise stresses these systems and can reveal abnormalities that may not be present at rest.

Methods of providing controlled exercise include the treadmill and bicycle ergometer. Subjects exercise at steadily increasing levels of work while a variety of measurements are made, including total ventilation, respiratory frequency pulse rate, blood pressure, electrocardiography, O_2 uptake, CO_2 output, respiratory exchange ratio, and arterial blood gases. These measurements can be used to quantify the degree of limitation and identify whether exercise is limited by deficits in cardiac function, ventilatory capacity, or the ability to exchange gases across the blood-gas barrier. As such, it can be very useful in the evaluation of chronic dyspnea when other tests have not revealed a clear etiology.

KEY CONCEPTS

1. The measurement of a single forced expiration is simple to perform and often very informative. Specific patterns occur in obstructive and restrictive lung disease.

2. Arterial blood gases can be quickly measured with blood-gas electrodes, and this information is often essential in the management of critically ill patients.

3. The degree of ventilation-perfusion inequality in a diseased lung can be assessed from an arterial blood sample by calculating the alveolar-arterial P_{O_2} difference.

4. Lung volumes and airway resistance can be measured in a body plethysmograph relatively easily.

5. Exercise testing can be valuable in identifying the cause of the patient's exercise limitation.

QUESTIONS

For each question, choose the one best answer.

1. A 66-year-old woman presents with a 9-month history of worsening dyspnea on exertion. Spirometry reveals an $FEV_{1.0}$ that is significantly lower than predicted based on her age, height, and sex; a lower than predicted FVC; and a decreased $FEV_{1.0}/FVC$ ratio. Which of the following could explain these results?
   A. Decreased lung elastic recoil
   B. Decreased number of pulmonary capillaries
   C. Fibrotic changes in the interstitial space
   D. Increased radial traction on the airways
   E. Thickening of the blood-gas barrier

2. A patient is administered a tidal volume of 600 ml·breath^{-1} while receiving invasive mechanical ventilation for acute respiratory failure. During morning rounds, you obtain the data contained in the table below.

pH	Arterial P_{O_2} (mm Hg)	Arterial P_{CO_2} (mm Hg)	End-tidal P_{CO_2} (mm Hg)	Mixed Expired P_{CO_2} (mm Hg)
7.33	69	42	36	21

Based on this information, what is the volume of the physiologic dead space in this patient?
   A. 85 ml
   B. 150 ml
   C. 250 ml
   D. 300 ml
   E. 450 ml

3. A 30-year-old otherwise healthy man is brought into the emergency department after an overdose of opiate pain medications. Upon arrival, he has an oxygen saturation of 85% breathing ambient air, which improves to 98% when he is put on oxygen by nasal cannula at a flow rate of 2 liters·min^{-1}. He is taking shallow breaths at a rate 6 breaths·min^{-1} and has a chest radiograph without lung opacities. Which of the following would you expect to find on additional investigations with this patient while if they are done while he is breathing ambient air?
   A. Decreased bicarbonate
   B. Decreased P_{ACO_2}
   C. Decreased pH
   D. Increased alveolar-arterial P_{O_2} difference
   E. Increased shunt fraction

4. An esophageal pressure monitor is used to estimate pleural pressure during the respiratory cycle in two subjects of equal age and stature. Before the start of inspiration, each subject has a functional residual capacity of 2.5 liters and estimated pleural pressure of -5 cm H_2O. Each individual pauses with an open glottis after inhaling a total of 0.5 liter of air. During this pause, Subject 1 has an estimated pleural pressure of -10 cm H_2O, while Subject 2 has an estimated pleural pressure of -15 cm H_2O. Which of the following could account for the estimated pleural pressure in Subject 2 compared to that measured in Subject 1?
   A. Airway mucosal edema
   B. Decreased elastic recoil
   C. Increased airway secretions
   D. Increased pulmonary vascular resistance
   E. Pulmonary fibrosis

5. Two patients take a vital capacity breath containing 100% oxygen. The changes in nitrogen concentration during exhalation are shown for each patient in the figure below. Which of the following is likely decreased in Patient 2 (blue line) compared to Patient 1 (black line)?

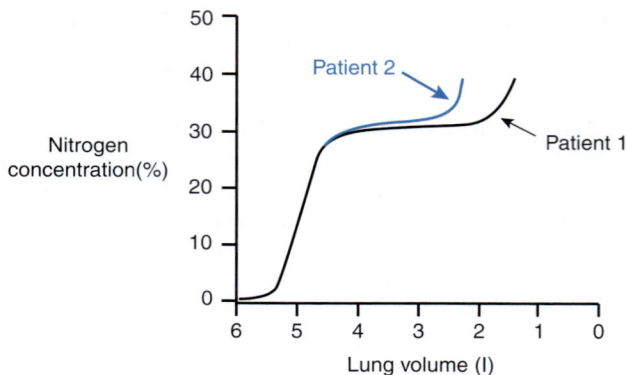

A. Anatomic dead space
B. Chest wall recoil
C. Hemoglobin concentration
D. Lung parenchymal compliance
E. Radial traction on the airways

6. A patient with a long history of heavy cigarette smoking undergoes pulmonary function testing as part of an evaluation for chronic dyspnea. Spirometry demonstrates an $FEV_{1.0}$ of 1.25 liters (45% predicted), FVC of 3.0 liters (65% predicted), and $FEV_{1.0}/FVC$ of 0.42. Lung volumes are subsequently measured using nitrogen washout and body plethysmography. Which of the following would you expect to find when comparing the results of these two measurements?
A. Higher value with nitrogen washout
B. Lower value with nitrogen washout
C. No difference between the two measurements

7. The multiple-breath nitrogen washout test is performed as part of the evaluation of a man with chronic dyspnea. The plot of log of the N_2 concentration versus the number of breaths reveals two distinct phases with the rate N_2 concentration declining quickly in the first phase and more slowly in the other. Which of the following could account for this observation?
A. Decreased hemoglobin concentration
B. Decreased peripheral chemoreceptor output
C. Decreased number of pulmonary capillaries
D. Nonuniform ventilation
E. Thickening of the blood-gas barrier

8. A 33-year-old woman develops severe hypoxemic respiratory failure as a complication of pneumonia and is treated with mechanical ventilation. The inspired oxygen concentration is increased to 100% shortly following intubation, and an arterial blood sample gives the following results: pH 7.32, P_{CO_2} 34, P_{O_2} 70 mm Hg, and HCO_3^- 16 mEq·liter^{-1}. Which of the following mechanisms is likely to be responsible for the patient's hypoxemia?
   A. Hypoventilation
   B. Diffusion impairment
   C. Shunt
   D. Ventilation-perfusion inequality
   E. Hypoventilation and ventilation-perfusion inequality

SYMBOLS, UNITS, AND EQUATIONS

SYMBOLS

Primary Symbols

C   Concentration of gas in blood
F   Fractional concentration in dry gas
P   Pressure or partial pressure
Q   Volume of blood
$\dot{Q}$ Volume of blood per unit time
R   Respiratory exchange ratio
S   Saturation of hemoglobin with O_2
V   Volume of gas
$\dot{V}$ Volume of gas per unit time

Secondary Symbols for Gas Phase

A   Alveolar
B   Barometric
D   Dead space
E   Expired
ET   End-tidal
I   Inspired
L   Lung
T   Tidal

Secondary Symbols for Blood Phase

a   Arterial
c   Capillary
c′   End-capillary
i   Ideal
v   Venous
$\bar{v}$ Mixed venous

Examples

O_2 concentration in arterial blood Ca_{O_2}

Fractional concentration of N_2 in expired gas $F_{E_{N_2}}$

Partial pressure of O_2 in mixed venous blood $P\bar{v}_{O_2}$

UNITS

Traditional metric units have been used in this book. Pressures are given in mm Hg; the torr is an almost identical unit.

In Europe, SI (Système International) units are commonly used. Most of these are familiar, but the kilopascal, the unit of pressure, is confusing at first. One kilopascal = 7.5 mm Hg (approximately).

EQUATIONS

Gas Laws

General gas law : $PV = RT$

where T is temperature and R is a constant. This equation is used to correct gas volumes for changes of water vapor pressure and temperature. For example, ventilation is conventionally reported at BTPS, that is, body temperature (37°C), ambient pressure, and saturated with water vapor, because it then corresponds to the volume changes of the lung. By contrast, gas volumes in blood are expressed as STPD, that is, standard temperature (0°C or 273 K) and pressure (760 mm Hg) and dry, as is usual in chemistry. To convert a gas volume at BTPS to one at STPD, multiply by:

$$\frac{273}{310} \times \frac{P_B - 47}{760}$$

where 47 mm Hg is the water vapor pressure at 37°C.

Boyle's law $\quad P_1 V_1 = P_2 V_2 \quad$ (temperature constant)

and

Charles' law $\quad \dfrac{V_1}{V_2} = \dfrac{T_1}{T_2} \quad$ (pressure constant)

are special cases of the general gas law.

Avogadro's law states that equal volumes of different gases at the same temperature and pressure contain the same number of molecules. A gram molecule, for example, 32 g of O_2, occupies 22.4 liters at STPD.

Dalton's law states that the partial pressure of a gas (x) in a gas mixture is the pressure that this gas would exert if it occupied the total volume of the mixture in the absence of the other components.

Thus, $P_x = P \cdot F_x$, where P is the total dry gas pressure, since F_x refers to dry gas. In gas with a water vapor pressure of 47 mm Hg,

$$P_x = (P_B - 47) \cdot F_x$$

Also, in the alveoli, $P_{O_2} + P_{CO_2} + P_{N_2} + P_{H_2O} = P_B$.

The *partial pressure of a gas in solution* is its partial pressure in a gas mixture that is in equilibrium with the solution.

Henry's law states that the concentration of gas dissolved in a liquid is proportional to its partial pressure. Thus, $C_x = K \cdot P_x$.

Ventilation

$$V_T = V_D + V_A$$

where V_A here refers to the volume of alveolar gas in the tidal volume.

$$\dot{V}_A = \dot{V}_E - \dot{V}_D$$

$$\dot{V}_{CO_2} = \dot{V}_A \cdot F_{A_{CO_2}} \quad \text{(both $\dot{V}$ measured at BTPS)}$$

$$\dot{V}_A = \frac{\dot{V}_{CO_2}}{P_{A_{CO_2}}} \times K \quad \text{(alveolar ventilation equation)}$$

If $\dot{V}_A$ is BTPS and $\dot{V}_{CO_2}$ is STPD, K = 0.863. In normal subjects, $P_{a_{CO_2}}$ is nearly equal to $P_{A_{CO_2}}$.

Bohr equation

$$\frac{V_D}{V_T} = \frac{P_{A_{CO_2}} - P_{E_{CO_2}}}{P_{A_{CO_2}}}$$

Or, using arterial P_{CO_2},

$$\frac{V_D}{V_T} = \frac{P_{a_{CO_2}} - P_{E_{CO_2}}}{P_{a_{CO_2}}}$$

This gives *physiologic dead space*.

Diffusion

In the *gas phase*, *Graham's law* states that the rate of diffusion of a gas is inversely proportional to the square root of its molecular weight.

In *liquid* or a *tissue slice*, *Fick's law** states that the volume of gas per unit time that diffuses across a tissue sheet is given by:

$$\dot{V}_{gas} = \frac{A}{T} \cdot D \cdot (P_1 - P_2)$$

where A and T are the area and thickness of the sheet, P_1 and P_2 are the partial pressure of the gas on the two sides, and D is a diffusion constant sometimes called the permeability coefficient of the tissue for that gas.

This *diffusion constant* is related to the solubility (Sol) and the molecular weight (MW) of the gas:

$$D \alpha \frac{Sol}{\sqrt{MW}}$$

When the diffusing capacity of the lung (D_L) is measured with carbon monoxide and the capillary Pco is taken as zero,

$$D_L = \frac{\dot{V}_{CO}}{P_{A_{CO}}}$$

D_L is made up of two components. One is the diffusing capacity of the alveolar membrane (D_M), and the other depends on the volume of capillary blood (V_c) and the rate of reaction of CO with hemoglobin, θ:

$$\frac{1}{D_L} = \frac{1}{D_M} + \frac{1}{\theta \cdot V_c}$$

Blood Flow

Fick principle

$$\dot{Q} = \frac{\dot{V}_{O_2}}{Ca_{O_2} - C\bar{v}_{O_2}}$$

---

*Fick's law was originally expressed in terms of concentrations, but partial pressures are more convenient for us.

Pulmonary vascular resistance

$$PVR = \frac{P_{art} - P_{ven}}{\dot{Q}}$$

where P_{art} and P_{ven} are the mean pulmonary arterial and venous pressures, respectively.

Starling's law of fluid exchange across the capillaries

$$\text{Net flow out} = K[(P_c - P_i) - \sigma(\pi_c - \pi_i)]$$

where i refers to the interstitial fluid around the capillary, π refers to the colloid osmotic pressure, σ is the reflection coefficient, and K is the filtration coefficient.

Ventilation-Perfusion Relationships

Alveolar gas equation

$$PA_{O_2} = PI_{O_2} - \frac{PA_{CO_2}}{R} + \left[PA_{CO_2} \cdot FI_{O_2} \cdot \frac{1-R}{R} \right]$$

This is only valid if there is no CO_2 in inspired gas. The term in square brackets is a relatively small correction factor when air is breathed (2 mm Hg when $Pco_2 = 40$, and $R = 0.8$). Thus, a useful approximation is

$$PA_{O_2} = PI_{O_2} - \frac{PA_{CO_2}}{R}$$

Respiratory exchange ratio
If no CO_2 is present in the inspired gas,

$$R = \frac{\dot{V}CO_2}{\dot{V}O_2} = \frac{PE_{CO_2}(1 - FI_{O_2})}{PI_{O_2} - PE_{O_2} - (PE_{CO_2} \cdot FI_{O_2})}$$

Venous to arterial shunt

$$\frac{\dot{Q}_S}{\dot{Q}_T} = \frac{Cc'_{O_2} - Ca_{O_2}}{Cc'_{O_2} - C\bar{v}_{O_2}}$$

where c' means end-capillary.

Ventilation-perfusion ratio equation

$$\frac{\dot{V}_A}{\dot{Q}} = \frac{8.63R\,(Ca_{O_2} - C\bar{v}_{O_2})}{PA_{CO_2}}$$

where blood gas concentrations are in $ml \cdot 100\ ml^{-1}$.
Physiologic shunt

$$\frac{\dot{Q}_{PS}}{\dot{Q}_T} = \frac{Ci_{O_2} - Ca_{O_2}}{Ci_{O_2} - C\bar{v}_{O_2}}$$

Alveolar dead space

$$\frac{V_D}{V_T} = \frac{Pi_{CO_2} - PA_{CO_2}}{Pi_{CO_2}}$$

The equation for *physiologic dead space* is on p. 22.

Blood Gases and pH

O_2 dissolved in blood

$$C_{O_2} = Sol \cdot P_{O_2}$$

where Sol is $0.003\ ml \cdot O_2 \cdot 100\ ml \cdot blood^{-1} \cdot mm\ Hg^{-1}$.
Henderson-Hasselbalch equation

$$pH = pK_A + \log \frac{(HCO_3^-)}{(CO_2)}$$

The pK_A for this system is normally 6.1. If HCO_3^- and CO_2 concentrations are in millimoles per liter, CO_2 can be replaced by Pco_2 (mm Hg) $\times$ 0.030.

Mechanics of Breathing

Compliance = $\Delta V/\Delta P$
Specific compliance = $\Delta V/(V \cdot \Delta P)$
Laplace equation for pressure caused by surface tension of a sphere

$$P = \frac{2T}{r}$$

where r is the radius and T is the surface tension. Note that for a soap bubble, P = 4T/r, because there are two surfaces.

Poiseuille's law for laminar flow

$$\dot{V} = \frac{P\pi r^4}{8nl}$$

where n is the coefficient of viscosity[†] and P is the pressure difference across the length l.

Reynolds number

$$Re = \frac{2rvd}{n}$$

where v is average linear velocity of the gas, d is its density, and n is its viscosity.

Pressure drop for laminar flow, PαV, but for turbulent flow, PαV$_2$ (approximately).

Airway resistance

$$\frac{P_{alv} - P_{mouth}}{\dot{V}}$$

where P_{alv} and P_{mouth} refer to alveolar and mouth pressures, respectively.

[†]This is a corruption of the Greek letter η for those of us who have little Latin and less Greek.

ANSWERS

B

CHAPTER 1

CLINICAL VIGNETTE

We might expect the volume to be reduced by 50%. However when one lung is removed, the alveoli of the other lung increase in size because of the large increase of available volume in the thoracic cavity. Another factor in this example is that the left lung is slightly smaller than is the right because the heart normally takes up some of the volume on the left side of the thorax.

The reduction in the ability of the blood-gas barrier to transfer gases can be explained by the removal of almost half of the capillaries. This greatly reduces the area of the barrier available for gas exchange.

The pulmonary artery pressure increased more on exercise than preoperatively because of the great reduction in the number of capillaries. At rest, these remaining capillaries undergo recruitment and distension (see Chapter 4) and so the pulmonary vascular resistance is almost normal. Because the pulmonary capillaries are already recruited and distended at rest following the pneumonectomy, when pulmonary blood flow increases on exercise, there is less opportunity for further recruitment and distention and pulmonary artery pressure rises.

The exercise capacity was reduced for at least two reasons. First as indicated above, the ability of the lung to transfer gases is reduced. Next with only one lung, the ventilatory capacity of the respiratory system is diminished.

1. D is correct. The capillary walls are exceptionally thin. If the pressure within the vessels rises too high, wall stress may increase to the point that ultrastructual changes occur in the wall of the vessel. This leads to leakage of plasma and even red blood cells into the alveolar spaces, a condition known as pulmonary edema. The pulmonary capillary pressure is higher in Subject A than in Subject B and, as a result, Subject A is at higher risk for development of pulmonary edema than Subject B.

2. A is correct. The airways are lined by a ciliated respiratory epithelium. The millions of tiny cilia beat in a coordinated manner and propel mucous and foreign material from the lower airways to the oropharynx where it is either expectorated or swallowed. Factors that impair ciliary function, such as inhaled toxins or genetic defects in ciliary structure and/or function impair this normal beating motion and, as a result, decrease mucous clearance, thereby exposing the affected individual to an increased risk of recurrent infection.

3. D is correct. Surfactant is a phospholipoprotein produced by Type II alveolar epithelial cells whose primary role is to decrease alveolar surface tension and prevent alveolar collapse. Its function is described further in Chapter 7. Production starts relatively late in gestation. As a result, fetuses born prematurely are at risk for having insufficient quantities of this important molecule which puts them at high risk for acute respiratory failure due to alveolar collapse and markedly increased work of breathing.

4. A is correct. As one moves from the distal to the proximal airways on exhalation, the cross-sectional area for air flow decreases as the total number of airways declines. As the cross-sectional area declines, the forward velocity of gas must increase in order to maintain expiratory flow. Gas moves by diffusion only in the respiratory zone whereas in the conducting zone, it moves by bulk flow, like water moves through a hose. Alveolar ducts are only present in the respiratory zone and, therefore, would not be increased in number with the transition from the respiratory to terminal bronchiole. Cartilage is not present in the respiratory bronchioles but becomes more prevalent as one moves to the very proximal airways (bronchi to trachea).

5. A is correct. The bronchial arteries branch off the aorta and provide blood flow to the conducting airways down to about the terminal bronchioles. As a result, blockage of bronchial arteries serving the right upper lobe through embolization would decrease blood flow to segmental bronchi in this lobe. The bronchial arteries are part of the bronchial circulation rather than the pulmonary circulation and, therefore, embolization does not affect the cross-sectional area of or flow through the pulmonary arteries. Because the bronchial circulation does not provide blood flow to the alveoli, embolization of the bronchial arteries would not affect alveolar epithelial cells.

6. B is correct. The thin side of the blood-gas barrier is 0.8 µm, which is much thicker than normal. This will slow the rate of diffusion of oxygen across the barrier but will not affect the volume of individual red cells, diffusion of gas in the distal airways, or alveolar surfactant concentrations. The risk of rupture of the blood-gas barrier should not be increased. In fact, if the thickening is caused by deposition of collagen, the risk of rupture might be reduced.

CHAPTER 2

CLINICAL VIGNETTE

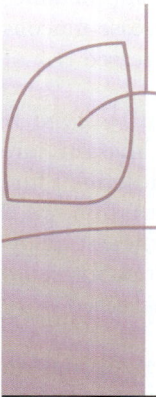

Her total ventilation is 8 breaths·min^{-1} × 300 ml·breath^{-1}, which corresponds to 2,400 ml·min^{-1} or 2.4 liter·min^{-1}. This is far below the normal level of 7 to 10 liter·min^{-1}. The reduced ventilation is due to depression of her normal impetus (i.e., "drive") to breathe. In this case, this could be caused by the ingestion of some substances presumably at a party. Assuming that her anatomic dead space is 150 ml, the dead space as a fraction of her tidal volume is 150 divided by 300, that is, 50%, far greater than the normal value of about 0.3 or 30%. Because her alveolar ventilation is grossly depressed and P_{CO_2} is inversely proportional to alveolar ventilation, when CO_2 production is assumed to be constant, we would expect to see a substantial rise in the arterial P_{CO_2}.

---

1. C is correct. Because of the effects of gravity, ventilation per unit volume is greatest in the most dependent portions of the lung. When an individual is in the supine position, as depicted in the figure, ventilation would be greatest in the most dependent portion of the lung, which would be the area near their back (position C).
2. C is correct. The alveolar ventilation is determined by the product of the volume of gas going to the alveoli (i.e., that portion of each breath that gets to the alveoli and participates in gas exchange) and the respiratory rate. The respiratory rate is given in this case, but the alveolar volume is not and, instead, must be calculated from the other information provided. If the dead space fraction is 0.3, we know that the dead space volume is 0.3 × 450 ml or 135 ml. As a result, the alveolar volume is 450 ml − 135 ml or 315 ml. Multiplying by the respiratory rate of 12 breaths·min^{-1}, we see that the alveolar ventilation is 315 ml·breath^{-1} × 12 breaths·min^{-1} or 3780 ml·min^{-1} or roughly 3.8 liter·min^{-1}.
3. C is correct. If the volume of the FRC is denoted as V, the amount of helium initially in the spirometer is 5 × 0.1, and the amount after dilution is (5 + V) × 0.06. Therefore, V = 0.5/0.06 − 5 or 3.3 liters.
4. D is correct. When the patient makes an expiratory effort, he compresses the gas in the lung so that airway pressure increases and lung volume decreases slightly. The reduction of volume in the lung means that the box gas volume increases and therefore, its pressure decreases according to Boyle's law.

5. B is correct. The alveolar ventilation equation states that if CO_2 production is constant, the alveolar P_{CO_2} is inversely related to the alveolar ventilation. Therefore, if the ventilation is increased 3 times, the P_{CO_2} will be reduced to a third of its former value, that is, 33%.

6. E is correct. Because the volume of the anatomic dead space remains largely the same, when the tidal volume is decreased, the dead space fraction increases. Minute ventilation is also unchanged with the new ventilator settings. Because the dead space fraction is higher, the alveolar ventilation is, therefore, reduced. The other choices are incorrect. Arterial P_{O_2} would actually increase, while CO_2 production and airway resistance would not change.

7. C is correct. Arterial P_{CO_2} is related to the ratio of CO_2 production and alveolar ventilation. With fever and a bloodstream infection, CO_2 production increases. Because minute ventilation is fixed, the patient cannot raise alveolar ventilation to compensate for the increase in CO_2 production and, as a result, arterial P_{CO_2} increases.

8. C is correct. In the figure, A represents functional residual capacity (FRC), the volume of air left in the lungs at the end of a tidal exhalation. B represents residual volume, the volume of air left in the lungs after a maximal exhalation. C represents the vital capacity, the volume of air exhaled in a maximum exhalation maneuver. D represents total lung capacity, the maximum volume of the lung. Of these volumes and capacities, the only one that can actually be measured by spirometry is the vital capacity. FRC, residual volume and total lung capacity can only be measured through measurements of lung volumes using either helium dilution or body plethysmography.

9. C is correct. Based on the alveolar ventilation equation, we can see that the arterial P_{CO_2} is determined by the balance between carbon dioxide production on the one hand and alveolar ventilation on the other. The fact that the arterial P_{CO_2} decreased from yesterday to this morning tells you that there must have been either a decrease in CO_2 production or an increase in alveolar ventilation. If the respiratory rate and tidal volume were not changed and the patient does not take any extra breaths on his own, then minute ventilation must have remained constant. If minute ventilation is constant and the dead space fraction is unchanged, then alveolar ventilation must have remained constant as well and the change in arterial P_{CO_2} must be due to a decrease in CO_2 production. Of all the remaining items on the list, only lowering of body temperature (hypothermia) will decrease CO_2 production. The remaining items all increase CO_2 production.

CHAPTER 3

CLINICAL VIGNETTE

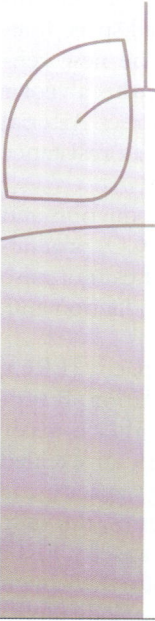

The diffusing capacity for carbon monoxide is decreased because of thickening of the blood-gas barrier as shown by the lung biopsy. As Figure 3.1 shows, the diffusion rate of gas through a tissue slice is inversely proportional to the thickness of the slice.

The arterial P_{O_2} decreased with exercise because this reduces the time spent by the red blood cells in the pulmonary capillaries. As Figure 3.3A shows, thickening of the blood-gas barrier slows the rate of rise of P_{O_2} in the pulmonary capillary and results in a reduced end-capillary P_{O_2}, and therefore arterial P_{O_2}, when red blood cell transit time in the pulmonary capillaries decreases during exercise.

The transfer of oxygen across the blood-gas barrier could be improved by raising the P_{O_2} of the inspired gas. This would increase the P_{O_2} in the alveolar gas and greatly raise the pressure differential responsible for oxygen diffusion across the blood-gas barrier.

We would not expect the arterial P_{CO_2} to be elevated because the diffusion rate for carbon dioxide is so much greater than are those for oxygen. In fact, these patients sometimes show a reduced arterial P_{CO_2} because the low oxygen in the blood stimulates ventilation as described in Chapter 8.

1. C is correct. The law states that the diffusion rate is proportional to the solubility but inversely proportional to the square root of the molecular weight. Therefore, the ratio of X to Y is $4/(\sqrt{4})$ or $4/2$, that is, 2.

2. E is correct. The equation is CO uptake divided by alveolar P_{CO}, or $30/0.5$, that is, 60 ml·min^{-1}·mm Hg^{-1}.

3. E is correct. The question is really asking for the conditions under which oxygen uptake or CO_2 output are diffusion limited. The only correct answer is maximal oxygen uptake at extreme altitude (see Figure 3.3B). None of the other choices refer to situations where gas transfer is diffusion limited. The only possible alternative choice is B, but resting oxygen uptake is unlikely to be diffusion limited when a subject breathes 10% oxygen. Furthermore, in all these questions, we are looking for the one best answer, and this is clearly E.

4. B is correct. The partial pressure of Gas A virtually reaches that of alveolar gas very early in the pulmonary capillary. As a result, the transfer of this gas is perfusion limited. By contrast, the partial pressure of Gas B changes very little as the blood moves through the pulmonary capillaries, and there is a large difference between the alveolar and end-capillary partial pressure.

This gas is, therefore, diffusion limited. The time course of Gas B resembles that of carbon monoxide.

5. E is correct. Under condition B, the rate of rise in the Po_2 as the red blood cells traverse the pulmonary capillaries is slower than under condition A. Of the items on the list, thickening of the blood-gas barrier is the most likely to cause this phenomenon. A decrease in minute ventilation and ascent to high altitude would also slow the rate of diffusion but in both of those cases, the alveolar Po_2 would be lower, whereas in the figure, the alveolar Po_2 is the same under condition A and B. Exercise would shorten the time available for diffusion to occur but would not affect the rate of rise in the Po_2. Increasing the inspired oxygen fraction would raise the alveolar Po_2 and, therefore, the pressure gradient driving diffusion and, as a result, lead to a faster rise in the Po_2 across the pulmonary capillaries.

6. A is correct. Emphysema, asbestosis, pulmonary embolism, and severe anemia all reduce the diffusing capacity by reducing the surface area of the blood-gas barrier, increasing its thickness, or reducing the volume of blood in the pulmonary capillaries. Diffuse alveolar hemorrhage can actually increase the measured diffusing capacity because the red blood cells that leak into the alveolar space due to damage to the pulmonary capillaries take up the carbon monoxide.

7. C is correct. The decreased diffusion capacity for carbon monoxide is consistent with the lung biopsy showing that the blood-gas barrier is thickened. This will slow the rate of diffusion of oxygen across the blood-gas barrier. At rest, the red blood cells spend enough time in the pulmonary capillaries to allow complete equilibration between the alveolar and end-capillary Po_2, but with exercise red blood cell transit time will decrease to the point that full equilibration may not occur and the end-capillary Po_2 will be lower than the alveolar value. The other choices are incorrect. The inspired Po_2 does not change with exercise, while the alveolar Po_2 remains largely constant through most of the exercise before increasing at the end of the test in most individuals. Anatomic dead space may actually increase slightly when the individual breaths at higher volumes during exercise.

8. A is correct. The diffusing capacity for carbon monoxide depends on the volume of blood in the pulmonary capillaries, or more strictly by the volume of red cells containing hemoglobin. Since this is reduced in severe anemia, diffusing capacity is decreased. This is the reason why the diffusing capacity is corrected for hemoglobin concentration.

9. A is correct. The histopathologic image on the right shows markedly thickened walls between alveoli compared to the normal lung. As a result, the diffusion distance between the alveoli and red cells in the pulmonary capillaries is increased, slowing the transfer of oxygen across the blood-gas barrier. While there may be sufficient time for full equilibration between the alveolar and end-capillary Po_2 while the patient remains at rest, with exercise, red cell transit time shortens and the end-capillary Po_2 is likely to

be lower than the alveolar value. The diffusion capacity for carbon monoxide would be reduced in this patient. The alveolar P_{O_2} would not increase. The reaction rate of oxygen with hemoglobin would not increase in this situation.

CHAPTER 4

CLINICAL VIGNETTE

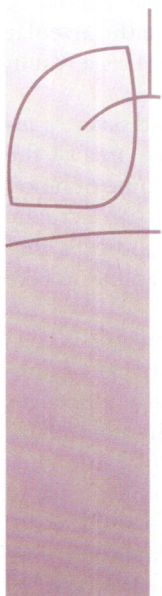

Although a substantial amount of the pulmonary circulation was blocked by the embolus, the increase in pulmonary artery pressure was small because blood is diverted from the vessels occluded by the pulmonary embolism to other areas of the lung where the resulting increase in capillary transmural pressure leads to recruitment and distention of capillaries. Nevertheless, pulmonary vascular resistance is increased, which explains the small increase in pulmonary artery pressure.

If the patient is sitting upright in bed, an increase in blood flow to the apex of the right lung would be expected because of the rise in pulmonary artery pressure.

By interrupting blood flow to ventilated units, pulmonary emboli create alveolar dead space and, as a result, increase dead space ventilation. An individual with normal ventilatory mechanics and respiratory drive will raise their total ventilation to compensate for the increase in dead space ventilation and, as a result, the arterial P_{CO_2} remains constant. If pain and anxiety associated with the pulmonary embolus cause the individual to raise their total ventilation by more than the increase in dead space ventilation, the arterial P_{CO_2} may actually fall.

1. E is correct. Pulmonary vascular resistance increases with the change in lung volume from Point A to Point B. This is due to stretching of the intra-alveolar capillaries, which decreases their diameter, thereby increasing resistance to flow. This counteracts any decrease in resistance associated with the increase in extra-alveolar vessel diameter due to increased radial traction on these vessels at higher lung volume. Recruitment and distention occurs with increases in pressure (e.g., during exercise) rather than increases in lung volume and is associated with decreased resistance. Decreased endothelin-1 concentration would lower pulmonary vascular resistance, as would increased nitric oxide concentration. Neither of these change with changes in lung volume.

2. E is correct (Figure 4.5). Pulmonary vascular resistance decreases during exercise due to recruitment and distention of the pulmonary capillaries in response to the increase in intravascular pressure and increase in blood

flow. This is the primary reason why pulmonary artery pressure increases to only a small extent with progressive exercise to maximum exercise capacity compared to systemic blood pressure. Although blood pH falls and sympathetic outflow increases in exercise, these factors are associated with vasoconstriction and increased resistance, as is an increase in endothelin-1 concentration. Zone 1 conditions are less prevalent during exercise due to the increase in pulmonary blood flow.

3. E is correct. The pulmonary vascular resistance is given by the pressure difference divided by the flow, or $(55 - 5)$ divided by 3, that is, approximately 17 mm $Hg \cdot liter^{-1} \cdot min$.

4. D is correct. The patient has experienced collapse, or atelectasis, of the left lower lobe because a mass lesion (possibly a lung cancer) is obstructing the bronchus traveling to that lobe. Because of the collapse, the alveolar Po_2 will be reduced throughout the lobe, leading to localized pulmonary arteriolar smooth muscle constriction (hypoxic pulmonary vasoconstriction) in an effort to direct blood flow away from this region to other, better ventilated regions of the lung.

5. C is correct. Under most circumstances, pulmonary blood flow equals cardiac output. The Fick principle can be used to calculate the cardiac output which is equal to the oxygen consumption divided by the arterial-venous oxygen concentration difference. The latter is $(20 - 16)$ ml$\cdot$100 ml^{-1} or $(200 - 160)$ ml$\cdot$liter^{-1}. Therefore, the cardiac output is equal to $300/(200 - 160)$ or 7.5 liters$\cdot$min^{-1}.

6. B is correct. In the preintervention period, $P_{arterial} > P_{venous} > P_{alveolar}$. The hierarchy of pressures corresponds to Zone 3 blood flow conditions, whereby blood flow is determined by the difference between arterial and venous pressure. Following the intervention, $P_{arterial} > P_{alveolar} > P_{venous}$, which corresponds to Zone 2 blood flow conditions in which blood flow is determined the difference between arterial and alveolar pressure. This pressure gradient is smaller than in the pre-intervention state and, as a result, flow will decrease.

7. C is correct. The key changes with the intervention are the decrease in pulmonary vascular resistance and pulmonary artery pressure. As a result, of these changes, cardiac output has increased. Of the items on the list, the only one that reduces pulmonary vascular resistance is intravenous administration of prostacyclin (PGI_2). Endothelin, histamine, and serotonin all cause pulmonary vasoconstriction and increase pulmonary vascular resistance. Inhalation of a gas mixture with a low inspired oxygen fraction would cause hypoxic pulmonary vasoconstriction and increase pulmonary vascular resistance.

8. A is correct. The movement of fluid between the capillary lumen and interstitium obeys Starling's Law. In the example given, the hydrostatic pressure difference moving fluid out of the capillary is $(3 - 0)$, and the colloid osmotic pressure tending to move fluid into the capillary is $(25 - 5)$ mm Hg. Therefore, the net pressure in mm Hg moving fluid into the capillaries is 17 mm Hg.

9. A is correct. The elevated pulmonary artery pressure on echocardiogram is most likely related to hypoxic pulmonary vasoconstriction. The stimulus for this is a decreased alveolar P_{O_2} rather than the arterial P_{O_2}. Increased pulmonary venous pressure can increase pulmonary artery pressure but would be expected in a patient with heart failure rather than a patient with pneumonia.

10. D is correct. The patient has impaired systolic function following a myocardial infarction. This leads to increased left heart end-diastolic and pulmonary venous pressures, which raise pulmonary capillary hydrostatic pressure. The result is an imbalance of the Starling forces and movement of fluid out of the capillaries. The decreased P_{O_2} is a consequence of pulmonary edema, while colloid osmotic pressure would be normal given her normal albumin concentration.

11. A is correct. Angiotensin-converting enzyme (ACE) catalyzes the conversion of angiotensin I to angiotensin II and is also responsible for most of the inactivation of bradykinin as it travels through the lung. Inhibition of this enzyme would therefore decrease inactivation of bradykinin. Angiotensin II is unaffected by passage through the lung and, therefore, degradation of this molecule would not increase with inhibition of ACE. ACE has no role in the processes described in the other answer choices.

CHAPTER 5

CLINICAL VIGNETTE

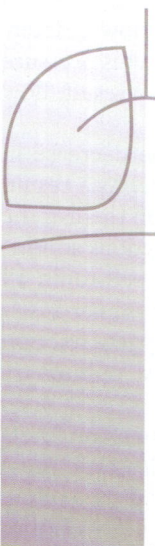

The alveolar-arterial oxygen difference is calculated from the alveolar gas equation. Since he is breathing air, the inspired P_{O_2} is 149 and we subtract the arterial P_{CO_2} of 45 divided by 0.8 giving an alveolar P_{O_2} of 93 mm Hg. The alveolar-arterial difference is therefore 20 mm Hg. This is abnormally high, and the probable cause is ventilation-perfusion inequality.

Using the same calculation, the alveolar-arterial oxygen difference in the emergency room is $80 - 45 = 35$ mm Hg. This increase indicates worsening of the ventilation-perfusion inequality.

The main reason P_{CO_2} is higher in the emergency department than in the clinic is because of increasing ventilation-perfusion inequality. In addition, there may be a reduction in the amount of ventilation going to the alveoli because of increasing airflow obstruction.

There was a substantial increase in arterial P_{O_2} from 55 to 90 mm Hg when this patient was given oxygen to breathe by nasal cannula. This is consistent with the cause of the hypoxemia being ventilation-perfusion inequality, rather than shunt.

1. D is correct. The P_{O_2} of moist inspired gas is given by $(P_B - P_{H_2O}) \times F_{I}O_2$. The arterial P_{O_2} and arterial P_{CO_2} are not needed to calculate this value, although, along with the respiratory exchange ratio, they can be used to calculate the ideal alveolar P_{O_2} and alveolar-arterial P_{O_2} difference. Using the data from the vignette, we get $P_{I}O_2 = (447 - 47) \times 0.2093$, which is about 84 mm Hg.

2. B is correct. To answer this question, we first use the alveolar ventilation equation, which states that if the carbon dioxide output is unchanged, the P_{CO_2} is inversely proportional to the alveolar ventilation. Therefore, since alveolar ventilation was halved, the arterial P_{CO_2} will increase from 40 to 80 mm Hg. Then we use the alveolar gas equation $P_{A_{O_2}} = P_{I_{O_2}} - (P_{a_{CO_2}} / R) + F$ and we ignore F because it is small. With no change in either carbon dioxide production or oxygen consumption, the respiratory exchange ratio remains 0.8. Therefore, which is approximately equal to 50 mm Hg.

3. A is correct. The last equation above shows that to return the alveolar P_{O_2} to its normal sea level value of about 100 mm Hg, we need to raise the inspired P_{O_2} from 149 to 199 mm Hg. Recall that the inspired P_{O_2} equals the fractional concentration of oxygen $\times (760 - 47)$. Therefore, the fractional concentration = 199/713 or approximately 0.28. Thus, the inspired oxygen concentration as a percentage has to be increased from 21 to 28, that is, by 7%. This example emphasizes how powerful the effect on oxygenation of increasing the inspired oxygen concentration is when hypoxemia is caused by hypoventilation. The more appropriate intervention, however, would be to fix the underlying cause of the hypoventilation.

4. C is correct. Despite the ventilation-perfusion inequality that develops when patients have pneumonia or other forms of respiratory failure, the arterial P_{CO_2} often remains normal and may even decrease. This is because the central chemoreceptors sense the rising P_{CO_2} and increase ventilatory drive. Because the CO_2 dissociation curve is linear in the physiologic range, the increase in ventilation increases CO_2 elimination from both high and low ventilation-perfusion ratio areas. This is contrast to the situation with oxygen, where increased uptake occurs only in units with low ventilation perfusion ratios. Due to the flat shape of the hemoglobin oxygen dissociation curve when the P_{O_2} is high, there is little-to-no increase in oxygen uptake from the high ventilation-perfusion ratio areas. The change in ventilation will not change the rate of diffusion across the alveolar capillary barrier. Any decrease in the alveolar P_{O_2} would lead to hypoxic pulmonary vasoconstriction and an increase in pulmonary vascular resistance.

5. B is correct. The inspired $P_{O_2} = 0.21 \times (253 - 47)$ or 43 mm Hg. Therefore, using the alveolar gas equation as stated above and neglecting the small factor F, the alveolar P_{O_2} is given by $42 - P_{CO_2}/R$, where R is equal to or less than 1. Therefore to maintain an alveolar P_{O_2} of 34 mm Hg, the alveolar P_{CO_2} cannot exceed 8 mm Hg.

6. C is correct. Patient 1 demonstrates the pattern typically seen in a healthy individual in which all ventilation and perfusion go to lung units with close to the normal ventilation-perfusion ($\dot{V}_A/\dot{Q}$) ratio of 1.0. In addition, no blood flow goes to unventilated compartments (shunt). In Patient 2, while much of the ventilation and blood flow goes to compartments with $\dot{V}_A/\dot{Q}$ near 1.0, there is considerable blood flow going to lung units high $\dot{V}_A/\dot{Q}$ ratios. This $\dot{V}_A/\dot{Q}$ inequality will widen the alveolar-arterial Po_2 difference and decrease the arterial Po_2, although the effects on these two variables will not be as extensive as would be seen if there was a lot of blood flow to low $\dot{V}_A/\dot{Q}$ units, as in Figure 5.15.

7. E is correct. Both ventilation and perfusion decrease with movement from the base to the apex of the lung. Because perfusion decreases to a greater extent than ventilation, the average $\dot{V}_A/\dot{Q}$ ratios are higher at the apex than at the base. As a result, the end-capillary Po_2 is higher and end-capillary Pco_2 is lower at the apex than at the base.

8. D is correct. A pulmonary embolism will decrease the perfusion to the affected lung segment. If alveolar ventilation remains constant, this will result in a high $\dot{V}_A/\dot{Q}$ ratio in the lung units served by the occluded pulmonary artery. As demonstrated in Figure 5.8, high $\dot{V}_A/\dot{Q}$ units are marked by increased alveolar Po_2 and decreased alveolar Pco_2. CO_2 elimination from those lung units because less CO_2-containing blood is delivered to the alveoli. The low Pco_2 in the alveoli and end-capillary blood will result in an increased pH. Hypoxic pulmonary vasoconstriction is triggered by a decrease, rather than an increase in the alveolar Po_2.

9. D is correct. First, we calculate the ideal alveolar Po_2 using the alveolar gas equation. This is $P_{A_{O_2}} = P_{I_{O_2}} - (P_{a_{CO_2}} / R) + F$, and we ignore the small factor F. The respiratory exchange ratio, R, is the ratio of carbon dioxide production to oxygen consumption which, in this case is 0.8. Therefore, the ideal alveolar $Po_2 = 149 - 48/0.8$ that is, 89 mm Hg. However, the arterial Po_2 is given as 49 so that the alveolar-arterial difference for Po_2 is 40 mm Hg.

10. C is correct. When the patient is placed on supplemental oxygen, the arterial Po_2 increases by only a small amount. This is consistent with shunt, which, in this case, may be the result of pneumonia. If the patient had predominantly ventilation-perfusion inequality, the arterial Po_2 would have risen to a much greater extent with supplemental oxygen. Hypoventilation is not present given the low arterial Pco_2, while diffusion impairment rarely causes hypoxemia in patients at sea level.

11. E is correct. In pneumonia, the alveolar space is filled with pus (largely neutrophils), leading to shunt physiology. The shunt as a fraction of cardiac output is given by (Cc' − Ca) / (Cc' − C$_{\bar{v}}$) where all the concentrations refer to oxygen. Calculated using the data provided in the vignette, the shunt fraction is (20 − 17) / (20 − 12) or 37.5%, markedly increased from the normal value of 5% to 10%. When the shunt fraction is increased, the response to supplemental oxygen is less than the response seen with oxygen administration in patients with other causes of hypox-

emia. Increases in the shunt fraction lead to increases in the alveolar-arterial oxygen difference but do not affect the alveolar P_{O_2}. Although a shunt tends to increase the arterial P_{CO_2}, the chemoreceptors increase ventilatory drive, such that P_{CO_2} often remains normal. The alveolar-arterial oxygen difference would only be normal if hypoventilation was the only cause of hypoxemia, which is not the case with this patient given the increased shunt fraction.

12. E is correct. With an arteriovenous malformation, pulmonary arterial blood finds its way into the pulmonary veins without going through ventilated regions of the lung, that is, it is a shunt. Since blood flow to the lower lobe where the shunt is located increases when the patient moves from the supine to the upright position, the shunt will increase. The other choices are incorrect. The alveolar P_{O_2} is not affected. The alveolar-arterial difference increases. There is no increase in the arterial P_{CO_2} due to the increase in ventilatory drive, and there is no change in the dead space.

CHAPTER 6

CLINICAL VIGNETTE

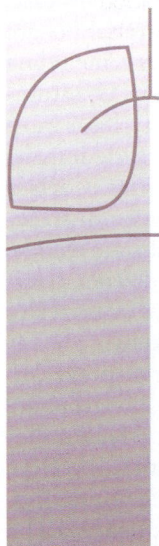

Because her lungs are apparently normal, we would expect the arterial P_{O_2} and oxygen saturation to be normal. These would not be altered by the severe anemia.

The arterial oxygen concentration would be expected to be very low, approximately one-third of the normal value because her hemoglobin concentration is reduced to about one-third of normal. We can neglect the amount of dissolved oxygen.

Her heart rate is increased because her cardiac output increases in response to the very low arterial oxygen concentration. This compensatory mechanism will help to raise the amount of oxygen being delivered to the tissues although, given the severity of the anemia, oxygen delivery will still be low.

The oxygen concentration of the mixed venous blood would be expected to be low. Because oxygen delivery, that is, the product of cardiac output and arterial oxygen concentration, is decreased while the amount of oxygen required to satisfy metabolic requirements (oxygen consumption) is unchanged, the oxygen concentration of the mixed venous blood must be reduced.

1. B is correct. The decrease in hemoglobin concentration decreases oxygen carrying capacity and, as a result, arterial oxygen concentration. In response to the decrease in oxygen delivery, there is an increase in O_2 extraction from the blood and, as a result, the mixed venous oxygen content ($C_{\bar{v}O_2}$) decreases as well. Hemoglobin-O_2 saturation is a function of the P_{O_2} only and, as a result, should not change with changes in hemoglobin concentration (Figure 6.2). Ventilation should not change in response to a change in hemoglobin concentration, as the chemoreceptors respond to changes in P_{O_2} rather than oxygen concentration (Chapter 8). As a result, the arterial P_{CO_2} should remain unchanged.

2. B is correct. The figure depicts a leftward shift in the hemoglobin-O_2 dissociation curve. This corresponds to a decrease in the P_{50} of hemoglobin and an increase in hemoglobin-O_2 affinity. Of the items on the list, the one that would cause such a shift would be a decrease in temperature (i.e., hypothermia). Hypoventilation is marked by an increase in P_{CO_2} which shifts the curve to the right, as does lactic acidosis. Heavy exercise is associated with increases in temperature and decreased blood pH, which would shift the curve to the right.

3. A is correct. Prior to being placed in the hyperbaric chamber, the arterial P_{O_2} was already 120 mm Hg, a level at which hemoglobin is nearly fully saturated with O_2. Even though the arterial P_{O_2} increases significantly in the hyperbaric chamber due to the high barometric pressure, there are no free hemoglobin binding sites and any further increases in O_2 content can only come by putting O_2 into solution (see Figure 6.1). CO_2, rather than O_2, binds to the terminal amine groups on the hemoglobin chains, while no information was provided to suggest a change in hemoglobin-O_2 affinity, nor would such changes account for the increase in O_2 content in this case.

4. A is correct. Even though the hemoglobin concentration and arterial P_{O_2} are normal, the patient has evidence of impaired tissue O_2 delivery, including an increased lactate concentration and a decreased mixed venous O_2 saturation. Given that he was exposed to car exhaust in a closed space, this is most likely related to carbon monoxide intoxication. Carbon monoxide impairs O_2 delivery by outcompeting O_2 for hemoglobin binding sites. Carbon monoxide also causes a leftward shift in the hemoglobin oxygen dissociation curve. Cyanide intoxication inhibits mitochondrial cytochrome oxidase and can cause lactic acidosis but is associated with a high mixed venous oxygen saturation and is not found in car exhaust. With a normal arterial P_{O_2} and chest radiograph, ventilation-perfusion inequality is unlikely.

5. D is correct. Carbon dioxide produced in the tissues is transported to the lungs by one of several means including in solution, as bicarbonate and bound to the terminal ends of hemoglobin chains (carbaminohemoglobin). As blood moves from the arterioles to the venules, the P_{CO_2} increases. As a result, you would expect to see increased carbaminohemoglobin formation as well as increased dissolved carbon dioxide and a rise in the bicarbonate concentration. Due to the increase in P_{CO_2}, the P_{50} for hemoglobin would increase, indicating a decreased affinity for oxygen. Because the P_{O_2} falls as blood traverse the tissue capillaries, the relationship between carbon dioxide concentration and P_{CO_2} shifts to the left (Haldane Effect, Figure 6.6).

6. B is correct. Between Time 1 and Time 2, both the quadriceps P_{O_2} and mixed venous oxygen content ($C_{\bar{v}O_2}$) fell. This suggests that something

occurred which either decreased tissue oxygen delivery and/or increased tissue oxygen utilization. Of the items on the list, the one that would decrease oxygen delivery would be a decrease in hemoglobin concentration, as this would decrease oxygen carrying capacity. Oxygen extraction increases in response to decreased oxygen delivery, which leads to a fall in the $C_{\bar{v}O_2}$. Cyanide intoxication causes tissue hypoxia, but the $C_{\bar{v}O_2}$ is increased due to decreased tissue oxygen utilization. Increases in cardiac output or the inspired oxygen fraction would increase oxygen delivery. Decreased temperature of the quadriceps muscle would decrease oxygen utilization and, other things being equal, lead to an increase in $C_{\bar{v}O_2}$.

7. C is correct. There is a respiratory acidosis because the PCO_2 is increased to 50 mm Hg and the pH is reduced to 7.20. However, there must be a metabolic component to the acidosis because as Figure 6.7A shows, a arterial PCO_2 of 50 will reduce the pH to only about 7.3 if the point moves along the normal blood buffer line. Therefore, there must be a metabolic component to reduce the pH even further. The other choices are incorrect because, as indicated above, an uncompensated respiratory acidosis would give a pH of above 7.3 for this PCO_2. Clearly, the patient does not have a fully compensated respiratory acidosis because then the pH would be closer to 7.4. There is not an uncompensated metabolic acidosis because the PCO_2 is increased, indicating a respiratory component. Finally, there is not a fully compensated metabolic acidosis because this would give a pH closer to 7.4.

8. B is correct. While a low arterial PCO_2 and normal HCO_3^- can be seen with acute respiratory alkalosis, the pH in such a case should be abnormally high rather than low. This can be appreciated in Figure 6.7A. Note also in this figure, that there is no way that the three given values can coexist on the diagram. Together, this information points to the fact that the blood gas values in this case are due to a laboratory error. Choice A is incorrect because the patient has a respiratory alkalosis rather than acidosis. Choice C is incorrect because a metabolic acidosis requires an abnormally low HCO_3^-, while Choice D is incorrect because a metabolic alkalosis requires an abnormally high HCO_3^-. Choice E is incorrect, as a compensated respiratory alkalosis would have a low arterial PCO_2, a low HCO_3^-, and a near normal pH.

9. C is correct. At high altitude, the fall in barometric pressure decreases the arterial PO_2, which, in turn, leads to an increase in ventilation. Assuming CO_2 production is unchanged, this causes a respiratory alkalosis. Because the individual has just arrived at the summit, there is no time for renal compensation. Note that the HCO_3^- has not changed significantly from normal and, as a result, the pH remains high. Choice D demonstrates a similar pattern but the arterial PO_2 is higher than would be the case at 4,000 m. Choice E demonstrates compensated respiratory alkalosis, which would be seen if the individual remained on the summit of the mountain for several days. The HCO_3^- has decreased and, as a result, the pH has decreased back toward normal. Neither Choice A (acute respiratory acidosis) or Choice B (normal blood gas at sea level) would be expected at high altitude.

10. B is correct. While smoke exposure in a fire should raise concern for carbon monoxide poisoning, the finding of an elevated mixed venous oxygen saturation is most consistent with cyanide intoxication, another complication of fire exposure in which inhibition of cytochrome oxidase in the mitochondrial electron transport chain leads to decreased tissue oxygen uptake. The oxygen saturation of mixed venous blood is decreased in carbon monoxide poisoning and methemoglobinemia due to decreased oxygen delivery. Hypovolemic shock and pulmonary edema would both also be associated with low mixed venous oxygen saturation.

11. E is correct. Fever causes a rightward shift (i.e., increased P_{50}) in the hemoglobin-oxygen dissociation curve such that at any given Po_2, there will be a lower oxygen saturation and, therefore, lower oxygen concentration. Fever is associated with increased carbon dioxide production and is not by itself associated with an increased shunt fraction.

12. E is correct. The patient has a primary metabolic alkalosis with a compensatory respiratory acidosis. The only item on the list that can cause this picture is vomiting, because the loss of hydrochloric acid during vomiting leads to the metabolic alkalosis. Anxiety attacks can cause an acute respiratory alkalosis, while an opiate overdose leads to an acute respiratory acidosis. Severe chronic obstructive pulmonary disease is often associated with a compensated respiratory acidosis, while uncontrolled diabetes mellitus and, in particular, diabetic ketoacidosis, can cause a primary metabolic acidosis with respiratory compensation.

CHAPTER 7

CLINICAL VIGNETTE

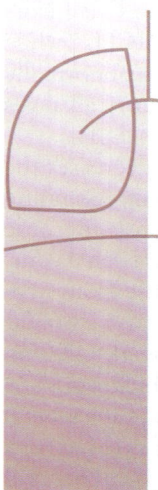

Flow in the small airways is laminar and therefore obeys Poiseuille's law, which states that resistance is inversely proportional to the fourth power of the radius of the tube. Therefore if the radius is reduced by one-half, the resistance is increased by 2 to the power 4, that is, 16 times.

Alveolar pressure will be abnormally low during inspiration and abnormally high during expiration. The reason is that because of the increased resistance of the airways, the pressure difference between the mouth and alveoli must increase to preserve flow.

The observed hyperinflation, that is, increased lung volume, will tend to reduce airway resistance because of the increased radial traction exerted by the alveolar walls on the airways. In spite of this, airway resistance will be higher than normal because of the airway constriction.

Overinflation, that is, a high lung volume, reduces the compliance of the lung, that is, makes it more stiff (see Figure 7.3).

1. C is correct. The results demonstrate that the patient has normal inspiratory muscle strength, as the measured value is nearly the same as the predicted value, but markedly decreased expiratory muscle strength. Of the items on the list, the one muscle group that is involved in expiration is the rectus abdominis. The diaphragm, external intercostals, scalene, and sternocleidomastoid muscles all play a role in inspiration, either at rest or as accessory muscles of respiration recruited during exercise.

2. C is correct. The pressure-volume relationship for Lung B is steeper than that seen with Lung A. Given that the slope of this relationship ($\Delta V/\Delta P$) represents the compliance of the lung, this indicates Lung B is more compliant than Lung A. Of the items on this list, the one that can cause an increase in lung compliance is a loss of elastic fibers, similar to that seen with emphysema or as part of normal aging. Increased fibrous tissue, decreased surfactant concentrations, and atelectasis (collapse) of lung segments would decrease compliance. A change in airway diameter would affect airways resistance but would not affect compliance.

3. A is correct. The Laplace relationship shown in Figure 7.4C states that the pressure is inversely proportional to the radius for the same surface tension. Since bubble X has three times the radius of bubble Y, the ratio of pressures will be approximately 0.3:1.

4. B is correct. Due to the effects of gravity, when an individual is in the upright position, intrapleural pressure is less negative, resting volume is smaller and ventilation is greater at the lung base than at the apex. In orbit in space, the effects of gravity are removed. As a result, intrapleural pressure at the lung base will be more negative because the downward acting forces of the lung in the upright position are decreased and less pressure is needed below it to balance these forces. As a result, the transpulmonary pressure is larger and the resting volume will be higher at the lung base. Regional heterogeneity in ventilation still persists in space, but it is less than at sea level so there is less variability in ventilation between the base and the apex in space. At sea level, regional differences in perfusion are due, in part, to the effects of gravity. As a result, one would not expect increased variability in a zero gravity environment.

5. C is correct. On fluoroscopy, the diaphragm descends into the abdomen. This is the expected pattern of diaphragm movement on inhalation and suggests that this patient's diaphragm, which is innervated by nerve roots from the 3rd through 5th cervical spinal levels, functions normally. Maximum expiratory pressure and cough strength are both decreased indicating that expiratory muscles, including the internal intercostals, rectus abdominis, transversus abdominis, and oblique muscles, do not function properly. These are innervated largely by nerve roots from the thoracic spinal cord. Therefore, if the diaphragm functions properly but expiratory muscles are impaired, the highest level of the spinal cord at which this patient could be injured would be C6.

6. B is correct. The arrow points to functional residual capacity. This is the equilibrium volume of the respiratory system where the elastic recoil of the lung is balanced by the elastic recoil of the chest wall (i.e., its tendency to spring out). Because of the elastic recoil of the lung, intrapleural pressure is −5 cm H_2O at FRC. Both the airways and the extra-alveolar vessels are affected by radial traction of surrounding alveoli. As a result, both airway resistance and resistance associated with the extra-alveolar vessels are at their minimum at high lung volumes, such as total lung capacity (TLC). Transmural pressure across the wall of the alveolus is at its maximum when the alveoli are at their maximum volume, as would be the case near TLC.

7. A is correct. Point B represents the end of inspiration. This is the point in the respiratory cycle at which lung volume is at its greatest. Due to the effects of radial traction exerted by the alveoli, airway resistance will be at its lowest at this point. Alveolar pressure must be lower than atmospheric pressure during inspiration to establish a driving pressure. There is no longer any driving pressure at the end of inspiration (Point B) as there is transiently no airflow. The driving pressure on expiration is positive at Point C and would be at its minimum (zero) at Point B. Intrapleural pressure is at its most negative at Point B when alveolar volume is at its highest and, therefore, the transpulmonary pressure is at its maximum.

8. D is correct. If the lung is held at a given volume, mouth and alveolar pressure must be the same because there is no airflow. Therefore, the answer is either C or D. Because the lung was expanded with positive pressure, all the pressures inside the thorax increase. Since the normal intrapleural pressure is about −5 cm H_2O, it cannot fall to −10 as shown in C. Therefore, the only possible answer is D.

9. C is the correct answer. The fact that the two lung units achieve the same change in volume with the same transpulmonary pressure indicates that they have the same compliance. The fact that inspiration takes longer in lung unit B despite an equal driving pressure implies that the flow rate on inhalation is lower and, therefore, the airway resistance must be higher. Increased parasympathetic activity causes bronchoconstriction and would increase airway resistance, thereby lengthening the time needed for inspiration. Fibrosis, pneumonia, pulmonary edema, and an increase in the number of elastic fibers would all decrease lung compliance.

10. D is correct. If the airway mucosa is 1 mm thicker around the entire circumference of an airway, an airway whose lumen is normally 4 mm in diameter will now be only 2 mm in diameter. According to Poiseuille's law during laminar flow, airway resistance is inversely proportional to the 4th power of the radius, other things being equal. Therefore, a reduction in the radius by a factor of 2 increases the resistance by 2^4, that is, 16.

11. B is correct. Infants born prematurely sometimes lack surfactant, which is necessary to overcome alveolar surface tension and prevent atelectasis. This puts them at risk for infant respiratory distress syndrome (also referred to as neonatal respiratory distress syndrome), which is associated with decreased

compliance. Increased airway mucus production and smooth muscle contraction and increased edema of the airway wall are all associated with increased airway resistance. Decreased alveolar macrophage concentrations might affect susceptibility to infection but would not affect compliance.

12. D is correct. During forced expiration tests, increased effort causes an increase in peak expiratory flow but has no effect on flow toward the end of exhalation (see Figure 7.16). This period of effort-independent flow is due to dynamic compression of the airways during forced exhalation. The other answer choices do not fit this pattern and are incorrect.

13. D is correct. The clinical features of this case, including the long smoking history, wheezes, and prolonged exhalation on examination, and a chest radiograph with large lung volumes and increased lucency of the lung are all suggestive of obstructive lung disease. A diagnostic hallmark is a low $FEV_{1.0}/FVC$ ratio. $FEV_{1.0}$ is typically reduced as is FVC. None of the other choices have a low $FEV_{1.0}/FVC$ ratio and, therefore, they are all incorrect.

CHAPTER 8

CLINICAL VIGNETTE

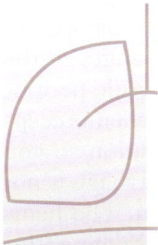

On arrival at high altitude, the arterial Po_2 is reduced because of a reduction of the inspired Po_2 due to the decrease in barometric pressure. Hypoxemia causes an increase in ventilation as a result of stimulation of the peripheral chemoreceptors, which accounts for the reduced Pco_2, the increased pH, and the reduced bicarbonate concentration.

After 1 week at high altitude, the Po_2 has increased because of a further rise in ventilation. This further increase is explained by the return toward normal of the pH values of the blood and CSF that result from renal compensation for the respiratory alkalosis in the blood, and a similar change in the CSF. As a result, their inhibiting effect on ventilation is decreased. The near-normal level of arterial pH is consistent with this. The further fall in the Pco_2 and bicarbonate reflect the increase in ventilation.

The hemoglobin concentration increased from 15 to 16.5 $g \cdot dl^{-1}$ over the week. Although the serum erythropoietin level has increased by this time, the change in hemoglobin concentration is too fast to be accounted for by this mechanism and must be caused, instead, by hemoconcentration, that is, a loss of plasma volume.

During the exercise test, the arterial Po_2 fell because of diffusion limitation of oxygen across the blood-gas barrier. This occurs because of the reduced alveolar Po_2 and the shorter red blood cell transit time in the pulmonary capillaries as a result of the increase in cardiac output during exercise (Chapter 5). Ventilation-perfusion inequality as a result of interstitial edema in the lung is another possible contributing factor. The fall in Pco_2 and pH can be explained by an increase in ventilation in response to the lactic acidosis seen in late exercise.

1. E is correct. The cerebral cortex is injured while the brainstem is uninjured. Of the answer choices, the only one located within the cerebral cortex is voluntary control of breathing. The central chemoreceptors are located in the ventral surface of the medulla while respiratory rhythm generation is handled by the Pre-Botzinger complex in the ventrolateral region of the medulla. The peripheral chemoreceptors reside in the carotid and aortic bodies while the Hering-Breuer reflex is mediated by stretch receptors in the lungs and the vagus nerve.

2. E is correct. The increase in respiratory frequency described in this scenario is referred to as the deflation reflex: inspiratory activity is initiated by lung deflation. This is the opposite response to the Hering Breuer inflation reflex, in which distention of the lung leads to a slowing of respiratory frequency due to an increase in expiratory time. These reflexes are mediated primarily by pulmonary stretch receptors located in airway smooth muscle. Arterial baroreceptors respond to changes in blood pressure. Bronchial C fibers respond to chemical changes in the bronchial circulation, while irritant receptors in the airways respond to noxious gases, cigarette smoke and other inhaled substances. J receptors respond to changes in the volume of pulmonary capillaries and interstitial fluid and would not play a role in this case.

3. E is correct. The gastrointestinal hemorrhage and decrease in hemoglobin concentration will lower the arterial oxygen concentration. Importantly, the oxygen saturation and arterial P_{O_2} are unchanged from before the hemorrhage. The peripheral chemoreceptors respond to changes in the P_{O_2} rather than the oxygen concentration of the blood. As a result, peripheral chemoreceptor output should not change. The central chemoreceptors do not respond to changes in P_{O_2} or oxygen concentration so you would not see a change in their output, given that the hemorrhage is not associated with changes in pH or bicarbonate concentration. The hemorrhage should not affect juxtacapillary receptor output. If anything, this output may decrease if overall blood volume is decreased due to the hemorrhage and subsequent decrease in pulmonary capillary blood volume.

4. A is correct. The data from the test shows that despite increases in her end-tidal P_{CO_2}, a marker of the arterial P_{CO_2}, there is no perceptible change in minute ventilation. This is in contrast to the healthy control who demonstrated a large rise in minute ventilation once the end-tidal P_{CO_2} rose above about 55 mm Hg. The central chemoreceptor is the component of the respiratory control system most responsible for responding to changes in the P_{CO_2}. The fact that her ventilation does not increase despite a rising P_{CO_2} indicates the central chemoreceptor is likely not functioning properly. The peripheral chemoreceptors also respond to changes in P_{CO_2} but their response is not as important as the central chemoreceptor. The juxtacapillary and stretch receptors and the pneumotaxic center do not play a role in the ventilatory response to changes in P_{CO_2}.

5. C is correct. This patient has severe COPD with chronic CO_2 retention, as indicated by her blood gas demonstrating a compensated respiratory

acidosis. Because the pH of the brain extracellular fluid has returned to near normal, she has lost most of the stimulus for ventilation from hypercarbia. In this situation, arterial hypoxemia is the primary stimulus to increased ventilation beyond the basic level set by the medullary respiratory centers. When she is placed on supplemental oxygen and the oxygen saturation increases, peripheral chemoreceptor stimulation decreases and, as a result, minute ventilation decreases. This will increase the arterial Pco_2. Supplemental oxygen will raise alveolar Po_2 and relieve hypoxic pulmonary vasoconstriction, thereby decreasing pulmonary vascular resistance. In and of itself, the increase in oxygen saturation does not affect the P_{50}, but the increase in arterial Pco_2 will shift the hemoglobin-oxygen dissociation curve to the right and raise the P_{50}. Increasing the oxygen saturation will not affect J receptor or ventral respiratory group output.

6. D is correct. This individual is experiencing a form of periodic breathing known as *Cheyne-Stokes respiration,* an abnormal pattern of breathing often seen in healthy individuals at high altitude. This occurs as a result of abnormalities in the ventilatory feedback control system with one of the major factors being abnormally strong ventilatory response to changes in arterial Pco_2. When breathing movements cease (apnea), the arterial Pco_2 rises. When the central chemoreceptor finally senses and responds, the increase in ventilation is excessive by which there is an overly large decrease in arterial Pco_2 and an overshoot of the equilibrium condition. Hypoxemia at this altitude is not sufficient to cause injury to the medullary respiratory center. The other factors do not play a role in this breathing pattern.

7. E is correct. The history of several days of nausea, vomiting and polyuria and the markedly elevated glucose, suggest this patient has diabetic ketoacidosis. This causes a metabolic acidosis, denoted by the markedly low bicarbonate concentration, which causes a fall in blood pH (acidemia). The peripheral chemoreceptors respond to decreases in pH, as well as decreased arterial Po_2 and increased arterial Pco_2 so you would expect the peripheral chemoreceptor output to increase. Central chemoreceptor output can also increase in response to metabolic acidosis, but the response is slower due to the relative impermeability of the blood-brain barrier to hydrogen ion. CSF Pco_2 should decrease because the metabolic acidosis will lead to a compensatory respiratory alkalosis. The Pre-Botzinger complex generates the respiratory rhythm and would not affect the response to changes in blood pH. The P_{50} will increase as decrease pH shifts the hemoglobin oxygen dissociation curve to the right (Chapter 6).

8. C is correct. Despite not receiving any sedative or neuromuscular blockade medications, this patient is not making any respiratory efforts. His arterial Pco_2 is also normal so the lack of effort cannot be attributed to the ventilatory depressant effects of respiratory alkalosis. The lack of respiratory effort would suggest that his stroke has affected the region of his central nervous system responsible for generating the respiratory rhythm. This center is located in the medulla, which receives its blood

flow from branches off the vertebral artery. The cerebellum and midbrain also receive blood flow from the vertebral artery but do not contain centers responsible for generating the primary respiratory rhythm.

9. C is correct. When the blood P_{CO_2} rises, CO_2 diffuses into the CSF. This increases CSF P_{CO_2}, leading to liberation of hydrogen ions and a decreased pH. If the CSF pH is displaced for a long period of time, as in a patient with chronic hypercarbia due to severe COPD, CSF bicarbonate concentration increases as a compensatory response. The pH will increase but will not usually return all the way to a normal CSF pH of 7.32.

10. A is correct. The most important peripheral chemoreceptors that mediate the hypoxic ventilatory response are located in the carotid bodies. Following bilateral carotid body resection, the patient would not experience the same increase in minute and alveolar ventilation following ascent to high altitude as individuals with intact carotid bodies and would have a higher arterial P_{CO_2}. With less increase in minute ventilation than a normal individual, the alveolar and arterial P_{O_2} would be lower. The pH would also be lower because of the higher P_{CO_2}.

11. E is correct. Ventilation increases in response to increases in arterial P_{CO_2}. When arterial P_{O_2} decreases, as would occur following ascent to high altitude, ventilation for a given P_{CO_2} is higher than in normoxia and the slope of the ventilatory response curve is steeper. The other choices are incorrect. Alveolar hypoxia would trigger hypoxic pulmonary vasoconstriction and increase pulmonary artery pressure, while hypoxemia increases peripheral chemoreceptor output. The decrease in P_{CO_2} that results from the increase in total ventilation will lead to a decrease in serum bicarbonate and an increase in pH.

CHAPTER 9

CLINICAL VIGNETTE

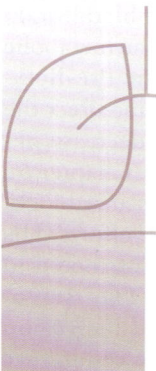

The maximum oxygen consumption reaches a plateau in late exercise because the oxygen delivery system including ventilation, cardiac output, and the diffusion properties of the lung and peripheral tissues are not able to deliver any more oxygen to the exercising muscles. The increase in work rate after the maximum oxygen consumption has been reached must be attributed to anaerobic glycolysis.

Initially, minute ventilation increases linearly with work rate. However, above a work rate of about 350 watts in this example, the ventilation increases much more rapidly. This can be explained by the accumulation of lactic acid in the blood and its stimulation of the peripheral chemoreceptors.

CLINICAL VIGNETTE

The alveolar-arterial P_{O_2} difference at rest and with mild exercise is small but may increase to about 30 mm Hg on maximum exercise. This is thought to be caused by ventilation-perfusion inequality that may develop as a result of interstitial edema in the lung. Fit individuals reaching very high levels of power output may possibly develop diffusion limitation of oxygen transport across the pulmonary blood-gas barrier, but this is uncommon at sea level.

The pH changes little at mild exercise but falls markedly at maximum exercise because of the formation of lactic acid in the blood.

1. **B is correct.** While hypoxemia can be seen at peak exercise in elite athletes, it would be not be expected in a sedentary, healthy individual at sea level. Heart rate increases with progressive exercise and is a big contributor to the increase in cardiac output. Minute ventilation also increases, as does systemic blood pressure. Because minute ventilation increases in late exercise more than is required to meet metabolic demands due to the developing lactic acidosis, arterial P_{CO_2} decreases in late exercise.

2. **D is correct.** After birth, the increase in P_{O_2} and decrease in circulating prostaglandin concentrations lead to closure of the ductus arteriosus. If the ductus remains open, blood flows through the ductus from the aorta to the pulmonary artery due to the decrease in pulmonary vascular resistance from levels seen in utero. This will increase blood flow in pulmonary circulation and eventually to the left atrium, leading to left atrial dilation and increased left atrial pressure. Increases in left atrial pressure following birth lead to closure of the foramen ovale. Further increases in pressure with a patent ductus arteriosus will increase the tendency toward closure.

3. **A is correct.** Complete occlusion of the airway feeding the right middle lobe will cause absorption atelectasis. The P_{O_2} of the alveoli in that lobe will exceed that of mixed venous blood and, as a result, oxygen will diffuse from the alveoli into the blood, leading to their collapse. This happens faster if the inspired oxygen fraction is 1.0 than if the patient was breathing ambient air. The decrease in alveolar P_{O_2} that results from atelectasis will cause hypoxic pulmonary vasoconstriction which will decrease blood flow to that lobe. Even though exchange of P_{CO_2} will not occur in the right middle lobe due to the atelectasis, which causes shunt, the arterial P_{CO_2} should not rise due to the expected response of the central chemoreceptor and the shape of the CO_2 dissociation curve. Pneumothorax results from entry of air into the pleural space which would not happen with right middle lobe atelectasis.

4. **E is correct.** Due to the streaming of blood in the right atrium, much of the blood that reaches the right atrium moves through the foramen ovale

into the left atrium and through the left ventricle to the aorta. Due to the high resistance of the pulmonary circulation in utero, blood flows from the pulmonary artery through the ductus arteriosus to the aorta. The placenta and the peripheral tissues are in parallel with each other rather than in series. Blood coming from the placenta will join with blood coming from the peripheral tissues and drain to the right atrium via the inferior vena cava. The foramen ovale sits between the atria rather than between the ventricles.

5. B is correct. In zero G, the deposition of inhaled particles by sedimentation is abolished. Both blood flow and ventilation to the apex of the lung are increased because the normal effects of gravity are abolished (see Figures 2.7, 4.7, and 5.8). Thoracic blood volume increases because blood no longer pools in dependent regions of the body as a result of gravity. The abolition of gravity results in a reduction of the $\bar{v}$ at the apex (see Figure 5.10).

6. D is correct. This individual suffered a seizure while being treated with hyperbaric therapy for what is most likely carbon monoxide poisoning given that he had been removed from a fire. Seizures are a complication of oxygen toxicity which can result when an individual is exposed to high barometric pressure either during diving or when breathing a high inspired oxygen fraction during hyperbaric therapy. The partial pressure of nitrogen increases during hyperbaric therapy but this causes altered mental status rather than seizures. Nitrogen bubbles can form in the blood when decompression occurs too quickly, while gas embolism occurs as a complication of decompression sickness or barotrauma.

7. D is correct. At low to moderate levels of exercise, ventilation increases at a rate sufficient to meet metabolic demand. At heavier levels of exercise, the slope of the ventilation versus work relationship steepens, as ventilation rises in response to the developing lactic acidosis. Bronchodilation occurs during exercise secondary to β_2 receptor stimulation, but this is not responsible for the increase in ventilation. The arterial Po_2 remains relatively constant through exercise, while the arterial Pco_2 typically decreases. The hemoglobin-oxygen-dissociation curve shifts to the right in exercising muscle, but this does not affect the ventilatory response.

8. A is correct. The development of joint pains, itchiness (pruritus), respiratory symptoms, and neurologic findings following a rapid ascent to the surface of the water is strongly suggestive of decompression sickness ("the bends"). This occurs because bubbles of nitrogen form in the tissues and expand further as ascent continues. Failure to exhale on ascent can lead to rupture of the lungs (barotrauma), while excessive partial pressures of carbon dioxide and oxygen may cause alterations in mental status rather than the findings seen in this patient. Middle ear and sinus compression are a consequence of changes in pressure while diving but are not the cause of the findings in this case.

9. A is correct. Spending 5 days at high altitude allows time for the acclimatization, a series of processes that help the body adjust to the low oxygen partial pressures. One of the most important of these is the hypoxic ventilatory response. Minute ventilation increases upon initial ascent and continues to do so over the following days. As a result, the P_{CO_2} will continue to decrease relative to the values seen immediately after ascent. Due to ventilatory acclimatization, the alveolar and arterial P_{O_2} should increase rather than decrease if she remains healthy. The serum bicarbonate decreases and the individual develops a base deficit as renal compensation occurs in response to the respiratory alkalosis. pH rises upon arrival at high altitude due to the respiratory alkalosis but declines back toward normal as renal compensation takes place.

10. E is correct. With ascent to high altitude, the rate of rise of the P_{O_2} in pulmonary capillary blood is decreased. If the individual remains at rest, there is still time for complete equilibration across the blood-gas barrier. With high levels of exercise however, red blood cell capillary transit time is decreased and, as a result, the end-capillary P_{O_2} does not rise to the alveolar value resulting in hypoxemia. The other choices are incorrect. The dead space fraction does decrease with exercise but does not contribute to hypoxemia. Hemoglobin concentration does not decrease with exercise and would be expected to rise over time at altitude. Individuals raise their ventilation during exercise, and the shunt fraction would not be expected to increase in a healthy individual at high altitude.

CHAPTER 10

1. A is correct. The low $FEV_{1.0}/FVC$ indicates the patient has airflow obstruction. Decreased lung elastic recoil contributes to airflow obstruction by decreasing the pressure gradient responsible for airflow on exhalation and reducing the radial traction on the airways. The other answers are incorrect. Decreased numbers of pulmonary capillaries and thickening of the blood-gas barrier may affect gas exchange but will not affect airflow. Fibrotic changes in the interstitial space increase lung elastic recoil, tether airways open and are not associated with airflow obstruction.

2. D is correct. The physiologic dead space fraction can be calculated using the following equation:

$$\frac{V_{D,phys}}{V_T} = \frac{P_a CO_2 - P_E CO_2}{P_a CO_2}$$

The term $P_E CO_2$ refers to the mixed expired P_{CO_2} rather than the end-tidal value. V_T refers to the tidal volume. Using this equation and the values provided in the equation, the physiologic dead space fraction is $[42 - 210] / 42 = 50\%$. When the dead space fraction is multiplied by the tidal volume of 600 ml, this yields a physiologic dead space volume of 300 ml.

3. C is correct. Opiate medications suppress ventilation, particularly when taken in excessive amounts. Based on this, as well as the fact that the patient is taking small breaths at a very low frequency, one would expect this patient to have hypoventilation. He would have an increased arterial P_{CO_2} and a decreased pH. The bicarbonate would increase due to dissociation of carbonic acid (see Chapter 6, Figure 6.7). The alveolar arterial P_{O_2} difference and shunt fraction are likely not increased. Hypoxemia due to hypoventilation is associated with a normal alveolar-arterial P_{O_2} difference. The lack of opacities on chest radiography suggests that there is no lung process that would cause ventilation-perfusion inequality, while the fact that the oxygen saturation increases readily with administration of a small amount of oxygen suggests that the shunt fraction is not increased.

4. E is correct. Subject 2 required a greater change in pressure to achieve the same change in volume as Subject 1. This indicates that Subject 2 has a lower lung compliance than Subject 1. Of the items on the list, pulmonary fibrosis is the one factor that would decrease lung compliance. Decreased elastic recoil would be associated with increased compliance, as is seen in emphysema. Airway mucosal edema and airway secretions would increase resistance. These issues would not affect the pressure measured during a pause in breathing nor affect compliance. Pulmonary vascular resistance would not affect the pressure required to inflate the lung.

5. E is correct. Late in exhalation, there is an abrupt increase in nitrogen concentration. The volume at which this occurs is the closing volume, which signals the closure of airways at the base of the lung and preferential emptying of airways at the lung apex. The closing volume is higher in Patient 2 than in Patient 1, indicating that airway closure occurs earlier. Of the items on the list, the one that could cause this would be decreased airway radial traction. Radial traction tends to keep airways open. If this is diminished, as occurs in emphysema, airways collapse earlier during exhalation. The dead space volume is the first, short portion of exhalation and is no different between the two patients. Decreased lung compliance would lead to later airway closure as the airways are tethered open to a greater extent. Closing volume is not affected by hemoglobin concentration or chest wall recoil.

6. B is correct. This patient has a long history of cigarette smoking and spirometry shows evidence of air flow obstruction, which make it likely they have chronic obstructive pulmonary disease. Due to a loss of elastic recoil, gas is often trapped behind closed airways on exhalation. When such air-trapping occurs, the nitrogen washout, as well as helium dilution, method of measuring lung volume may yield a lower value than body plethysmography, as nitrogen washout and helium dilution measure only ventilated lung, whereas body plethysmography accounts for the gas trapped behind closed airways.

7. D is correct. The presence of two distinct phases in the plot of nitrogen concentration versus number of breaths indicates that lung units have their

nitrogen diluted at different rates, and, therefore, the individual has non-uniform ventilation (see Figure 10.2). The other choices are incorrect. The nitrogen washout test is not affected by hemoglobin concentration, peripheral chemoreceptor output, or the thickness of the blood-gas barrier. The nitrogen washout test assesses inequality of ventilation, rather than perfusion, and would not be affected by the number of pulmonary capillaries.

8. C is correct. The patient has a large alveolar-arterial P_{O_2} difference despite inspiring 100% O_2. This is consistent with the presence of shunt. The other choices are incorrect. Because the P_{CO_2} is 34, she does not have hypoventilation. Diffusion impairment is rarely a cause of hypoxemia at sea level. Ventilation-perfusion inequality causes hypoxemia, but the P_{O_2} would increase to a much greater extent with supplemental oxygen administration than seen here.

INDEX

Note: Page numbers followed by "*f*" indicates figures; those followed by "*t*" indicates tables and those followed by "*b*" indicates boxes.